Immunochemistry
of Proteins

Volume 3

Immunochemistry of Proteins

Volume 3

Edited by

M. Z. Atassi

Mayo Medical School
Rochester, Minnesota
and
University of Minnesota
Minneapolis, Minnesota

PLENUM PRESS • NEW YORK AND LONDON

Library of Congress Cataloging in Publication Data
Main entry under title:

Immunochemistry of proteins.

Includes bibliographies and indexes.
1. Immunochemistry. 2. Proteins — Analysis. 3. Antigens — Analysis. I. Atassi, M. Z. [DNLM: 1. Antigens — Analysis. 2. Immunochemistry. 3. Proteins — Analysis. QU55 I32 1977]
QR182.I47   574.1'9245   76-25956
ISBN-13: 978-1-4613-2924-4   e-ISBN-13: 978-1-4613-2922-0
DOI: 10.1007/ 978-1-4613-2922-0

© 1979 Plenum Press, New York
Softcover reprint of the hardcover 1st edition 1979
A Division of Plenum Publishing Corporation
227 West 17th Street, New York, N.Y. 10011

Contributors

N. J. Calvanico · Department of Immunology, Mayo Medical School, Rochester, Minnesota 55901. Present address: Department of Medicine, Woods VA Hospital, Medical College of Wisconsin, Milwaukee, Wisconsin

A. F. S. A. Habeeb · Department of Biochemistry and Nutrition, University of Puerto Rico, Medical Sciences Campus, San Juan, Puerto Rico 00936

J. Michael Kehoe · Department of Microbiology and Immunology, Northeastern Ohio Universities College of Medicine, Rootstown, Ohio 44272

Thomas F. Lint · Department of Immunology, Presbyterian-St. Luke's Hospital, Chicago, Illinois 60612

Shigeharu Nagasawa · Faculty of Pharmaceutical Sciences, Hokkaido University, Sapporo, 060, Japan

Frank F. Richards · Department of Internal Medicine, Yale University School of Medicine, New Haven, Connecticut 06510

Rochelle Seide-Kehoe · Department of Microbiology and Immunology, Northeastern Ohio Universities College of Medicine, Rootstown, Ohio 44272

Robert M. Stroud · Division of Clinical Immunology and Rheumatology, The University of Alabama in Birmingham, Birmingham, Alabama 35294

T. B. Tomasi, Jr. · Department of Immunology, Mayo Medical School, Rochester, Minnesota 55901

John E. Volanakis · Division of Clinical Immunology and Rheumatology, The University of Alabama in Birmingham, Birmingham, Alabama 35294

Richard B. Weininger · Department of Internal Medicine, Yale University School of Medicine, New Haven, Connecticut 06510

Preface

The structural features responsible for the immunogenicity of certain parts of native protein molecules have been of interest to immunochemists and protein chemists for over three decades. However, until recently no concerted effort was (or could be) devoted to the elucidation of the complete antigenic structure of a protein. In order for these endeavors to be successful and meaningful, knowledge of both the amino acid sequence and the detailed three-dimensional structure of the protein is necessary. Such information was not available for a protein until early in the 1960s. This and the fact that protein chemistry was not in fact sufficiently developed early in the 1960s to enable the successful unraveling of the entire antigenic structure of a protein were major reasons for the slow progress in this field. Determination of the antigenic structures of proteins, therefore, posed a chemical challenge of enormous proportions. For these reasons, many investigators diverted their attention to study of the immunochemistry of amino acid polymers in the hope that the information derived from these systems might prove useful in the understanding of the immunochemistry of proteins. A great many data on these systems were accumulated that have provided valuable information on the immune mechanism. Unfortunately, it has now become clear the information from amino acid polymers has not helped in understanding the immunochemistry of proteins. Proteins represent the majority of antigens associated with the control and normal regulation of the immune system at the molecular-cellular interface and with many immunological disorders. Knowledge of the antigenic sites of these protein antigens lies at the basis of elucidating these phenomena at the molecular level. From a purely chemical perspective, the reaction of protein antigens with their antibodies remains one of the most fascinating and little-understood phenomena in biochemistry.

The last decade has witnessed a great deal of activity carried out by many workers to investigate the immunochemistry of several protein antigens. A great wealth of information in chemistry, immunochemistry, and technology has accumulated. The entire antigenic structures of sperm whale myoglobin and hen egg-white lysozyme were determined in 1975 and 1978, respectively, culminating studies that spanned in each case over 10 years of intensive research. It is surprising that there has been little awareness of the magnitude of the progress achieved in protein immunochemistry. Many recent immunological treatises have barely touched on this subject while amino acid polymers, haptens, polysaccharides, etc., have been reviewed frequently and extensively. Therefore, critical analysis of the knowledge available in protein immunochemistry appears timely and should serve as a valuable guide for present and future undertakings.

The various chapters are written by leading and highly active workers in the field. In view of the fact that methods and techniques employed in immunochemistry and immunology have been the subject of many excellent texts, the present work does not propose to duplicate these aspects. Only certain approaches that are, by the very nature of the subject, of particular relevance to immunochemical studies of proteins will be reviewed in this series. Volume 1 dealt with the approaches and the chemical strategy employed in studying the immunochemistry of proteins, the influence of conformation on immunochemical properties of proteins, investigation of immunochemical reactions by fluorescence polarization, in vitro immune responses to proteins and peptides, autoimmune antigens, histocompatibility antigens, and the immunochemistry of some well-characterized protein systems. Volume 2 discussed immunoadsorbents, which have proven to be a very powerful tool in immunochemistry, and presented a comprehensive critical account of the precise determination of the entire antigenic structure of myoglobin and a detailed analysis of the antigenic structure of lysozyme, the influence of antigen structure on humoral and cellular immunogenicity, the immunochemistry of tobacco mosaic virus protein, the effect of evolutionary amino acid replacements on protein immunochemistry, and the evolution of the immunogenic and subunit interaction sites of oligomeric enzymes, and finally a treatment of the structure and specificity requirements of concanavalin A, a protein which is being extensively employed as reagent in immunology.

Volume 3 is devoted primarily to the antibody aspect of the immune recognition and the immunochemistry of the complement system. The structure of antibodies is discussed and correlated with our present knowledge of antibody effector sites, antigenic features, and combining sites. This is followed by a chapter on the immunochemistry and biology of complement proteins and finally by a review of our current knowledge of the immunochemistry of serum albumin.

The treatise is intended to be a major reference work for those engaged in research in protein immunochemistry. One of the cruel shortcomings of review articles and books is that any work inadvertently overlooked by the reviewer may tend to be less cited and studied by others. It is my hope that the meticulous effort of the authors has minimized, if not completely avoided, this hazard.

M. Z. Atassi

Rochester, Minnesota

Contents

Chapter 1

Effector Sites on Antibodies

   N. J. Calvanico and T. B. Tomasi, Jr.

Chapter 2

Antigenic Features of Immunoglobulins

   J. Michael Kehoe and Rochelle Seide-Kehoe

Chapter 3

Combining Regions of Antibodies

Richard B. Weininger and Frank F. Richards

Chapter 4

Biochemistry and Biological Reactions of Complement Proteins

Robert M. Stroud, John E. Volanakis, Shigeharu Nagasawa, and Thomas F. Lint

Chapter 5

Immunochemistry of Bovine Serum Albumin

A. F. S. A. Habeeb

Contents of Volume 1

Contents of Volume 2

1

Effector Sites on Antibodies

N. J. Calvanico and T. B. Tomasi, Jr.

I. Introduction

Antibodies are bifunctional molecules. Their primary function is to specifically bind other molecules at their antigen-binding sites. Secondary functions which may arise as a consequence of antigen binding can be one of any number of important biological events such as the fixation of complement or the binding to one of several types of cells. These secondary properties are usually referred to as "physiological" or "effector" functions, and the mechanism of how the immunoglobulin molecule mediates them is of great importance to immunology and medicine.

In his Nobel Prize lecture in 1972, R. R. Porter commented on the fact that some aspects of the structural studies of immunoglobulins have reached completion (Porter, 1973). Indeed, the complete structures of several human heavy and light chains are known (Edelman et al., 1969; Putnam et al., 1973; Kratzin et al., 1975; Titani et al., 1966, 1967). Porter stated that the role of structural studies should now be involved in solving problems such as the interaction of antibodies with complement. It is to these types of studies that this chapter is addressed. The purpose is to examine what progress has been made in identifying the sites on immunoglobulins responsible for their various effector functions.

N. J. Calvanico and T. B. Tomasi, Jr.   ·   Department of Immunology, Mayo Medical School, Rochester, Minnesota, 55901. Present address of N. J. C.: Department of Medicine, Woods VA Hospital, Medical College of Wisconsin, Milwaukee, Wisconsin. This investigation was supported by Grant No. CA 09127, awarded by the National Cancer Institute, DHEW, and U.S. Public Health Research Grant AM 17554.

A brief account of immunoglobulin structure will be given here in as much detail as is necessary to discuss their effector functions. Also, in the following sections certain aspects of structure will be covered as they relate to the functions under discussion. A thorough review of the structure of immunoglobulins is beyond the scope of this chapter, and the reader is directed to the review of Gally (1973) for a detailed account of general immunoglobulin structure. In addition, several reviews are available on isolated areas such as structure and function of IgA (Tomasi and Grey, 1972) and the chemistry and biology of IgE (Ishizaka, 1973).

Finally, it should be noted that the major interest of this account is human immunoglobulins, but the studies done in other species will also be cited where they provide additional significant information concerning structure–function relations.

II. General Structure and Organization of Immunoglobulins

A. General Structure

All immunoglobulins have a generally similar basic four-polypeptide chain structure with the monomeric unit having a sedimentation rate of approximately 7 S. Two types of chains, heavy chains (55,000 daltons) and light chains (22,500 daltons), are, with a few exceptions, linked by disulfide bonds. A single immunoglobulin molecule has two identical heavy chains and two identical light chains (either κ or λ). There are five major *classes* of immunoglobulins in the human defined by the chemical and antigenic nature of the heavy chains (IgG, IgA, IgM, IgD, and IgE).

In addition to the major classes and types, there are subclasses and subtypes. These are determined by more subtle changes in the chemical structure of the heavy and light chains, respectively. Thus the IgG class has four subclasses while IgA has two and the other classes have one each, although there is some evidence that IgM may also have subclasses (Franklin and Frangione, 1968). There are subtypes of λ chains but not κ. There is yet a further chemical and antigenic subdivision of immunoglobulins based on genetically inherited variants of subclasses and subtypes. Thus, while normal individuals have all subclasses and subtypes, they may possess molecules which are allotypically different from those of another individual. This means that there is a polymorphism of the genes at a locus directing the synthesis of a given subclass or subtype. At present, allotypes are known for the four subclasses of IgG, one of the IgA subclasses, and κ chains. Although much of the chemical basis is known, these are, for the most part, serologically defined, and the relationships of these allotypic markers form the basis of a complicated area of genetics. For a review of this subject, the reader is directed to the article by Mage *et al.* (1973).

In addition to amino acid sequence, the classes and subclasses differ in the size of their heavy chains, carbohydrate content, arrangement of interchain disulfide bonds, and tendency to polymerize. Thus, while IgG shows little tendency to polymerize, IgM is nearly always found as a pentamer of the basic 7 S subunit and by electron microscopy has been shown to be a closed ring structure having a spiderlike appearance (Chesebro *et al.*, 1968). Low molecular weight IgM (7 S) has been found in trace amounts in normal human serum (Killander, 1963), and large quantities are usually indicative of disease (Stobo and Tomasi, 1967). The μ chain (heavy chain of IgM) is larger than the γ chain (heavy chain of IgG) and has more carbohydrate (Metzger, 1970). The major molecular form of human IgA is a 7 S protein, but significant amounts of a variety of polymers are usually found in addition to the monomer (Vaerman *et al.*, 1965). In other animals the polymeric forms, particularly the dimer, may predominate (Grey *et al.*, 1970). The γA polymers (dimers, trimers, tetramers) do not have the closed ring structure of IgM but are linked via disulfide bridges with little noncovalent interaction existing between these subunits (Beale and Feinstein, 1969; Miller and Metzger, 1965). The molecular weight of the α chain (heavy chain of IgA) is greater than the molecular weight of the γ chain because of higher carbohydrate content.

Fewer data are available concerning the structure of IgD and IgE. The ϵ chain (H chain of IgE) is similar in size to the μ chain and contains slightly more carbohydrate (Kochwa *et al.*, 1971). IgD is unusual in that it has a molecular weight close to that of IgE but its sedimentation rate is much lower. The size and carbohydrate content of its H chain (δ chain) appear also to be similar to those of IgE (Rowe *et al.*, 1969).

In addition to H and L chains, two other types of polypeptide chains, J chain and secretory component, have been found to be associated with the polymeric forms of IgA and IgM. The J chain (Halpern and Koshland, 1970; Mestecky *et al.*, 1971) is covalently linked by disulfide bonds to the penultimate cysteine residue in α and μ chains (Mestecky *et al.*, 1977). It contains 129 amino acids and a single carbohydrate moiety. The molecular weight calculated from the sequence is approximately 15,000, which agrees well with the previously reported molecular weight (Kang *et al.*, 1974). There is one J chain per polymer of IgA or IgM (Halpern and Koshland, 1973). The physiological role of J chain is not clear, but there is evidence that it may in some way control intracellular polymerization mechanisms (Della Corte and Parkhouse, 1973). It has been suggested that the presence of J chain is necessary for the association of the polymers with secretory component (SC) (Eskeland and Brandtzaeg, 1974), although IgA myeloma proteins have been described whose polymers lack J chain (Eskeland and Brandtzaeg, 1974; Brandtzaeg, 1976; Tomasi and Czerwinski, 1976) and are capable of binding SC in vitro. SC is a single chain with a molecular weight of 80,000 (Labib et al., 1976) and is primarily associated with the polymeric forms of IgA and IgM in secretions (Tomasi and Grey, 1972). Its function is unknown, but it has been postulated to be involved in the selective glandular transfer of these two classes of immunoglobulins. The observation that secretory IgA is more resistant to proteolysis than serum IgA polymers has led to the suggestion (Tomasi and Bienenstock, 1968; Lindh, 1975) that SC may protect secretory IgA from degradation in the "hostile" environment of the luminal secretions where it exerts its biological action.

The subclasses of IgG and IgA are similar to each other in size, with the exception of the IgG3 subclass which has a larger H chain than the other subclasses because of an unusually large "hinge" region (Michaelsen and Natvig, 1974a; Adlersberg et al., 1975). However, the number and arrangement of interchain disulfide bonds vary considerably between classes and subclasses, and this variability is the basis of a chemical method of distinguishing subclasses by autoradiography (Frangione and Franklin, 1972). Table I is a summary of the properties of the classes and subclasses of immunoglobulins.

B. Domain Theory

The primary structures of heavy chains and light chains from several sources have been completely or partially sequenced (Gally, 1973). The most salient characteristic of these primary structures is the fact that they can be divided into homology regions composed of 110–115 amino acids containing one intrachain disulfide bond formed by two cysteine residues separated by approximately 60 amino acid residues. There are two such regions in light chains and four in IgG and IgA heavy chains. IgM, IgD (Bennich and von Bahr-Lindstrom, 1974), and probably IgE have five homologous regions. The first, or amino-terminal region, is referred to as the "variable region" in both H and L chains because its sequence varies from molecule to molecule. This region contains the antibody site. Three stretches where variation in sequence is more pronounced have been localized in the NH_2-terminal region of both H and L chains. These regions are intimately involved in binding of the antigen

Table I. Properties of Classes and Subclasses of Immunoglobulins

	IgG₁	IgG₂	IgG₃	IgG₄	IgA₁	IgA₂	IgM	IgD	IgE
Formula	$\gamma 1_2 L_2$	$\gamma 2_2 L_2$	$\gamma 3_2 L_2$	$\gamma 4_2 L_2$	$\alpha 1_2 L_2$ $(\alpha 1_2 L_2)_2$-J $(\alpha 1_2 L_2)_2$-J-SC	$\alpha 2_2 L_2$ $(\alpha 2_2 L_2)_2$-J $(\alpha 2_2 L_2)_2$-J-SC	$(\mu_2 L_2)_5$-J $(\mu_2 L_2)_5$-J-SC	$\delta_2 L_2$	$\epsilon_2 L_2$
Light-chain (L) κ/λ ratio	2.4	1.1	1.4	8.0	1.4	1.6	3.2	0.3	—
Sedimentation rate (S)	6.6	6.6	6.6	6.6	6.2–17 (10–11 in secretions)	6.2–17	18–32	6.6	8.0
Molecular weight of heavy chain (with CH_2O)	52,000–54,000	52,000–54,000	60,000	52,000–54,000	56,000–58,000	52,000–54,000	65,000–70,000	70,000	71,000
Carbohydrate (%)	2–3	2–3	2–3	2–3	5–10	5–10	7–12	10	12
Polymers	Rare	Rare	Aggregates	Rare	Dimers primarily (multimers also)		Formed from pentamer		
Serum concentration mg/ml[a]	5–12	2–6	0.5–1.0	0.2–1.0	0.5–2.0	0–0.2	0.5–1.5	0.03	0.0003
approximate % of total[b]	50	15	5		15	1.5	10	Negligible	Negligible
Synthesis (mg/kg/day)	25.4	—	3.4	—	24	4.3	2.2	0.4	0.002
Fractional turnover (% per day)	8.0	6.9	16.8	6.9	24	34.0	10.6	37.0	72
Half-life (days)	21	20	7	21	5.9	4.5	5.1	2.8	2.4
Number of domains in H chain	4	4	4	4	4	4	5	5	5

[a] J chain (molecular weight = 15,000).
[b] Secretory component (molecular weight = 80,000) (Labib et al., 1976).

and are referred to as the "hypervariable regions" (or, more recently, the "complementarity regions") (Kehoe and Capra, 1971; Kabat and Wu, 1972, Wu and Kabat, 1970). These regions are associated with the individual antigenic determinants of the molecule referred to as "idiotypic markers." The rest of the variable region is sometimes referred to as the "framework" and is relatively less variable.

The remaining homology regions have sequences which are essentially invariant within a subclass, except for genetic substitutions at certain positions. These regions are referred to as the "constant regions" and are numbered starting at the amino-terminal end. Thus, while a light chain has one variable region and one constant region, a γ chain has one variable region and three constant regions (V_H, C_H1, C_H2, C_H3). Between C_H1 and C_H2 is an 18–20 amino acid "hinge region" which is not analogous in structure to the rest of the chain and contains most of the inter-heavy-chain disulfide bonds. This hinge peptide usually has a high content of proline and is susceptible to attack by several proteolytic enzymes, an important property in the studies of immunoglobulin structure and function, as we shall discuss later.

The variable (V) region sequences can be grouped into subgroups by certain criteria such as invariability at certain positions, linked amino acid substitutions, length, and sequence homology. Thus, while two proteins from two different subgroups may differ in sequence by as much as 40%, the homology within a subgroup is much greater, and a high proportion of the amino acid interchanges present can be accounted for by a single base change in the codon (Gray et al., 1967; Milstein, 1967). At present, there are three V region subgroups for κ chains, five for λ chains, and three for heavy chains. V_κ regions associate only with C_κ regions and V_λ regions with C_λ regions, whereas heavy-chain variable regions can associate with any class or subclass constant region. These observations led to the theory that at least two genes (V and C) code for each of the polypeptide chains in immunoglobulins (Dreyer and Bennett, 1965). The questions of (1) how does the diversity of the variable genes arise? and (2) how do the V and C genes unite? are areas of continuing controversy and the subject of several reviews (Capra and Kindt, 1975; Todd, 1972; Smith et al., 1971; Gally and Edelman, 1972).

Edelman (1970) proposed that each of the homology regions was separately folded into compact globular domains joined by relatively linear stretches of amino acids. Moreover, these domains evolved for specific funtions. Thus the V_H and V_L domains interact to form the antigen-combining site. The functions of the constant domains are the subject of this chapter.

C. Fragmentation of Immunoglobulins

A key to studies on the localization of sites of biological activities on immunoglobulins is the extent to which segments of their polypeptide chains can be isolated. The classicial work of Porter (1959) demonstrated that by treating rabbit antibody with papain two types of fragments were produced: a Fab fragment composed of a light-chain disulfide bonded to the amino-terminal half of the heavy chain, and the Fc (because of its crystallizability) composed of the two carboxyl-terminal halves of the heavy chains. The Fab fragments contain the antibody-combining site, and the Fc is responsible for the majority of the effector functions of immunoglobulins. Each antibody molecule on cleavage yields two identical Fab fragments and one Fc fragment. An analogous cleavage of human immunoglobulins with papain was later achieved by other investigators (Edelman, 1970; Porter, 1959; Franklin, 1960; Hsiao and Putnam, 1961; Deutsch et al., 1961).

The success of Porter was fortuitous in that it provided a method of easily dividing the molecule into its two major functional parts. This led many investigators to examine the effect of other enzymes on immunoglobulins with the hope of further localizing these functions more precisely.

Pepsin at pH 4.5 releases a fragment composed of two Fab-like fragments joined by disulfide bonds (Nisonoff et al., 1960; Heimer et al., 1967). The pepsin F(ab')$_2$ fragment is divalent and, although able to precipitate with polyvalent antigen, does not participate in most effector functions since it lacks the Fc fragment which is degraded by pepsin into smaller but antigenically active fragments (Goodman, 1963). One of these fragments, the Fc', precipitates with antisera and can be shown to be immunologically deficient to the Fc but of greater anodal electrophoretic mobility (see Fig. 1) (Turner and Bennich, 1968; Utsumi and Karush, 1965; Prahl, 1967; Heimer and Schnoll, 1968). A similar type of fragment is released by prolonged papain cleavage (Poulik, 1966; Irimajiri et al., 1968; Grey and Abel, 1967) and by several other enzymes (Calvanico and Tomasi, 1971; Schrohenloher, 1963; Gall and D'Eustachio, 1972). Fc' fragments have been extensively studied by Turner and his associates (Turner and Rowe, 1966; Bennich and Turner, 1969; Turner et al., 1969a,b; Turner and Berggard, 1969; Natvig et al., 1971), who have established the point of pepsin cleavage on the heavy chain as being between the C_H2 and C_H3 domains at Ile-336 (Eu numbering). The peptic Fc' subunit (pFc'), therefore, is a dimeric subunit of the C_H3 domain held together by noncovalent interaction. The C_H2 domain is completely de-

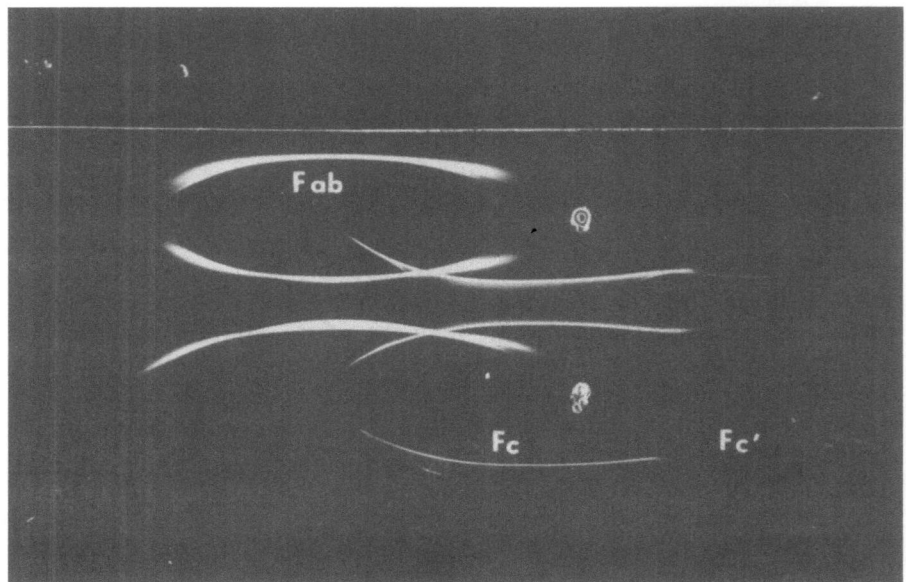

Figure 1. Immunoelectrophoretic pattern of Fab, Fc, and Fc' fragments. Both wells contain papain-digested human IgG. The upper trough contains antiserum made against the Fab fragment, the middle trough contains antiserum made against the undigested native IgG, and the bottom trough contains antiserum made against the Fc fragment. The mobility of the undigested native IgG is not shown, but it migrates to a position between the Fab and Fc fragments. The anode is to the right.

graded to dialyzable peptides in the course of peptic digestion. Papain further reduces the pFc' fragment by six amino acids on the amino terminus and 14 amino acids on the carboxyl terminus, while prolonged (> 10 hr) digestion of this subunit results in further degradation to dialyzable peptides. In contrast to this, prolonged digestion of the Fab fragment by pepsin at pH 4.5 does not reduce its size. However, at pH 2.5, pepsin digestion completely destroys antibody activity, reducing the native molecule to 90% dialyzable peptides in 8 hr. In 1 hr almost half of the antigen-binding capacity is lost (Haber and Stone, 1967). Papain at pH 7.0 also produces a 100,000 molecular weight fragment from normal IgG. The nature of the fragment differs with the amount of cysteine used to activate the enzyme (Michaelsen and Natvig, 1972). In no case, however, is a F(ab')$_2$ fragment obtained. The sites of pepsin and papain digestion of IgG are shown diagrammatically in Fig. 2.

The mouse IgA myeloma 315, which has antibodylike activity for the 2,4-dinitrophenyl (DNP) group, on treatment with pepsin at pH 3.8

releases a fragment composed of only the V_H and V_L domains, termed the "F_V fragment," capable of binding DNP (Inbar *et al.*, 1972; Hochman *et al.*, 1973). This provides direct and conclusive evidence that the antigen-binding site is located in the variable domains. A similar cleavage of human IgG with trypsin has also been reported (Medgyesi *et al.*, 1973). In this case, however, a fragment containing the C_H1 and C_L domains linked by a disulfide bond was obtained (called "t Fab' fragment") instead of the F_V fragment, which is apparently degraded. Peptic digestion at pH 4.5 of a Waldenstrom IgM has been reported to liberate a F_V fragment (Kakimoto and Onoue, 1974). The C_H1 domain may also be prepared by chemical cleavage of fully reduced and aminoethylated Fd fragment (V_H plus C_H1 domains) with CNBr (Zegers *et al.*, 1975).

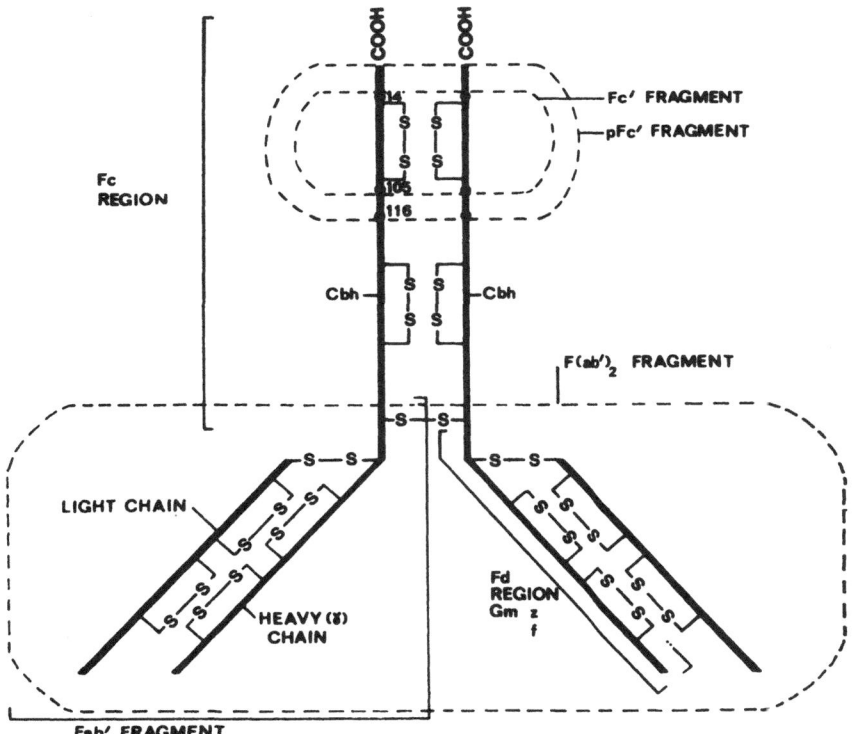

Figure 2. Human IgG, showing the location of the sites of cleavage of F(ab')₂ and Fc fragments as well as the Fc' (papain) and pFc' (pepsin) fragments (numbered from COOH-terminal ends of γ chains). Carbohydrate is denoted by Cbh. Reproduced from Turner *et al.* (1969*a*) by courtesy of Dr. M. W. Turner and *Nature*.

The C_H2 region of IgG has proved to be the most labile of the domains. It is extremely susceptible to proteolysis, in contrast to the C_H3 homology region. The C_H2 region has now been isolated in good yield by exposing the molecule to pH 2.5, then readjusting to pH 8.0 and treating with immobilized trypsin for short periods of time (Connell and Porter, 1971; Ellerson et al., 1972, 1976). In addition, a second method based on peptic digestion at elevated temperatures has been reported for the isolation of this domain (Seon and Pressman, 1975).

The IgG subclasses vary in their susceptibility to papain (Jeffries et al., 1968; Gergely et al., 1970; Virella and Parkhouse, 1971). The order of increasing resistance to papain digestion is IgG3 < IgG1 < IgG4 < IgG2. It is not clear whether or not papain releases a Fc' fragment from all subclasses. Thus, while the IgG3 subclass is readily degraded to Fab and Fc fragments, the Fc appears to be stable to further degradation. Similar studies have been carried out on the effect of pepsin digestion of the four IgG subclasses (Turner et al., 1970a,b,c; Michaelsen and Natvig, 1971). The results indicate that IgG1 and IgG2 are resistant to degradation into smaller peptides while the IgG3 and IgG4 subclasses are more sensitive. However, there are also some qualitative differences. For example, it was found that no Fc' fragment was obtained from the IgG4 subclass unless the enzyme–substrate ratio was lowered to 1/200 (instead of the 1/100 used with the other subclasses). Also, the F(ab')$_2$ fragment of the IgG2 subclass was sensitive to further breakdown, but the nature of the end product was not determined. Taken together these results indicate that Fab, Fc, and Fc' fragments can be obtained from all the subclasses but the conditions required vary.

Fab and Fc fragments have now been isolated from all classes and subclasses of immunoglobulins. Several investigators have examined the effect of papain on IgM. In general, the results have shown that a Fab-type fragment was obtained in good yields while the yield of the Fc_μ fragment was poor (Inman and Hazeu, 1968; Onoue et al., 1968; Mihaesco and Seligmann, 1968a). Peptic digestion yields initially a F(ab')$_2$-like fragment which, on further hydrolysis, degrades to a Fab-type fragment and finally completely into small peptides (Mihaesco and Seligmann, 1968b; Kishimoto et al., 1968). Other enzymes have also been investigated and have given similar results in that small amounts, if any, of the Fc_μ fragment can be isolated, while F(ab)$_2$ or Fab-type fragments are recovered in good yields (Miller and Metzger, 1966; Chen et al., 1969). A significant advance came with the finding that treatment of IgM with trypsin at elevated temperatures resulted in the release of Fab and Fc_μ fragments in excellent yields (Plaut and Tomasi, 1970). This has facilitated sequence studies of IgM as well as the location of functional sites. The "hot trypsin" technique, as it is now called, has proved useful in obtaining limited proteolysis of other immunoglobulins as well as fragments of other unrelated proteins. As mentioned earlier, there are five homology regions in IgM, with the inter-H-chain disulfide bond between the C_H2 and C_H3 domains. This inter-H-chain disulfide bond joins the two μ chains of a given 7 S subunit, while the inter-subunit-H-chain disulfide which connects H chains of two different 7 S subuits is in the C_H3 domain at position 414 (Ou numbering). Hydrolysis with the hot trypsin technique cleaves the Arg-325–Gly-326 peptide bond (Ou numbering), just 11 amino acids NH_2-terminal to the inter-H-chain cysteine (Cys-337). This treatment also results in the degradation of the C_H2 domain (Putnam et al., 1973), between residues 214 and 325. A similar tryptic cleavage of IgM has recently been obtained by the use of 4–5 M urea instead of heat to obtain the conformational changes necessary for accessibility of the bond to trypsin (Shimizu et al., 1974). These results are summarized diagrammatically in Fig. 3.

Human IgA has proved to be resistant to papain digestion (Underdown and Dorrington, 1974). Under conditions in which 90% of IgG1 proteins are cleaved to Fab and Fc fragments, IgA (serum and secretory) is undigested. This is not true of mouse IgA (Fahey, 1963) and rabbit s-IgA (Hanly et al., 1973), which readily yield Fc fragments. Mild reduction and alkylation of human IgA render it susceptible to digestion with papain (as with IgG2 and IgG4), which results in Fab fragments and peptides derived from the Fc. Various degrees of cleavage of IgA with pepsin have been reported, but in no case had the Fc_α been successfully isolated. The major product is either a $F(ab')_2$ or Fab-type fragment, or, most commonly, both. The more susceptible IgA proteins appear to belong to the IgA2 subclass (Zegers et al., 1974; Wilson and Williams, 1969; Bernier et al., 1965; Shuster, 1971). Recently, an enzyme, IgA protease, has been discovered in bacteria which specifically cleaves only IgA (Mehta et al., 1974) into Fab and Fc_α. This enzyme acts only on molecules of the IgA1 subclass (Plaut et al., 1974a) and splits at the Pro-227–Thr-228 bond (Frangione and Wolfenstein-Todel, 1972). It should be pointed out that the same sequence in other proteins and even in the synthetic peptide Ac-Pro-Thr-Pro-Thr is not cleaved by IgA protease (Labib et al., 1978). This unique enzyme has now been found in other organisms (Plaut et al., 1974b, 1975; Genco et al., 1975). The Fc_α liberated by this enzyme shows size heterogeneity reflecting the monomer-polymer content of the starting IgA substrate. Reduction and alkylation give a preparation homogeneous in size and similar to the Fc produced by papain digestion of IgG. Another method which has been used to prepare human IgA Fc fragments is based on the hot trypsin technique but with the addition of relatively high

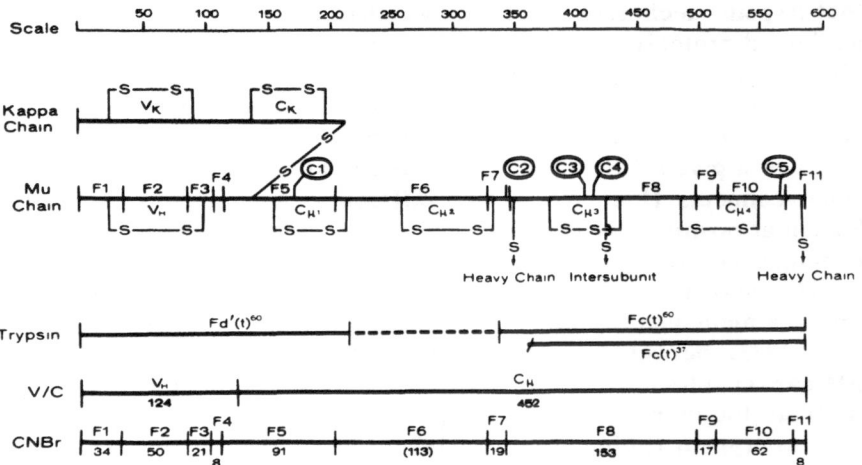

Figure 3.   Structure of the μ heavy chain and the κ light chain of IgM Ou, showing (1) the interchain and intrachain disulfide bridges, (2) the two homology regions of the light chain (V_κ and C_κ), and (3) the five homology regions of the μ heavy chain (V_H and $C_\mu1$–$C_\mu4$). The figure for the μ chain also shows the location of the five oligosaccharides (C1–C5), the points of cleavage by trypsin with the respective fragments (Fd and Fc), and the sites of cleavage by CNBr and the respective fragments (F1–F11). The scale indicates the number of amino acid residues in each chain and fragment. The Fc sequence has 251 residues joined in a single polypeptide chain. Ten such chains are linked through intrachain and intersubunit bridges to form the decameric Fc fragment derived by cleavage of intact IgM with trypsin at 60°C [sometimes designated $(Fc)_5\mu$]. The molecular weight of a single Fc chain, calculated from the amino acid composition and exclusive of the carbohydrate, is 27,600; thus $(Fc)_5\mu$ has a molecular weight of 276,000. Reproduced from Putnam *et al.* (1973); copyright 1973 by the American Association for the Advancement of Science, reprinted with permission.

concentrations of neutral salts (Calvanico and Tomasi, 1976). This technique produces Fc_α fragments from both IgA1 and IgA2. The exact point of cleavage is unknown. Similar results have now been obtained by using guanidine hydrochloride in place of heat and neutral salts (N. J. Calvanico and T. B. Tomasi, unpublished observations). The cleavage of IgA is illustrated in Fig. 4.

    Fab and Fc fragments have also been prepared from IgD and IgE immunoglobulins. IgD is very susceptible to proteolysis and is often degraded during storage (Griffiths and Gleich, 1972). Incubation with various enzymes including papain, trypsin, and plasmin causes the rapid production of Fab and Fc_δ (Spiegelberg *et al.*, 1970). Prolonged incubation results in complete degradation of these fragments. Surprisingly, high-temperature trypsinolysis of IgD produces a stable Fc_δ fragment with concomitant destruction of the Fab fragment (Wolcott *et al.*, 1975). The IgE myeloma proteins ND and PS have both been cleaved to Fab, Fc, and Fc' by papain digestion (K. Ishizaka *et al.*, 1970*a*; Bennich *et al.*, 1968; Ito *et al.*, 1971). Pepsin produces a $F(ab')_2$ fragment.

From the preceding discussion on the fragmentation of immunoglobulins, it is obvious that the primary site of attack of the proteolytic enzymes is most commonly within the hinge region. The other sites of attack are between the V_H and C_H1 domains and between the C_H2 and C_H3 domains. The most resistant parts of the molecule are the domains themselves. This is also true of the light chains where cleavage by a number of enzymes results in liberation of the two domains (Cioli and Baglioni, 1968; Karlsson *et al.*, 1969, 1972; Fraser *et al.*, 1972). These studies support the idea that the domains or homology regions of immunoglobulin polypeptide chains are tightly packed globular regions connected by relatively linear stretches of amino acids which are more susceptible to enzymatic attack. The ability to excise a given domain from the polypeptide chain by proteolytic techniques has greatly aided our knowledge of the location of various effector functions.

Another point evident from these studies is that there is little noncovalent interaction between domains on the same polypeptide chain since simple proteolysis causes their separation. This is in contrast to the domains that are aligned with each other or paired in the native molecule, such as the V_H and V_L domains or the C_H3 domains on separate H chains,

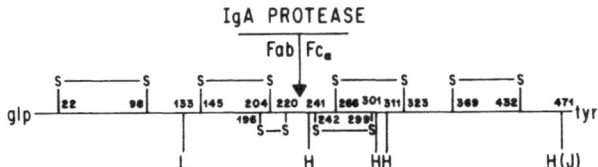

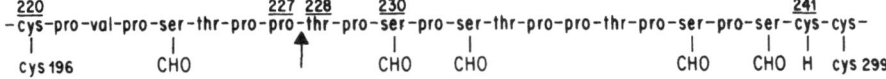

Figure 4.   Structure of α chain and the site of cleavage of IgA protease. Numbering refers to positions of cysteine residues according to the BUR sequence (Liu *et al.*, 1976). H refers to heavy chains and L to light chains. The J in parentheses indicates that this cysteine may be joined to either the J chain or another heavy chain. The arrow marks the position of cleavage by IgA protease. The lower half of the diagram shows the sequence of the hinge region from residues 220 to 242 and the position of IgA protease cleavage. Carbohydrate is denoted by CHO.

which may show considerable noncovalent interaction, and denaturing conditions are usually required to effect their separation. However, this is not always true since noncovalent interactions have not been found in the Fc region of IgM (Hester *et al.*, 1975). In contrast to this, it has been found that after reduction of 19 S IgM by a method which selectively cleaves intersubunit disulfide bonds, pentamers of IgM may be maintained solely by noncovalent forces (Tomasi, 1973). Apparently bonds other than the intersubunit disulfides must be reduced before noncovalent association is lost. It should be noted that the μ chain does not have a typical hinge region. The inter-H-chain disulfide bond is situated between C_H2 and C_H3 domains, but this region lacks the proline-rich sequence. A list of the fragments obtained by proteolysis of immunoglobulins is given in Table II together with the domains which they comprise.

D. Shape of Immunoglobulins

1. General Conformation

In considering the sites associated with specific functions, the contribution of the shape of the protein must be taken into account. In the last 2 or 3 years a considerable amount of information has been obtained concerning the three-dimensional shape of immunoglobulins and their subunits (see reviews by Poljak, 1975a; Davies *et al.*, 1975). In addition, the conformational changes of immunoglobulins resulting from their interaction with antigen have been explored. It is commonly held that the binding of antigen with the F_V region of antibody triggers conformational changes in the Fc fragment, thereby exposing sites for effector functions which are ordinarily hidden or unavailable in the native molecule. However, considerable controversy exists regarding this theory, as discussed below.

The antibody molecule is composed of three globular regions representing the two Fab fragments and one Fc linked by the more flexible hinge region. This model was first proposed by Noelken *et al.* (1965) from hydrodynamic data, supplanting the earlier prolate ellipsoid model of Edelman and Gally (1964). The major characteristics are the compactness of the Fab and Fc fragments and their ability to behave independently of each other through the flexible hinge region. The conformation of isolated Fab and Fc fragments is indistinguishable from their conformation in the native molecule (Steiner and Lowey, 1966; Ikeda *et al.*, 1968; Cathou *et al.*, 1968; Ross and Jirgensons, 1968). A variety of physicochemical techniques have been used to measure the angle between the two Fab fragments (Werner *et al.*, 1972; Cathou and O'Konski,

Table II.   Proteolytic Fragments

Nomenclature	Structure	Reference	Method
Fc_γ	$C_\gamma 2$, $C_\gamma 3$	Porter (1959)	Papain
Fc_α	$C_\alpha 2$, $C_\alpha 3$	Mehta et al. (1974), Calvanico and Tomasi (1976)	IgA protease; HTT^a + high salt
$(Fc)_5\mu$ and Fc_μ	$C_\mu 3$, $C_\mu 4$	Plaut and Tomasi (1970), Shimizu et al. (1974)	HTT^a; trypsin + urea
Fc_ϵ	$C_\epsilon 2$, $C_\epsilon 3$, $C_\epsilon 4$	Ishizaka et al. (1970a)	Papain
Fab	V_H, $C_H 1$, V_L, C_L	Porter (1959)	Papain
Fab_2'	$(V_H, C_H 1, V_L, C_L)_2$	Nisonoff et al. (1960)	Pepsin
Fd	V_H, $C_H 1$	Frangione et al. (1967)	Pepsin
Fc', pFc', tFc'	$C_H 3$	Turner and Bennich (1968), Calvanico and Tomasi (1971), Matthews et al. (1971)	Papain+; chymotrypsin C+; trypsin
Facb	$(V_H, C_\gamma 1, C_\gamma 2, V_L, C_L)_2$	Colomb and Porter (1975)	Low pH + trypsin^c
F_V	V_H, V_L	Inbar et al. (1972)	Pepsin at pH 3.6
Fd_V	V_H	Dammacco et al. (1972)	Papain
Fb(s), tFab'	$C_H 1$, C_L	Gall and D'Eustachio (1972), Medgyesi et al. (1973)	Subtilisin; trypsin
Fb_2'	$(C_H 1, C_L)_2$	Parr et al. (1976a)	Pepsin + urea
upFc	$C_\gamma 2$, $C_\gamma 3^d$	Parr et al. (1976b)	Pepsin + urea
Fh	IgG3 hinge region	Michaelsen et al. (1974)	α-Chymotrypsin
Fch	Fh, $C_{\gamma 3}2$, $C_{\gamma 3}3$	Michaelsen and Natvig (1974b)	Papain
$C_H 2$	$C_H 2$	Ellerson et al. (1972), Seon and Pressman (1975)	Low pH + trypsin^c; HTP^b
$F(ab)_2$	$(Fab)_2$ noncovalent	Michaelsen and Natvig (1972)	Papain
$F(c)_2$	$(Fc)_2$ disulfide linked	Michaelsen and Natvig (1972)	Papain
Fab/c	Fc, Fab	Michaelsen and Natvig (1972)	Papain

[a] HTT, high-temperature trypsinolysis.
[b] HTP, high-temperature pepsinolysis.
[c] Substrate immunoglobulin is exposed to low pH for short periods of time prior to incubation with enzyme at readjusted pH.
[d] Residues 337–410 (Eu numbering) missing.

1970; Pilz et al., 1970; Valentine and Green, 1967). It appears to vary between 0° and 180°, the larger angles existing in the unliganded molecule.

Optical rotatory dispersion (ORD) of immunoglobulins demonstrated a lack of α helix in earlier studies (Imahori and Momoi, 1962; Jirgensons, 1961; Winkler and Doty, 1961) and suggested the presence of some degree of β structure (Imahori, 1963; Jirgensons, 1965). These observations were later confirmed by circular dichroism studies in several laboratories (Sarkar and Doty, 1966; Ross and Jirgensons, 1968; Dorrington and Smith, 1972). CD spectra showing β structure have now been found in all classes, subclasses, L chains, γ chains, and Fab and Fc fragments (Johnson *et al.*, 1974; Dorrington and Tanford, 1968; Underdown and Dorrington, 1974; Kincaid and Jirgensons, 1972; Ghose and Jirgensons, 1971; Bjork and Tanford, 1971*a*; Dorrington and Bennich, 1973; Johnson *et al.*, 1975). CD spectra for V and C regions of L chains have been found to be distinct, but theoretical spectra calculated from an equimolar mixture of the two "add up" to the spectrum obtained with intact L chains (Bjork *et al.*, 1971). These data are taken as evidence in support of the domain theory, since each region supposedly behaves independently of the other. In contrast to this, however, the CD spectra of C_H2 and C_H3 do not "add up" to that found for the Fc of IgG, suggesting significant interactions between these two domains (Isenman *et al.*, 1977). The C_H3 domain appears to be the only one lacking the 217-nm negative band (Dorrington *et al.*, 1972).

In contrast to the experimental CD spectrum for the heavy chain, which is similar to that calculated from Fd and Fc fragments (Huston *et al.*, 1972), the spectrum for the native molecule differs from that calculated from spectra of H and L chains (Dorrington and Smith, 1972; Stevenson and Dorrington, 1970; Welter, 1972; Bjork and Tanford, 1971*b*). This is also true of spectra of the Fab fragment and its constitutive Fd and L chains and would be expected on the basis of the strong, noncovalent interaction between H and L chains (Smith and Dorrington, 1972). This has been shown by several techniques. Zimmerman and Grey (1972) studied this interaction in mildly reduced immunoglobulins by determining the amount of urea necessary to disrupt the secondary forces between H and L chains on starch gel electrophoresis. They found that dissociation of IgA2 required a higher urea concentration (approximately 3 M) than that required by IgM (approximately 1 M), while that for IgA1 and IgG was somewhat less than that for IgA2. Bigelow *et al.* (1974) estimated the association constant (K_a) between H and L chains to be greater than 10^9 M^{-1} by difference spectroscopy. The enthalpy of interaction for eight proteins was determined in a calorimeter as being -5.6 to -112.5 kJ/mole of heavy-light chain pairs at 25°C (Dorrington and Kortan, 1974). The wide range of values obtained is surprising but could not be related to L-chain type. It was suggested that the differences reflect interactions in the variable regions. On the assumption that the entropy change (ΔS^0) was negligible, a K_a was calculated from these data in the range of 10^1–10^{20} M^{-1}. The lower values are inconsistent with the values reported by Bigelow *et al.* (1974) and other available information, suggesting that H-L chains associate with significant entropy changes. The relative importance of the entropy and enthalpy terms in the H-L interactions clearly differs between individual proteins. It is also clear that while H and L subunits strongly interact, little interaction occurs between the domains of a given chain with the possible exception of a moderate interaction between the C_H2 and C_H3 domains.

Results of X-ray crystallography have supported the domain hypothesis. The early low-resolution (6 Å) crystallographic studies on the human IgG1 protein Dob (Terry *et al.*, 1968; Labaw and Davies, 1971; Sarma *et al.*, 1971) showed three globular regions, but the polypeptide backbone could not be traced at this level. The first evidence for individual domains came from studies on the Mcg λ-type Bence Jones dimer at 6 Å resolution (Schiffer *et al.*, 1970; Edmundson *et al.*, 1972). The results indicated the presence of two globular regions of unequal size having little interaction with each other, but having considerable interaction with homologous regions between chains. More recently, studies at a higher resolution (3.5 Å) have defined the path of the polypeptide backbone of this dimer (Schiffer *et al.*, 1973) and a β structure was found in both the V and C domains. Interestingly, the two light chains, although identical in sequence, are conformationally different and form a three-dimensional structure similar to the Fab. One monomer plays the structural role of the Fd fragment while the other behaves as a light chain, thereby resembling a Fab fragment. This Bence Jones dimer has been shown to bind several haptens, and the residues providing the binding site for each hapten have been determined (Edmundson *et al.*, 1974).

Poljak *et al.* (1973, 1974) examined the structure of the Fab′ fragment of the human IgG1 (λ) myeloma protein NEW, first at 2.8 Å and then at 2.0 Å. Their results showed four globular subunits (V_L, V_H, C_L, C_H1) arranged in a tetrahedral configuration. All the homology subunits showed the same type of folding (an antiparallel β-pleated sheet structure) referred to as the "immunoglobulin fold" (Poljak, 1975b) as shown in Fig. 5. Interestingly, the enzyme superoxide dismutase, which shows no homology in sequence with immunoglobulins, has a very similar fold (Richardson *et al.*, 1976). This structure consists of two sheets of antiparallel peptide chains connected by the interchain disulfide bond in the interior, which is filled by hydrophobic side chains (Fig. 6). The globular domains are formed by two "immunoglobulin folds" in contact with each other (V_H with V_L and C_H1 with C_L) to make a single globular unit. The two globular units (V_H/V_L and C_H1/C_L) are separated by an internal space accessible to solvent and, consistent with enzymatic studies, to attack by proteolytic enzymes (the switch region).

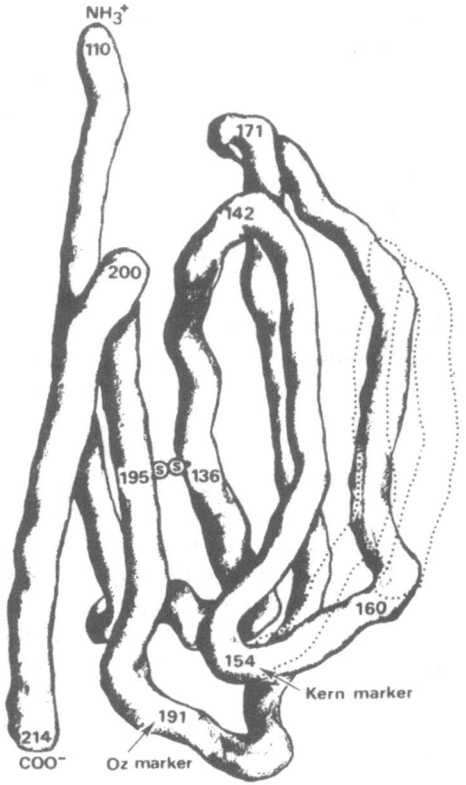

Figure 5. Basic "immunoglobulin fold." Solid trace shows the folding of the polypeptide chain in the constant sub-units (C_L and C_H1). Numbers designate L(λ)-chain residues, beginning at "NH_3^+," which corresponds to residue 110 for the L chain. Broken lines indicate the additional loop of polypeptide chain characteristic of the V_L and V_H subunits. Reproduced from Poljak (1975a) with permission of Dr. Poljak and *Nature*.

Studies by Epp *et al.* (1972, 1974) on the dimeric variable region unit of the K-type Bence Jones protein Rei (Palm, 1970) also indicated a structure with two cylindrical-shaped homology regions forming one globular unit. This variable region dimer forms a primitive antibody-like molecule having spatial relationships similar to the V unit of the BJ dimer Mcg (Epp *et al.*, 1975), again indicating the conformation of the variable domain is independent of the constant domain. The subsequent report of a similar structure in the McPC 603 mouse IgA myeloma Fab fragment suggests the universality of this globular domain arrangement for immunoglobulin polypeptide chains (Rudikoff *et al.*, 1972; Padlan *et al.*, 1973).

Information concerning the binding site of antibodies has recently been obtained from the X-ray studies (Amzel *et al.*, 1974; Segal *et al.*, 1974). Both the human myeloma NEW and the mouse myeloma IgA McPC603 are known to bind haptens. In both cases the antigen-binding site is at the end of the Fab fragment exposed to solvent and formed by the V_L and V_H domains. The cavities formed by these domains are entirely lined by the hypervariable regions which were predicted to be the contact points of the combining site by Wu and Kabat (1970) and Kabat and Wu (1972). It was also found that close interactions between the V_L and V_H domains occur through positions on both chains which are occupied by framework residues or conservative substitutions thereof. It is interesting to note in both studies of the structure of the antigen-combining site complexes at 3.1 Å (mouse) and 3.5 Å (human) that no major changes were observed in the Fab fragments on binding to hapten. However, such changes may be subtle, and higher-resolution studies are needed to confirm this important point.

Analogous information concerning the conformation and interaction of the Fc domains is lacking. This is due to the inability to obtain suitable crystals of Fc fragments (in particular, their heavy atom derivatives) (Colman *et al.*, 1974) or intact molecules (Davies *et al.*, 1971; Edmundson *et al.*, 1971). Recently, an attempt to rectify this problem with the IgG1 myeloma protein Dob has been made by Sarma and Zaloga (1975). This protein is known to be extremely sensitive to X-radiation (Davies *et al.*, 1971), thereby preventing high-resolution structure analysis. By growing the crystals in the presence of styrene monomers which subsequently polymerize to polystyrene by radiation, the authors found that they could stabilize the crystals and thus increase their resolution to 4 Å. Colman *et al.* (1976) have recently reported their findings on the intact myeloma IgG1 protein Kol at 5 Å resolution. The Fab part of the molecule is similar to those reported for NEW and McPC 603 but the Fab angle

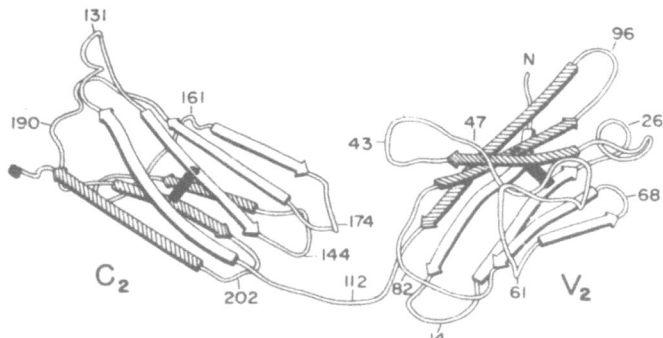

Figure 6.   A variable (V_2) and a constant (C_2) region of a Bence Jones protein. The arrows represent chain directions of some of the segments but do not represent accurate chain lengths. The white and striped arrows correspond to different layers (see text), and the numbers denote approximate positions of certain residues. Reproduced with permission from Schiffer *et al.* (1973); copyright by the American Chemical Society.

differs. The authors speculate that this may be due to the presence of the Fc part of the molecule and make note of the fact that the switch region between V and C domains may act similarly to the hinge region in being a point of flexibility for the ligand-binding sites. The Fc density map is hard to interpret, but there appears to be a flex point here as well. A recent report on the crystallographic structure of a human Fc fragment at 4 Å resolution indicates that whereas the $C_H 3$ unit shows close inter-action between the individual domains (as with the $C_H 1/C_L$ and V_L/V_H units), the $C_H 2$ domains of the individual chains are completely separated and do not interact at all (Deisenhofer *et al.*, 1976*a*). These authors also report very little interaction between $C_H 2$ domains at 3.5 Å resolution (Deisenhofer *et al.*, 1976*b*). These data are consistent with the recent report by Isenman *et al.* (1977), who have found a greater degree of aromatic chromophore exposure in the $C_\gamma 2$ domain than in the $C_\gamma 3$ by solvent perturbation difference spectroscopy.

Electron micrographs of IgA (Svehag and Bloth, 1970; Dourmashkin *et al.*, 1971; Munn *et al.*, 1971) indicate that the general organization of the molecule (serum dimeric IgA) is that of an end-to-end union through the Fc segment by a flexible linkage. The more recent data of Bjork and Lindh (1974) with two types of IgA (IgA dimers and secretory IgA) are consistent with an extended shape ($f/f_0 = 1.95$). These workers also found the ORD and CD spectra of IgA monomers and dimers as well as those of a secretory IgA to be very similar, indicating that the presence of J and SC does not greatly affect the conformation of IgA. Riesen *et al.* (1976) examined the CD spectra of IgA1 and IgA2 subclasses and found only minor differences except for the IgA2 allotype A2m(2) (van Loghem *et al.*, 1973), which had a reduced negative ellipticity at 217 nm. No data are available on the X-ray crystallography of IgA other than the work on the mouse IgA myeloma McPC603 referred to above.

The spiderlike arrangement (Chesebro *et al.*, 1968) of IgM has al-ready been mentioned. The CD spectrum of the isolated Fab fragment is similar to that of the IgG Fab, but the Fc fragments of the two classes differ (Ghose, 1971), the Fc_μ CD spectra showing greater amounts of β structure than Fc_γ.

In summary, the X-ray studies have confirmed the domain model and shown that significant interaction occurs between heavy and light chains, but not between domains. The structure of the Fc fragment is less clear, and the question of whether or not binding of a ligand in the Fab fragment affects the conformation of the Fc portion of the molecule awaits the results of X-ray studies on intact antibodies before and after binding antigen at resolutions below 3.5 Å.

2. Shape Changes Due to Ligand Binding

The subject of shape change due to ligand binding has recently been reviewed by Metzger (1974), who considered three possible models to account for the exposure of functional sites as a consequence of antigen binding. The first is the allosteric model, which has been favored historically. This model proposes a conformational change in the Fc fragment as a result of secondary force perturbations following antigen binding by the Fab fragment. The second model is the distortive model and suggests that because of the binding of antigen, the molecule is "stretched" so as to reveal or cover up critical sites. Third is the associative model, which considers the reaction of antibody with antigen as a means of bringing together or aggregating antibodies. This "polymerization" of antibody can then result in the formation of a new site or the creation of a polyvalent site from several monovalent ones. Metzger points out that the data provide no clear-cut conclusion but that the associative model explains much of the available information. The allosteric model is considered unlikely on the hypothesis that most of the available evidence indicates little or no change in conformation of the Fc or Fab fragments on binding to antigen. Similarly, the distortive model is not favored because of evidence suggesting limited flexibility between Fab arms. However, essentially the same experimental evidence (Werner *et al.*, 1972; Cathou and O'Konski, 1970; Yguerabide *et al.*, 1970; Green, 1969) has been used by others (Cathou and Dorrington, 1975) to suggest a significant degree of flexibility between the Fab fragments. Accordingly, therefore, no clear-cut conclusion can really be made as to the extent of freedom of rotation between the Fab arms.

There is also disagreement as to whether or not antibodies undergo conformational changes on binding with antigen. Earlier studies by Grossberg *et al.* (1965) indicated some change in conformation, at least in the Fab region. These workers found that the binding of hapten reduces chymotryptic digestibility of the antibody or its Fab fragment with little or no effect on the digestion of heterologous antibody. The results suggested some stabilization of the Fab region. These results were supported by ORD studies showing the stabilization of anti-2,4-dinitrophenyl antibodies by ϵ-DNP-lysine to denaturation with 4 M guanidinium chloride (Cathou and Haber, 1967). In contrast, other workers (Cathou *et al.*, 1968) have shown, using CD, that anti-2,4-dinitrophenyl Fab fragment possessed the same conformational parameters in the presence or absence of molar excess of ϵ-DNP-lysine. This has also been found for a human monoclonal IgM and its Fab fragment, which binds *p*-nitrophenyl-

ε-aminocaproate (Ashman *et al.*, 1971). However, studies on the susceptibility to proteolysis of the same paraprotein with chymotrypsin and
subtilisin did reveal differences between liganded and unliganded antibody, although no significant changes occurred with trypsin and pronase.
The changes in susceptibility to proteolysis were thought to be restricted
to the Fab fragment (Ashman and Metzger, 1971).

The significance of results involving hapten-antihapten systems is
open to question, since it is known that such complexes generally fail to
exhibit important biological activities. In the case of polyvalent antigens,
which do induce physiological effects, however, the information is more
difficult to interpret. Some studies do indicate that a conformational
change occurs on binding antigen. These include titration of free sulfhydryl groups in human serum albumin–equine antibody complexes (Robert
and Grabar, 1957), volume changes with dinitrophenylated bovine IgG–
anti-DNP antibody complexes (Ohta *et al.*, 1970), and hydrogen exchange
studies with a synthetic polypeptide system (Liberti *et al.*, 1972a,b). In
addition, antigenic changes (Henny *et al.*, 1965; Henny and Stanworth,
1966) and aggregation (Henny and Ishizaka, 1968) have been reported.

Most recently, Schlessinger *et al.* (1975) investigated the interaction
of antibodies to ribonuclease, poly-D-alanine, and the "loop" of lysozyme by circular polarization of luminescence (CPL) studies. The emission spectrum (as opposed to absorption in CD and ORD) shows changes
accompanying the binding of antigen to antibody in antigen excess. When
the Fab fragments alone were studied, the results observed were not the
same as for the total molecule, indicating that some of the changes took
place in the Fc region. The McPC 603 mouse myeloma IgA, which binds
phosphorylcholine, did not change its CPL on binding to the hapten. In
contrast to this, antibody to the "loop" of lysozyme did show spectral
changes when liganded to its antigen. The differences between these two
monovalent antigen systems is unclear, but it suggests that antigen size
may be an important factor in conformational change. Another interesting
result of this study was the finding that reduction of the inter-H-chain
disulfide bonds of the antibodies abolished the putative Fc spectral
changes but not the Fab changes. The authors suggest that the hinge
region disulfides may, therefore, be required for the proper propagation
of the conformational change.

Polysaccharide antigens are better suited for studies involving absorption or emission techniques because they lack bands in the relevant
spectral regions of proteins. It had been shown that antibodies to type
III pneumococcal polysaccharide (SIII), in the presence of a hexasac-
charide hapten, undergo changes in CD spectra between 260 and 310 nm
(changes in asymmetrical environments of aromatic groupings) (Holowka

et al., 1972). More recently, these studies were repeated and confirmed (Jaton *et al.*, 1975*a*). In addition, essentially the same spectral changes were observed with Fab fragments or with intact rabbit antibodies (three different homogeneous populations), suggesting little or no involvement of the Fc part of the molecule in these changes. Fluorescent quenching experiments on this system by the same investigators (Jaton *et al.*, 1975*a*) were reported to give similar results. However, when CPL was employed, additional changes attributed to the Fc were detected (Jaton *et al.*, 1975*b*). By using oligosaccharides of different sizes as well as the SIII polysaccharide, it was found that the larger the hapten, the greater the changes attributed to the Fc region. The greatest changes were observed with the intact SIII polysaccharide. Reduction of the interchain disulfide bonds abolished the Fc-dependent changes, confirming the findings of Schlessinger *et al.* (1975). That the conformational changes reflected antigen-antibody interactions and not aggregation by antibodies was indicated by the finding that ultracentrifugation of the complex between the 16-residue oligosaccharide and excess antibody revealed a major peak of 6.9 S ($s_{20,w}$) with an 8.5 S shoulder, consistent with a mixture of monomers and only small amounts of dimers. Pertinent in this regard are recent data (Jaton *et al.*, 1976) indicating that oligosaccharide ligands (up to 16 sugar residues) do not trigger complement fixation (CF), in spite of the demonstrated conformational changes. It appears that CF begins when haptens of at least 21 residues are used, and they result in complexes greater than trimers (Table III).

Good evidence for a conformational change has been presented in the case of bovine IgM antibody to *S. flagella* employing electron microscopy (Feinstein and Munn, 1969; Feinstein *et al.*, 1971), in which the Fab arms bound to the flagella are perpendicular to the plane of the Fc part of the molecule. In unliganded IgM, the arms appear to be more in the plane of the Fc. The effect of this change on the conformation of the Fc portion itself is unknown.

Taken collectively, the data indicate that while monovalent haptens have little or no effect on the conformation of immunoglobulins, polyvalent antigens do have a significant effect on conformation. Although association between molecules plays a key role in effector functions (two or more molecules of IgG are needed for complement fixation), the conformational changes may also be a factor. For example, IgM, which is already "associated," fixes complement more efficiently after binding univalent antigen (Brown and Koshland, 1975). It may, indeed, be possible to distinguish between the associative and allosteric models if functional sites can be localized on the three-dimensional structure of the Fc part of the molecule, thereby revealing whether the site is exposed in the

Table III.   Physical and Biological Properties of Antigen-Antibody Complexes[a]

Oligosaccharide antigens	Sedimentation values of Ag/Ab complexes ($s_{20,w}$)	Size of complexes	Complement fixation	CPL[b] changes in [c]	
				Fab	Fc
740 (tetra-)	ND[d]	ND	−	+	±
1110 (hexa-)	6.3	Monomers	−	+	±
1500 (octa-)	6.2	Monomers	−	+	±
2200 (dodeca-)	6.5; 8.7; 10.3 (ratio 1:1:1)	Mono + dimers	−	ND[d]	
3000 (16-)	6.3; 8.5; 10.2 + 11.1	Mono + dimers + trimers?	−	+	±
5000 (28-)	6.5; 9.3; 10.6; 12–16	Mono + dimers + higher oligomers	++	ND	
9000 (48-)	6.9; 10; 11–20	Dimers + higher oligomers	+++	ND	
SIII	ND	ND	++++	+	++

[a] Reprinted from Jaton et al. (1976) with permission of authors and publisher (Williams and Wilkins, Baltimore).
[b] Circular polarization of luminescence.
[c] CPL spectral changes; the amplitude of CPL changes in Fc moiety was small for small haptens (±), intermediate for the 16-sugar unit (+), and maximal for the intact polysaccharide (++); see Jaton et al. (1975b) for details.
[d] ND, not done.

unliganded molecule. It should also be kept in mind that the three mechanisms proposed by Metzger need not be mutually exclusive and may each play a role to a different extent with various antigens and effector functions.

III. Effector Functions Mediated by Antibodies

The effector functions mediated by antibodies range from the lysis of cells (through the initiation of the complement cascade) to the release of pharmacologically active substances (histamine and serotonin) by fixation to tissue mast cells. A complete list of these functions can be divided into (1) activities mediated by the interaction of immunoglobulins with other molecules and (2) activities mediated by the interaction of immunoglobulins with cells. In some cases questions exist as to which of these functions are of biological significance and which are purely phenomenological. While it is easy to understand the role of complement fixation as a defense mechanism, the significance of the binding of protein

A by the Fc of IgG is not easily visualized. Nevertheless, all functions represent properties peculiar to immunoglobulins, and the sites responsible for the interaction have been investigated to some extent. These properties have been found to be associated with the Fc fragment, and in some cases the localization has been further defined. Table IV lists the effector functions and the classes and subclasses they are associated with.

It should be mentioned at this point that no definitive function has been found to be associated with the carbohydrate moieties of immunoglobulins, most of which are associated with the Fc fragment. Hinrichs and Smyth (1970) have obtained some evidence that a portion (40%) of rabbit IgG molecules bear a C_H2 oligosaccharide, and these are not transferred across the placental membrane. It is interesting that in human IgM, which is also known not to cross the placental membrane, the C_H2 oligosaccharide occupies a similar position, i.e., close to the inter-H-chain disulfide bond. Moreover, carbohydrate has been reported (Swenson and Kern, 1967; Melchers and Knopf, 1967) to play a role in the

Table IV.   Biological Properties of Human Immunoglobulins

	IgG1	IgG2	IgG3	IgG4	IgA1	IgA2	IgM	IgD	IgE
Complement fixation									
1. Classic	+	+	+	−	−	−	+	−	−
2. Alternate	+	+	+	+	+	+	+	+	+
Protein binding									
Staphylococcal protein A	+	+	−	+	(+)[a]	(+)[a]	+	−	−
Secretory component	−	−	−	−	+	+	+	−	−
CFF[d]	+	+	−	−	−	−	−	−	−
IBF[e]	(+)[a]	(+)[a]	(+)[a]	(+)[a]	−	−	−	−	−
Homologous cell binding									
Lymphocytes	±	+[b]	±	−	−	−	−	−	+[b]
K cells[c]	±	+[b]	±	+[b]	−	−	+	−	−
Macrophage	+	±	+	±	−	−	−	−	−
Neutrophils	+	+[b]	+	±	+	+	−	−	−
Monocytes	+	+[b]	+	+	−	−	−	−	−
Platelets	+	+	+	+	−	−	−	−	−
Mast cells									
1. Homologous	(+)[a]	(+)[a]	(+)[a]	(+)[a]	−	−	−	−	+
2. Heterologous	+	−	+	+	−	−	−	−	−
Placental transfer	+	+	+	+	−	−	−	−	−

[a] Parentheses indicate activity demonstrated for class, but activity of individual subclasses is unknown.
[b] Positive only after aggregation.
[c] Antibody-dependent cellular cytotoxicity (ADCC).
[d] Cystic fibrosis factor.
[e] Immunoglobulin-binding factor.

transport and secretion of immunoglobulins, although this has not been firmly established in our view. In the sections to follow, it will be seen that certain interactions require the C_H2 domain in which the carbohydrate of the IgG is located.

A. Protein-Binding Properties of Immunoglobulins

Some of the effector functions of immunoglobulins are mediated by the binding of other proteins to the Fc fragment. The prime example of this is the fixation of complement. Other examples of binding of proteins to immunoglobulins are also known. However, the biological significance of these is less clear. Among the latter are the binding of rheumatoid factor, staphylococcal protein A, and certain serum proteins.

1. Complement Fixation

Complement is a group of 11 serum proteins which act on cells through a sequence of events initiated by fixation to antigen-antibody complexes. The classical complement pathway is started by the fixation of the first three complement components as a complex. These three components (Clq, Clr, and Cls) are referred to collectively as "C1" and are associated with each other noncovalently in the presnce of Ca^{2+} ion. Clq represents the recognition unit of the aggregate which is bound by the antigen-antibody complex and in turn causes the conversion of Cls (conformational change?) into a proteolytic enzyme. Cls then activates the next component (C4) of the sequence. For a full review of the complement system, the reader is directed to the chapter by Stroud in this volume.

Human Clq is a collagenlike molecule with a molecular weight of 409,000 (Reid et al., 1972). It consists of three distinct parts (Shelton et al., 1972): (1) a central core, (2) connecting strands, and (3) terminal subunits. There are six terminal subunits, each composed of two polypeptides of similar molecular weight and bound to each other by disulfide bonds. The terminal subunits, which are connected to the central subunit by the connecting strands, appear to be involved in the interaction with the Fc fragment of antibodies (Yonemasu and Stroud, 1972; Isliker et al., 1974). This would agree with Scatchard plot data which indicate six binding sites for IgG per Clq molecule (Müller-Eberhard, 1975).

Complement fixation via the classical pathway may be mediated by IgG1, IgG2, IgG3, or IgM (Ishizaka et al., 1967) but not by IgG4, IgA, IgD (Henny et al., 1969), or IgE (Ishizaka et al., 1972). As stated previously, earlier studies have indicated a need for two molecules of IgG acting in concert to fix complement while only a single molecule of IgM is required (Borsos and Rapp, 1965; Cohen, 1968). Other differences also exist in the complement-fixing properties of these two classes of immunoglobulins. Thus IgM is more efficient in complement fixation at 37°C with particulate antigens while IgG is more effective with soluble antigens at lower temperatures (Ishizaka et al., 1968; Cunniff and Stollar, 1968; Fauci et al., 1970). An essential requirement for IgG is multivalent antigens, and no complement fixation occurs when monovalent haptens are used since association of this class of antibodies is required for complement fixation. For IgM a monofunctional antigen of high molecular weight is needed since it exists as a pentamer in its native state (Brown and Koshland, 1975). In either case, aggregation always increases efficiency of complement fixation. The association of antibody molecules may be brought about without antigen by physical (heating) or chemical means (Ishizaka and Ishizaka, 1960; Ishizaka et al., 1961) or, as in the case of IgM, polymers of the 19 S pentamer occur naturally (Augener et al., 1971). Urea has been found to irreversibly inactivate IgM complement fixation but not that of IgG (Cunniff et al., 1968).

Recent studies have indicated that the bimolecular requirement for IgG to fix complement may not be valid. Hyslop et al. (1970), using rabbit antibody and a divalent hapten, has found that the smallest antibody polymer which will fix complement is a tetramer. In addition, it appears that this aggregation is unstable since the higher polymers readily dissociate to inactive dimers and trimers on simply standing at room temperature. To add to the confusion, Augener et al. (1971) have shown that monomeric IgG also fixes C1q, but approximately 100 times less efficiently than heat-aggregated IgG, as measured by the C1 fixation assay (Borsos and Rapp, 1963). Further, it was also found that IgM_s (7 S subunit of 19 S IgM prepared by gentle reduction and alkylation) (Stone and Metzger, 1968) had the capacity, similar to monomeric IgG, to fix C1. This capacity was 15 times lower than that of native 19 S IgM and about a hundredfold less than that of natural polymers of IgM having a sedimentation rate greater than 35 S. While heat-aggregated IgM does not fix complement (Frommhagen and Fudenberg, 1962; Murray et al., 1965), IgM cross-linked by bis-diazotized benzidine (BDB) is very efficient (Ishizaka et al., 1967). These studies indicate that while unliganded, monomeric forms of IgM and IgG show low levels of C1 fixation, the efficiency is greatly increased by conditions or agents which cause the molecules to associate without denaturation.

Several laboratories reported that the Fc fragment of IgG contains the site involved in the fixation of complement (Amiraian and Leikhim,

1961; Taranta and Franklin, 1961; Ishizaka *et al.*, 1962). It was found that while the monomeric Fc of IgG is capable of fixing some C1, cross-linking by BDB increases its efficiency. Heating of Fc fragment has no effect on C1 binding, probably because aggregation of IgG by this method occurs via the Fab fragment, at least for IgG1 and IgG2 (Augener and Grey, 1970). The isolated Fab fragment does undergo thermal aggregation but fails to fix C1 even in the associated form. The $(Fc)_5\mu$ of IgM prepared by the high-temperature trypsin technique fixes human complement more efficiently than the native molecule, but is a relatively poor fixer of guinea pig complement (Plaut *et al.*, 1972). Surprisingly, it was found that when the pentameric $(Fc)_5\mu$ was reduced and alkylated to the Fc, the resulting monomeric fragment was equally efficient in complement fixation. BDB-cross-linked $(Fc)_5\mu$ was also a better fixer of human than guinea pig complement, but was not as efficient as the non-cross-linked pentamer. Another surprising finding of this study was the inefficiency of the unfractionated digest of IgM to fix complement, indicating some influence of the Fab fragment. We shall return to this point at a later time. Sledge and Bing (1973) compared the abilities of IgG, IgM, and the $(Fc)_5\mu$ to inhibit C1q binding to IgM and also found the $(Fc)_5\mu$ fragment to be the most efficient. While heat treatment of the IgM and IgG increased their effectiveness, it did not affect the ability of the $(Fc)_5\mu$ to bind C.

A number of investigators have attempted to elucidate the nature of the complement-binding site by amino acid modification studies. Early studies by Schur and Christian (1964) indicated that the fixation of complement by rabbit IgG was lost by reduction of the inter-H-chain disulfide bond. It has also been shown that reduced, aggregated human IgG does not fix complement but still reacts with rheumatoid factor (Wiedermann *et al.*, 1963). These studies were subsequently confirmed and extended to human IgG1 proteins (Isenman *et al.*, 1975a). The reduction of hinge region disulfide bonds produces little or no change in the conformation of the molecule, but, as discussed previously, Schlessinger *et al.* (1975) and Jaton *et al.* (1975a,b) have provided evidence that this linkage may be required for conformational changes in the Fc associated with ligand binding in the Fab.

Basic amino acids appear to play a central role in the fixation of complement. Labeling of rabbit γ-globulin with 2-hydroxy-5-nitrobenzylbromide (NBB), a tryptophan-specific reagent (Horton and Koshland, 1965), has been shown to destroy complement-fixing capacity, leaving the antibody site unaffected (Griffin *et al.*, 1967). Cohen and Becker (1968a,b) have studied the effects of amidination, carbamylation, and benzylation of rabbit antibody on complement fixation. They found that amidination of 54% of the amino groups (lysine) with ethyl acetimidate hydrochloride, or carbamylation of 32% with potassium cyanate, causes a loss of 55% of the complement-fixing ability of the molecule with little effect on antigen binding. At higher levels of conjugation, greater losses occurred caused by nonspecific changes in the molecule, although this was not a result of failure to aggregate since conjugation with these reagents did not affect the association of antibody molecules. The combination of amidination and benzylation of tryptophans (with NBB) gave the greatest decrease in complement-fixing capacity (92%), with little effect on antigen-binding properties. Fluorescein conjugation, another lysine reagent, also suppresses complement fixation but not antigen binding (Thrasher *et al.*, 1975). These results are consistent with the findings that diamino compounds effectively inhibit the C1q-antibody interaction (Sledge and Bing, 1973; Wirtz, 1965) presumably because of the anionic character of the site on C1q (Bing, 1971). There may also be a contribution of hydrophobic groups to this interaction since diamines separated by long carbon chains or aromatic groups are more effective inhibitors than the shorter homologues.

Earlier attempts to further localize the C1 interaction site in the Fc fragment indicated that it was in the C_H2 domain on the NH_2-terminal half of the Fc fragment since isolated (C_H3) fragments were inactive (Irimajiri *et al.*, 1968). Confirmation of this finding by testing the C_H2 domain directly has not been possible until recently because of the lability of this region to proteolytic attack. The technique of Connell and Porter (1971), which entails exposure of rabbit antibody to pH 2.5 before proteolysis, renders the C_H2 region temporarily less susceptible and allows cleavage between the C_H2 and C_H3 domains with plasmin. The resulting C_H2-containing fragment was shown to retain its complement-fixing ability and, therefore, was designated the "Facb" (fragment antigen- and complement-binding) fragment (MacLennan *et al.*, 1974; Stewart *et al.*, 1973). The Facb fragment represents the entire molecule devoid of the C_H3 domain, and the position of the plasmin split has been ascertained between Lys-110 and Ala-111, numbered from the inter-H-chain disulfide bond in rabbit Fc. Treatment with acid causes a loss of 35–40% in CF ability of the native molecule, but there is no further loss due to plasmin cleavage (Colomb and Porter, 1975). In contrast to rabbit Ig, the human antibody molecule is split by similar treatment in the hinge area as well as between the C_H2-C_H3 region and the Facb fragment is not obtained (Connell and Painter, 1966).

Ellerson *et al.* (1972) replaced plasmin with trypsin in the acid exposure proteolysis treatment of human IgG1 Fc fragment and isolated the C_H2 domain. They were then able to demonstrate CF with this fragment.

These studies were later extended when it was found that trypsin cova-lently bound to Sepharose gave higher yields and more stable preparation of this fragment, presumably because free trypsin can remain bound to the isolated C_H2 and cause further degradation during storage (Ellerson *et al.*, 1976). The fragment which these workers isolated contains the sequence between Thr-223 and Lys-338 (Eu numbering) and therefore retains the inter-γ-chain disulfide (Cys-229). It was further characterized as lacking noncovalent affinity since it behaves as a monomer in phy-siological buffers after reduction. This is in contrast to the C_H3 domain, which, as previously stated, exhibits strong noncovalent interaction and exists as a dimer under similar conditions.

When the isolated C_H2 fragment was tested for its ability to fix complement by the classical hemolytic assay using the fragment aggre-gated on polystyrene latex beads, only small amounts of activity were obtained (about 15% of Fc fragment on a molar basis). However, when tested for its ability to fix isolated C1, there was no difference between C_H2 and Fc fragments on a molar basis; both were only slightly less active than native IgG1 (Fig. 7). Reduction and alkylation had no effect on the C1-fixing ability, indicating that the monomer was equally as

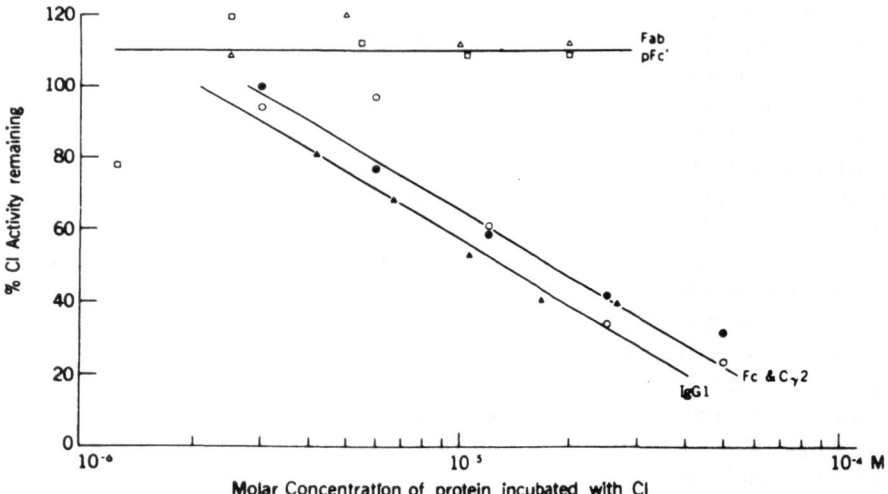

Figure 7.   Interaction between C1 and IgG (▲), Fc (●), $C_\gamma2$ (III) (○), Fab (△), or pFc' (□). C1 activity remaining after preincubation with the test protein is expressed as a percentage of the C1 measured in the absence of the test protein. Reproduced with per-mission from Yasmeen *et al.* (1976); copyright 1976 by the Williams and Wilkins Co., Baltimore.

effective as the dimer (Yasmeen *et al.*, 1976). Painter *et al.* (1974) reported that β_2-microglobulin, a component of histocompatibility antigens and structurally similar to the constant domains of immunoglobulins (Grey *et al.*, 1973; Cunningham and Berggard, 1974), was also able to fix complement and retained this ability even after reduction and alkylation (Isenman *et al.*, 1975b). These studies suggest that the CF site is formed by a linear sequence of amino acids and is not dependent on conformation since the native conformation of this fragment is dependent on the intrachain disulfide bond. In addition, it has been shown that C reactive protein (CRP), which appears to be unrelated to immunoglobulin structure (although the sequence has not yet been reported), can fix complement (Kaplan and Volanakis, 1974; Siegel *et al.*, 1974) as well as carry out other biological processes associated with the Fc part of the immunoglobulin molecule (Mortensen *et al.*, 1976). This suggests sequence similarity unrelated to conformation.

Allan and Isliker (1974a,b) studied the ability of pepsin fragments of rabbit IgG to fix complement. Although peptides of the Fc are inactive in the classicial hemolytic assay (Mayer, 1961), these workers found that by using polystyrene latex particles to aggregate the peptides (Utsumi, 1969) complement fixation could readily be detected. The active peptide, Pep V, actually consists of a mixture of peptides from the NH_2-terminal (C_H2) region of the Fc fragment (Utsumi and Karush, 1965). None of these peptides exceeds 5000 in molecular weight. Pep V was also found to inhibit complement fixation by aggregated IgG when added to a mixture with guinea pig complement, but only when the peptides were present at relatively low concentration. At higher concentrations, Pep V augmented CF. The blocking of a single tryptophan with NBB eliminates the enhancement effect which is due to the clustering of Pep V on the surface of the immunoglobulin, probably analogous to the effect obtained with latex particles. It was also found that the blocking of only two tryptophan residues with NBB is all that is required to cause a 60% decrease in CF capacity of the IgG and 100% of the Fc (see Fig. 8). However, the modification of the tryptophans decreased the ability of IgG1 to fix purified human C1q only by 20% and had even less of an effect on Fc (Fig. 9) and Pep V. Furthermore, Pep III (C_H3) was as effective as Pep V in inhibiting the reaction of the purified C1q with aggregated IgG1. The authors interpret these findings to indicate that (1) the loss of complement-fixing activity is due to impairment of C1 *activation* and not the failure to bind C1q and (2) tryptophan residues are not necessary for C1q binding. A recent report (Johnson and Thames, 1976) has shown that certain synthetic peptides having tryptophan and tyrosine in juxtaposition (similar to positions 277 and 278 of human IgG1

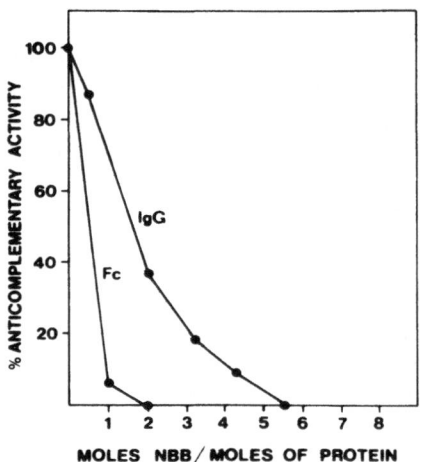

Figure 8. Effect of tryptophan modification by NBB (2-hydroxy-5-nitrobenzylbromide) on anticomplementary activity of rabbit IgG and its Fc fragment. IgG was first modified and then heat-aggregated. Modified Fc was tested as such. Results refer to 100 μg of each preparation. Reproduced with permission from Allan and Isliker (1974a); copyright 1974, Pergamon Press, Ltd.

and rabbit IgG) exhibit significant total activation (consumption of CH_{50} units).

Additional support for the CF site being present on the C_H2 domain comes from studies done with the McPC 173 IgG2a, a murine myeloma protein (Kehoe and Fougereau, 1969; Kehoe et al., 1974). A CNBr fragment (H-5) from the NH_2 terminus of the Fc was found to have CF activity. This fragment comprises 62 residues from Ile-253 to Met-314 (Eu numbering). The sequence of this fragment is shown in Fig. 10 and compared with the same region of the human IgG1 protein, Eu. It contains one of the cysteines involved in the intrachain loop (Cys-261) as well as the carbohydrate attachment site (Asx-297). The effect of carbohydrate on CF is unknown. No correlations were found between the carbohydrate composition of IgG myeloma proteins of all four subclasses and CF capacity in one study (Tomana et al., 1974). Although periodate oxidation caused the loss of 50% of the CF activity, the significance of this is not clear since 40% of the tryptophan was also lost in addition to carbohydrate. Another study (Williams et al., 1973) reported loss in CF ability of rabbit antipneumococcal antibody after removal of carbohydrate with a bacterial endoglycosidase, although negative results were obtained with other bacterial antibodies (S. aureus, E. coli, etc.).

As previously discussed, amidination and carbamylation cause the loss of CF activity (Cohen and Becker, 1968a). In addition, diamino compounds can inhibit the C1-antibody interaction (Sledge and Bing, 1973). Yasmeen et al. (1976) have, in fact, shown that diaminobutane reacts with C1 and had a dose curve parallel to that of Fc fragment but shifted by 4 log intervals. In contrast to this apparent involvement of amino groups, the H-5 fragment (Fig. 10) has been found to be devoid of lysine residues. It appears, therefore, that conflicting data exist which hinge on the point of whether or not fixation of C1q is equivalent to complement activation. The work of Allan and Isliker (1974a,b) suggests that the two processes can be separated. In addition, it has now been shown that the Fc fragments of IgG4 fix C1 when the intact molecule does not (Isenman et al., 1975a). Whether or not the rest of the complement sequence is activated as well is unknown. It has recently been

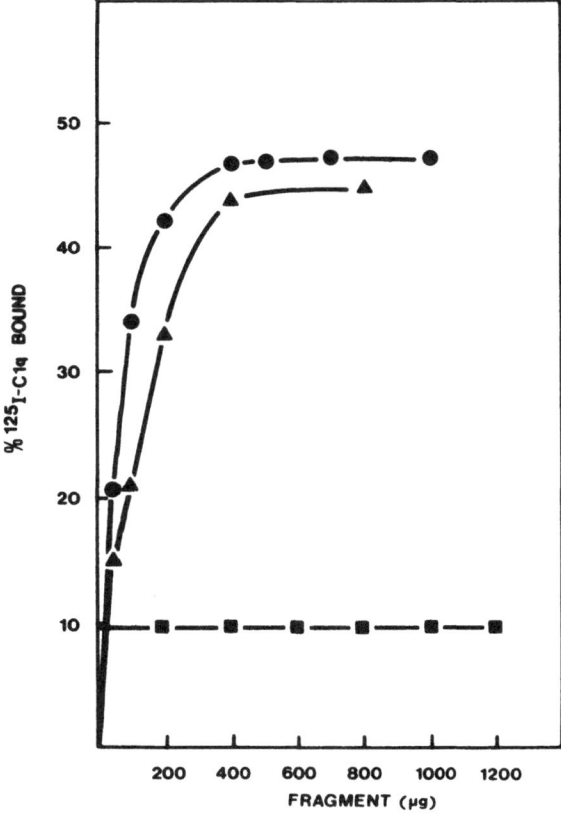

Figure 9.   Binding of [^{125}I]-C1q to Fc and F(ab')$_2$. One microgram of [^{125}I]-C1q was incubated at 0°C with increasing amounts of unmodified Fc (●), Fc containing four modified tryptophans (▲), and F(ab')$_2$ (■). Fc was an insoluble precipitate, and F(ab')$_2$ was aggregated by dioxan precipitation. Reproduced with permission from Allan and Isliker (1974b); copyright 1974, Pergamon Press, Ltd.

```
                                          260
Eu        Ile  Ser  Arg  Thr  Pro  Glu  Val  Thr  Cys  Val  Val  Val  Asp  Val  Ser  His  Glu
MOPC 173  ———  Leu  Ser  ———  Ile  ————————————————————————————————————————————  Glu  Asp
              270                        280
Eu        Asp  Pro  Gln  Val  Lys  Phe  Asn  Trp  Tyr  Val  Asp  Gly  Val  Gln  Val  His  Asn
MOPC 173  ———  Asp  ———  ———  Gln  Ile  Ser  ———  Phe  ————————  Asn  ———  Glu  ———  ———  Gln
                                                    cho
                    290                             300
Eu        Ala  Lys  Thr  Lys  Pro  Arg  Glu  Gln  Gln  Tyr  Asx  Ser  Thr  Tyr  Arg  Val  Val
MOPC 173  ———  ———  ———  His  Thr  Thr  Arg  ———  Asn  ———————————————————  Leu  ———  ———  ———
                         310
Eu        Ser  Val  Leu  Thr  Val  Leu  His  Gln  Asn  Trp  Leu
MOPC 173  ———  Ala  ———  Pro  Ile  Gln  ——————————————————  Met
```

Figure 10. Comparison of sequence of complement-fixing fragment (H-5) of murine γG2a (MCPC 173) (Kehoe and Fougereau, 1969) with comparable segment of human γG1 (Eu) (Edelman *et al.*, 1969).

reported that reduced and alkylated $C_\gamma 2$ loses the ability to fix C1 while a similar treatment of $C_\gamma 3$ causes it to gain this capacity (Yasmeen *et al.*, 1976). In both cases the fragments appear to be random coils. In the case of IgA, it has been shown that the Fc_α is able not only to fix the first component but also to activate the rest of the hemolytic sequence (Burritt *et al.*, 1977). In addition, treatment of $C_H 3$ with pepsin results in a fragment which fixes C1 (K. J. Dorrington, personal communication). It therefore appears that while the physiological site for C1 fixation is probably on the $C_H 2$ domain, other sites may also fix C1, probably nonspecifically, although a physiological role for these sites under certain conditions has not been excluded. Isenman *et al.* (1975a) suggest that these results reflect the fact that the Fab part of the molecule acts as a negative modulator in those classes and subclasses which do not activate C1q, perhaps by sterically hindering access to the CF site. This thesis is supported by the sensitivity of CF of IgG1 (which does fix complement) to reduction of hinge interchain disulfides (Richardson *et al.*, 1976). These bonds presumably maintain the rigidity of the molecule, preventing the Fab steric hindrance. Additional support for this theory comes from the observation that digestion of IgM without subsequent isolation of the $(Fc)_5\mu$ is relatively inefficient in CF (Plaut *et al.*, 1972). This indicates that Fab is somehow able to block the interaction of Fc fragment with C1, although the mechanism for this observation is unknown since there are supposedly few or no noncovalent interactions between the Fab and Fc. The Fab fragments of guinea pig antibodies to rabbit $C_H 3$ reported by Ovary *et al.* (1976) as inhibiting CF may mimic a modulator. In this case a Fab fragment (of anti-$C_H 3$) placed close to the CF site acts similar to a flexible Fab modulator by sterically hindering it.

In contrast to the situation with IgG1, the site for CF on IgM is in the terminal ($C_\mu 4$) domain (Hurst *et al.*, 1974, 1975). The $C_H 4$ fragment was obtained by limited tryptic cleavage at 37°C (Hester *et al.*, 1975) and shown to be composed of two stretches of amino acids (Ou numbering, Glu-468–Arg-491 and Tyr-515–Arg-546) joined by a disulfide bond. In effect, this represents the $C_\mu 4$ domain from which 23 amino acids (492–514) have been removed. The fragment was shown to be an efficient fixer of C1 (and subsequently C4). Reduction and alkylation in 6 M guanidine hydrochloride cause a 400-fold loss in this activity. It should be noted that this fragment represents a monomeric domain since noncovalent interactions appear to be absent in the Fc_μ region (Hester *et al.*, 1975). The effect of the position of the site of CF on the mechanism of the reaction is not known. As previously discussed, several characteristics of the CF pathways of IgG and IgM differ. It should also be noted that the $C_H 4$ fragment lacks lysine, similar to the H5 fragment of the mouse

(McPC 173) myeloma protein, again contrary to the putative importance of amino groups of IgG in this interaction.

It has been reported that human Waldenström IgM proteins can be divided into two groups depending on their ability to interact with isolated C1q (MacKenzie et al., 1971). The native protein is the principal reactor, and aggregation is not required. This finding was not supported by the work of Augener et al. (1971), who showed that all IgM proteins examined, including four of the putative non-complement-fixing group supplied by MacKenzie, interacted with highly purified C1q as assessed by analytical ultracentrifugation. A recent report (Füst et al., 1976) has found that the C1-fixing ability of the $(Fc)_5\mu$ fragment was lost after gel filtration at pH 3.0 and recovered in a low molecular weight peptide fraction released from the Fc fragment. Moreover, the peptide recombined with the $(Fc)_5\mu$, restoring the C1-fixing capacity. These results warrant closer examination since they suggest that the division of IgM into C1-fixing and non-C1-fixing could be an artifact due to the method of isolation. Alternatively, this small peptide may be a functional part of certain IgM molecules.

Schur and Becker (1963) reported that rabbit and sheep $F(ab')_2$ fragments with antibody activity against albumin retained a small amount of CF ability measured by the hemolytic assay. Reid (1971) later showed that such fragments utilize only the later components of complement (C3–C9) and thus activate via the alternate pathway (Osler et al., 1969; Sandberg et al., 1971; Götze and Müller-Eberhard, 1971). The mechanism of initiation of this pathway is unknown, but aggregation of the proteins (by antigen or BDB) is required. IgE (Ishizaka et al., 1972) and the four subclasses of IgG, IgM, and IgA (both subclasses and secretory IgA) have all been shown capable of activating the alternate pathway (Frank et al., 1976; Boackle et al., 1974). Although Henney et al. (1969) reported that IgD (aggregated with BDB) was unable to fix complement by the hemolytic assay with three different preparations, Konno and Hirai (1975) reported that, with one of two samples tested, BDB-IgD was able to fix C3–C9 but not the early components. Interestingly, these workers found that the BDB-aggregated Fc fragments of both the active and inactive IgD preparations were able to activate C3–C9. In addition, they found that the $F(ab')_2$ fragment (peptic fragment) was also active but not so active as the Fc. These results are similar to those obtained by Ishizaka et al. (1970a) for IgE, i.e., both $F(ab')_2$ and Fc activate. What is missing from both these studies is whether Fab fragments from papain digests activate. It is not certain, therefore, whether there are two sites on different domains or if a single domain contains both sites and an overlap occurs between the sites of cleavage by the two different enzymes. The latter appears to be true for IgE since both the pepsin $F(ab')_2$ and the papain Fc contain the C_H2 domain (Ishizaka and Ishizaka, 1975). The mechanism by which these fragments activate the alternate pathway is unknown, but it is currently thought that initiation occurs through a serum protein referred to as the "nephritic factor analogue." This 150,000 molecular weight protein has been shown to activate C3 in normal serum independent of C1, C2, and C4 (Arroyave et al., 1974).

2. Staphylococcal Protein A

Protein A was originally known as "Jensen's antigen" since it was initially isolated by this investigator from the cell wall of *Staphylococcus aureus* (Jensen, 1958). It was shown to be the antigen responsible for the agglutination of this strain by normal human sera (Yoshida et al., 1963; Löfkvist, 1966). The agglutination was found to be due to the presence of γ-globulin in the serum, and it was therefore hypothesized that all humans have "natural antibodies" to this cell wall protein (Löfkvist and Sjoquist, 1962; Oeding and Hankenes, 1963). It was subsequently demonstrated that the reaction was due to the interaction of protein A with the Fc part of the antibody molecule and not the antigen-binding site (Forsgren and Sjoquist, 1966), thereby giving a pseudoimmune reaction with human γ-globulin.

"Protein A," as it was subsequently named to distinguish it from polysaccharide A (Grov et al., 1964), has been isolated by several techniques from *S. aureus* cell walls. The molecular weight of this protein has varied with the technique of preparation. Yoshida et al. (1963) obtained a molecular weight of 13,200 by ultracentrifugation (assuming a $\bar{v}$ of 0.745) for their preparation isolated by pancreatic deoxyribonuclease digestion of cell walls. Heat extraction with buffer (pH 5.9) at 100°C was used by Grov (1967) and Forsgren and Sjoquist (1969) to obtain their preparations. Grov obtained a molecular weight of 12,000 on what appeared to be a homogeneous preparation while Forsgren and Sjoquist reported a molecular weight of 15,000 for a somewhat heterogeneous preparation. More recently, studies by Bjork et al. (1972) indicate that protein A is a single polypeptide chain of 42,000 molecular weight as determined by sedimentation equilibrium analysis and gel filtration in 6 M guanidine hydrochloride. It has a very extended shape with a frictional ratio of 2.1–2.2. The sample was obtained by digestion of cell walls with the bacteriolytic enzyme lysostaphin (Sjoquist et al., 1972a), indicating that the protein is covalently linked to the peptidoglycan structure of the cell wall (Sjoquist et al., 1972b). This apparently gentle method of preparation accounts for the higher molecular weight value obtained as opposed to those of earlier studies on preparations obtained by more drastic procedures, e.g., heat extraction.

Protein A has an unusual structure in many respects. It lacks cysteine, tryptophan (Sjoholm, 1975a), and carbohydrate (Sjoquist et al., 1972a), and it has four tyrosine residues, all of which appear to be completely exposed. Another unusual feature of the structure is the high degreee of α-helix content. Whereas soluble proteins often contain less than 30% α-helix, protein A contains about 50%, which is more compatible with insoluble proteins. Furthermore, the conformation of the protein is extremely stable to wide changes in pH and temperature. CD studies show that some tertiary structure is maintained even in 6 M guanidine hydrochloride, and the protein regains its native conformation entirely after the removal of the guanidine hydrochloride. This stability is even more remarkable in view of the lack of disulfide bonds.

The significance of protein A binding to immunoglobulins is not clear. Protein A is present in the cell walls of most (90%) strains of S. aureus but absent in S. epidermis strains (Kronvall et al., 1971). It is essentially always (98.9%) present in coagulase-positive (pathogenic) S. aureus strains (Forsgren, 1970; Forsgren et al., 1971) and absent from coagulase-negative strains (largely nonpathogens). Its presence also correlates with the ability of the strains to resist phagocytosis (Dossett et al., 1969). There are approximately 80,000 molecules per organism present in the cell wall (Kronvall et al., 1970b), but the protein is also found extracellularly (Forsgren, 1969). For these reasons protein A is thought to be a factor contributing to the pathogenicity of the organisms possessing it.

An important characteristic of protein A is its ability to bind the Fc portion of IgG. The binding usually, although not always, results in precipitation. Forsgren (1969) found that seven out of ten IgG myeloma proteins were precipitated by protein A, but all bound it, as determined by an inhibition test. The Fc fragment itself, although capable of binding protein A, does not precipitate it (Kronvall and Frommel, 1970). Furthermore, all subclasses of IgG, except IgG3, bind protein A (Kronvall and Williams, 1969; Kronvall et al., 1970a). In an extensive phylogenetic study (Kronvall et al., 1970c) it was found that immunoglobulin of all 62 species of mammals tested, except the oppossum, reacts with protein A. The only nonmammals showing reactions were two species of birds, Rhea americana and Pterocnemia pennata (Kronvall et al., 1974). Most but not all mammalian IgGs which bind protein A also precipitate it. The two phases of the reaction, combination and precipitation, thus represent separate events. It has been shown that immunization of rabbits with protein A results in the formation of antibodies to the protein A–immunoglobulin complex which subsequently precipitates as a three-component system (the so-called star phenomenon) even when F(ab')₂ fragments of the antibody are prepared. This is believed to be due to the unmasking of new antigenic sites on the Fc part of nonantibody immunoglobulin following combination with protein A (Kronvall and Williams, 1971; Lind and Mansa, 1974) since F(ab')₂ fragments of rabbit antisera to protein A are completely inhibited from hemagglutination of SRBC sensitized with protein A–rabbit anti-SRBC complexes only by protein A-modified rabbit IgG. Antigen-antibody complexes, protein A, and rabbit IgG Fc fragments are ineffective inhibitors in this assay system. This is supported by CD studies which show considerable conformational changes in both protein A and the Fc subsequent to their interaction (Sjoholm, 1975b). Immunization of rabbits with strains lacking protein A does not result in the formation of antibodies to "masked" sites, but most animals, including humans, have natural antibodies to this hidden antigenic determinant (Lind, 1974).

Recent investigations indicate that certain IgM and IgA myeloma proteins also bind protein A (Harboe and Folling, 1974). The binding to monoclonal IgM proteins is thought to represent a subclass of IgM, and a fraction of all normal (polyclonal) IgM also shows the same binding (Lind et al., 1975). The reaction with IgM was also found to occur via the Fc_μ fragment, and reduction of the pentameric fragment to the monomeric Fc_μ did not alter its binding to protein A linked to Sepharose (Grov, 1975).

Although the interaction of protein A with immunoglobulins occurs via the Fc rather than the antibody site, the complex may manifest biological activities resembling normal antigen-antibody reactions. Thus cutaneous hypersensitivity in nonimmunized guinea pigs (Gustafson et al., 1968) and immediate hypersensitivity in humans (Martin et al., 1967) have been demonstrated. In addition, it can be shown that rabbits given human IgG intravenously will develop an Arthus reaction with protein A given intradermally (Gustafson et al., 1967). This reaction requires the activation of complement (Cochrane, 1967), and it has been found that protein A–IgG complexes do fix guinea pig complement (Sjoquist and Stalenheim, 1969; Stalenheim and Sjoquist, 1970). Furthermore, it has been reported that the complement fixation results in C3 conversion (C3 convertase activation), suggesting that complete activation of the classical complement pathway by protein A–IgG complexes occurs (Stalenheim and Castensson, 1971). This is surprising in view of the aforementioned studies showing that protein A completely blocks opsonic uptake of bacteria by phagocytes (Dossett et al., 1969). The antiphagocytic effect of protein A was produced by the reaction of protein A with the Fc piece of IgG, thus preventing the attachment of the opsonin to phagocytic cells. It might be expected, therefore, that most functions involving sites on the Fc would be impaired or lost by the binding of protein A. It has been shown, however, that complement fixation by the protein A–IgG complex occurs only in IgG excess and that at equivalence or excess of protein A, inhibition of complement fixation occurs. It therefore appears that at least some of the complement fixation sites on the Fc may still be available in the active protein A–IgG complexes when IgG is present in excess (Kronvall and Gewurz, 1970).

It can be argued on the basis of the requirement of at least two binding sites on protein A for the precipitation of IgG that there must be a repeating structure within the molecule. Recently, structural evidence has been presented to support this view (Hjelm et al., 1975; Sjodahl, 1976). This work suggests the presence of three binding regions. The four tyrosine residues are apparently intimately involved in binding (Sjoholm et al., 1972, 1973; Sjoholm and Sjodin, 1974) while lysine, methionine, and histidine are not (Sjoholm and Ljungdahl, 1973).

Two reports indicate that the site of the Fc fragment responsible for interaction with protein A is on the C_H2 domain (Kronvall, 1967; Kronvall and Frommel, 1970). However, these reports show only the lack of activity in C_H3 domain, and studies were not carried out with isolated C_H2 fragments or with peptides obtained from the peptic digests. It is unlikely that the complement-fixing site and protein A-fixing site are the same since the subclasses involved in these two functions differ. However, similar to complement fixation, reduction and alkylation of the Fc fragment do not affect its binding to protein A. The role of the carbohydrate moiety of the C_H2 domain in protein A binding has not been studied. It is obvious that studies on the nature of the Fc-binding site constitute a fertile area for future research.

3. Other Proteins

There are several other examples of proteins which bind to sites on the Fc part of immunoglobulins, but these have not been studied in much detail, and the significance of these reactions is, in most cases, obscure. One group of proteins which are themselves antibodies are the antiglobulins. These include rheumatoid factor (or "Raggs" for rheumatoid agglutinators) and normal serum agglutinators (or "Snaggs") (Grubb, 1956; Ropartz et al., 1958; Steinberg, 1962). There are also serum agglutinators for sites exposed by several proteolytic enzymes (Osterland et al., 1963; Waller, 1967), but they reside on Fab fragments. Since all of these are antigenic sites which react with natural antibodies, they will not be covered here. The reader is referred to the chapter by Kehoe in this volume. Suffice it to say here that the Fc antigenic sites which react with "Raggs" and "Snaggs" are distributed in both C_H2 and C_H3 domains and in certain cases require both (Natvig et al., 1972; Okafor and Turner, 1974; Stewart and Stanworth, 1975).

A variety of other proteins may also bind to immunoglobulins, but the significance and mode of binding are largely unknown. IgA is a notorious binder of certain serum proteins such as albumin (Heremans, 1960), α_1-antitrypsin (Tomasi and Hauptman, 1974a), α_1-glycoproteins (Lewis and Page, 1965), and antihemophilic globulin (Glueck and Hong, 1965). IgM may also bind albumin and α_1-antitrypsin (Mannik, 1967; Tomasi and Hauptman, 1974b). The binding varies with the proteins, and the linkage may be through disulfide bonds and/or noncovalent interaction. Certain enzymes have also been found to bind IgA. Among these are lactic dehydrogenase (Biewenga and Thijs, 1970; Biewenga and Feltkamp, 1975) and amylase (Friedhandler et al., 1974). IgG has also been shown to bind both of these enzymes (Hansen et al., 1972; Kindmark, 1969). Light chains of the κ type, but not λ, have been found to complex proteins in sera of patients with myeloma (Laurell and Thulin, 1975). These complexes involve disulfide linkages through the C-terminal cysteine of κ chains.

Another protein associated with the Fc region of immunoglobulin is the epithelial glycoprotein, secretory component (Weicker and Underdown, 1975; Mehta et al., 1974). The structure and function of this protein have been covered previously (Section IIA). Briefly, it appears to afford the IgA and IgM molecules, with which it is usually associated, some degree of protection from proteolysis and may also facilitate their transport into the lumen of mucosal glands. The nature of the binding of SC to IgA dimer and IgM pentamer in vitro is at first noncovalent and apparently with roughly similar association constants in both classes, but in the case of IgA it subsequently becomes a covalent linkage through an unknown mechanism (Mach, 1970; Brandtzaeg, 1973; Lindh and Bjork, 1976). Some evidence has been presented indicating that J chain is necessary for the noncovalent attachment of SC to the Fc of polymeric IgA and IgM (Eskeland and Brandtzaeg, 1974; Brandtzaeg, 1976), although controversy exists with regard to this point (Tomasi and Czerwinski, 1976).

A serum factor from patients with cystic fibrosis (called "cystic fibrosis factor") has been found to bind to IgG1 and IgG2 immunoglobulins (Danes et al., 1973). However, this factor binds only to intact heavy chains of immunoglobulins and not Fab or Fc fragments, suggesting that the hinge area is involved in the binding. Another protein which binds to

IgG is the lymphokine, IBF (immunoglobulin-binding factor). This has been reported to be a T-cell product which binds the Fc region of IgG close to the complement-binding site (Fridman and Golstein, 1974). Its biological significance is unknown.

Finally, it should also be mentioned that certain segments of the Fc fragment of IgM and IgG obtained after proteolytic digestion appear to promote certain biological functions such as chemotaxis and phagocytosis (Takakazu *et al.*, 1976; Higuchi *et al.*, 1975, Constantopoulos *et al.*, 1973). Tuftsin (or leukokinin) is a tetrapeptide (Thr-Lys-Pro-Arg) obtained from the γ-chain C_H2 domain which stimulates PMN phagocytosis. Other examples of these immunoglobulin-derived factors have not been as well characterized but appear to be derived from the Fc part of the heavy chains. Their biological significance requires further exploration.

B. Cell-Binding Properties of Immunoglobulins

In this section we will review the effector functions mediated through the interaction of the Fc fragment with cells. These interactions may occur through one of two mechanisms. In the one case the Fc fragment is embedded in the lipid bilayer of the membrane (an integral membrane protein) while in the second it is not as tightly bound and is referred to as a "peripheral protein" (Singer, 1974). The classification of a protein as integral or peripheral depends on whether or not it can be extracted from cells with aqueous salt solutions (peripheral) or requires dissociating agents such as detergents, organic solvents or urea (integral). The solubility of integral proteins requires the continued presence of dissociating agents.

For reasons discussed in detail by Singer (1971) the current concept of membrane structure is that of a lipid bilayer intercalated with proteins, referred to as the "fluid mosaic model" (Fig. 11). It is based primarily on thermodynamic arguments (Tanford, 1973) concerned with the fact that it is energetically favorable for the ionic portion of an amphipathic substance to be in direct contact with water while its hydrophobic tail is sequestered from water and interacts with other nonpolar molecules. The role of hydrophobic interactions in protein conformation was first emphasized by Kauzman (1959). It is not our purpose here to review the area of membrane structure (see articles by Singer, 1971; Tanford, 1973), but certain points are important to the discussion of effector functions.

The average amino acid composition of membrane proteins does not show a clear difference from that of soluble proteins (Woodward and Munkres, 1966; Engelman and Morowitz, 1968), and yet membrane pro-

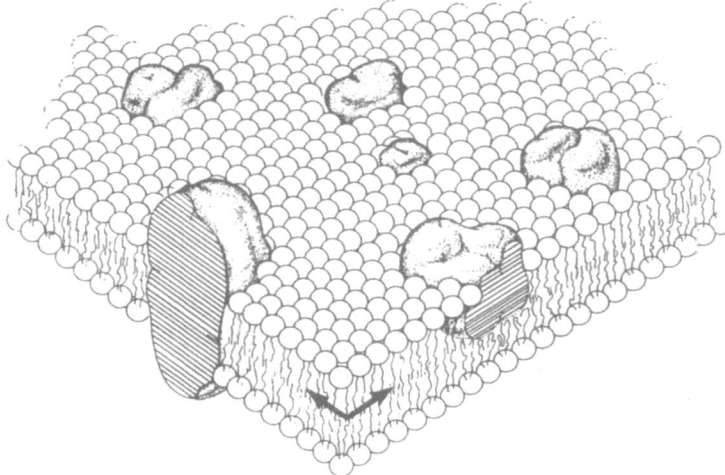

Figure 11. Fluid mosaic model of membrane structure. The solid bodies with stippled surfaces represent the globular integral proteins, with their hydrophilic ends protruding from the membrane and their hydrophobic ends embedded in the membrane (as seen in cross section). At long range, the integral proteins are randomly distributed in the plane of the membrane; at short range, some form subunit aggregates as shown. The spheres represent the ionic and polar head groups of the lipids and the wavy lines their fatty acid chains. The arrows denote the plane of cleavage in freeze-fracture experiments. Reproduced from Singer and Nicolson (1972); copyright 1972 by the American Association for the Advancement of Science.

teins aggregate in the absence of detergents or denaturants (Richardson *et al.*, 1963), suggesting the presence of unique structural features allowing them to complex with lipids within the membrane. There is evidence that the segments of integral membrane proteins embedded in the membrane have an amino acid sequence which allows hydrophobic side chains to associate with the lipid environment and thereby minimize free energy. Also, the CD spectra of several solubilized membranes from various cells are quite similar and indicate that little or no β conformation is present in most membrane proteins; approximately 30–40% is α helical, suggesting a globular nature of the proteins (Singer, 1971).

The lipid layer exhibits a fluidity allowing molecules to diffuse laterally in the plane of the membrane but not to rotate from one surface of the membrane to the other. This fluidity is temperature dependent, diminishing at lower temperatures. Membranes vary in their protein, lipid, and carbohydrate content, and it appears that the protein content in particular increases as the specialization of the membranes increases (Guidotti, 1972). In general, the percentage of protein varies from 18%

in the simplest membranes (myelin) to approximately 76% in the more complicated mitochondrial inner membrane. In the latter case the protein and not the lipid represents the greater part of the membrane and the protein may in fact be the continuous phase.

1. Integral Lymphocyte Membrane Immunoglobulins

There are two populations of lymphocytes differing in function and mode of development: bursal derived, or B cells, and thymic dependent, or T cells. In general, B cells are responsible for humoral immunity, and the T cells mediate cellular immunity (delayed hypersensitivity), although T cells also cooperate with B cells in antibody formation (Katz and Benacerraf, 1972).

B cells are easily detected by the presence of immunoglobulins on their surface (Pernis et al., 1970; Raff et al., 1970; Rabellino et al., 1971). These cell-surface immunoglobulins are thought to be the primary antigen receptors which, after combination with their specific antigens; initiate the chain of events leading to B-cell differentiation into plasma cells. These cells produce antibodies of the same specificity as that of the surface immunoglobulin, as first suggested by Burnet (1959). These surface immunoglobulins (SIg) are homogeneous with respect to light-chain type and idiotype (Wernet et al., 1972; Salsano et al., 1974; Fu et al., 1975), as would be predicted by clonal selection theory. Also, several workers have shown that SIg is closely associated with the membrane and behaves as an integral protein by several criteria (Melcher et al., 1975). This should not be confused with cytophilic antibodies, which are peripheral proteins (Section IIIB2). SIgs are primarily of the IgM and IgD classes (Vitetta and Uhr, 1975), and both are present in the monomeric form (H_2L_2) on human as well as mouse lymphoid cells (Rowe et al., 1973; Melcher et al., 1974; Abney and Parkhouse, 1974).

Several hypotheses have been suggested to explain the occurrence of IgM and IgD as both secreted (aqueous-soluble) and membrane-bound proteins. Any explanation must account for the fact that membrane immunoglobulins which have been extracted with detergent are insoluble in physiological buffers in the absence of detergents (or some other denaturant); i.e., membrane IgM and IgD are to a degree hydrophobic (Melcher et al., 1975) while the secreted form is not. Possible explanations which have been suggested are that (1) the two forms differ in sequence, (2) a separate "insertional" piece is added to the membrane form, or (3) the conformation of the membrane-associated position of the molecule differs from that of its soluble counterpart. The membrane-favored conformation would have to be maintained in a polar medium to explain the insolubility of the membrane immunoglobulin in aqueous media. This could be accomplished through disulfide pairing which differs from the soluble form. It would be interesting to study the reduction and reoxidation of membrane-bound IgD and IgM to determine if they can become water soluble if allowed to re-form disulfide bonds in a polar medium. The existence of two proteins with the same sequence but different conformation is difficult to reconcile with the principle that sequence alone determines tertiary structure. However, recently it has been shown that kinetic factors may also be involved (Wetlaufer *et al.*, 1974; Rose *et al.*, 1976), and according to this hypothesis "nucleation" occurs early in the biosynthesis of the protein which directs the subsequent folding. It could be argued that a membrane protein is synthesized at a different intracellular site or environment than a secreted protein (both having the same sequence), and therefore will have a different kinetic pathway and hence a different stable conformation.

It has been shown that most of the SIg can be labeled with the [^{125}I]lactoperoxidase system (Vitetta *et al.*, 1971; Baur *et al.*, 1972) and essentially all of the molecule is available to react with antisera (Fu and Kunkel, 1974). This would suggest that very little, if any, of the molecule is buried within the membrane. However, it appears that a long sequence of hydrophobic amino acids is not needed to anchor a protein in the membrane (Segrest and Feldman, 1974) (a minimal length of ten amino acids can penetrate a membrane of 30–35 Å). An examination of the sequence of IgM (Putnam *et al.*, 1973) in the Fc region does not disclose any areas abundant in hydrophobic residues as has been shown to be the case in the COOH-terminal region of the HLA antigen heavy chain (Springer and Strominger, 1976). A similar situation exists with the MN glycoprotein (glycophorin) of human erythrocytes. While the total amino acid composition of this protein is more polar than that of most water-soluble proteins (Capaldi and Vanderkooi, 1972), one segment of about 20 amino acids known to be associated with the membrane is composed primarily of hydrophobic amino acids (Segrest *et al.*, 1973; Segrest and Feldman, 1974). These arguments do not preclude a tight association between the SIg and another protein which is itself an integral protein. In this case it might be expected that the interaction between the two proteins would be primarily hydrophobic since solutions of high ionic strength do not release SIg (Kennel and Lerner, 1973).

There is some evidence to support the thesis that the soluble and membrane-bound immunoglobulins may have sequence or other structural differences. Studies have shown SIg and secreted immunoglobulins are synthesized at different rates and that SIg turnover occurs at a slower rate (Choi, 1976). These findings have been interpreted to indicate that different pathways exist for the synthesis of soluble and membrane-bound immunoglobulins and that SIg is not a precursor of secreted antibody. If this is the case, a more reasonable explanation for the two forms of IgM and IgD would be that immunoglobulins destined to be SIg may have an additional segment of hydrophobic amino acid chain attached to the COOH terminus, while the secreted form does not. There are in fact data to indicate that this may be the case. A comparison of SIg heavy chains of murine lymphocytes with those of the secreted counterpart has recently been made (Finkelman *et al.*, 1976; Melcher and Uhr, 1976). Membrane μ chain is slightly larger than the secreted μ chain, by approximately 1700 daltons. This suggests an extra piece of μ chain which could be involved in SIg binding to the membrane. It will be interesting to see a comparison of amino acid analysis of the two forms of μ chain. Other experiments also suggest themselves to determine if there is a different end piece on the SIg μ chain, e.g., COOH-terminal analysis of the internally labeled molecule. Also, it would be interesting after ^{125}I-labeling of the exposed SIg and extraction with detergent to relabel with ^{131}I to determine if any part of the molecule not exposed to radiolabeling initially becomes exposed after extraction from the membrane. Further experiments could be designed to determine the position of any additional label in the molecule. No mouse IgD myeloma is available for comparison with the IgD-like SIg. A comparison of this H chain with the human δ chain, however, indicates that the mouse SIg δ chain may be somewhat smaller by SDS-PAGE (Melcher and Uhr, 1976; Perry and Milstein, 1970). It appears that mouse is the only species examined in which the SIg μ and δ chains are not approximately the same in molecular weight (Finkelman *et al.*, 1976) by SDS-PAGE. In the murine SIg system, the δ chain moves faster than μ chain on electrophoresis. It is possible that these investigations are dealing with a cleavage product of the intact murine SIg δ chain since there is evidence for degradation in their preparations (Finkelman *et al.*, 1976). Recently, antisera have been prepared to the murine SIg IgD (Abney *et al.*, 1976; Goding *et al.*, 1976).

Whatever the mode of attachment of SIg to cell membranes, the major portion of the Fc part of the molecule is not embedded in the phospholipid bilayer. This is also supported by the fact that CD spectra of all membrane proteins (not lymphocytes specifically) show little β conformation, which, as previously mentioned, is the conformation of immunoglobulin domains. Experiments with reconstituted lymphocyte plasma membranes (Chavin and Holliman, 1975) and model membrane systems (Weissman *et al.*, 1974) have not, in general, been very revealing. With reconstituted membranes, very little of the original membrane immunoglobulin becomes reincorporated. Liposome models were tested by

Weissman *et al.* (1974) for the ability of immunoglobulins to perturb the model membranes. Release of small molecules was used to measure the degree of interaction. It was found that altered (heat-aggregated) immunoglobulins were better able to perturb the liposomes than native molecules. The significance of these studies is unclear, especially since IgM was inactive.

The presence of intact immunoglobulins on T lymphocytes is controversial (Marchalonis, 1975). If present, their number is probably less than the 10^5 per cell usually quoted for B cells (Singer, 1974; Vitetta *et al.*, 1972). While there is considerable functional evidence for their presence, methods similar to those used for detection of SIg on B cells have not been so successful for T-cell SIg (Grey *et al.*, 1972; Vitetta *et al.*, 1972). The contradictory reports by various workers in the field indicate that technical problems may account for the varied results (Haustein *et al.*, 1975). There are reports that immunoglobulins with heavy chains differing in size from the μ and δ of B cells are present on murine T lymphoma cells, T lymphocytes, and thymocytes and that most of the Fc part is buried within the membrane (Haustein *et al.*, 1975; Haustein and Goding, 1975). It has been shown that the T-cell SIg is antigenically related to IgM but does not appear to be completely exposed (Hammerling *et al.*, 1976a,b).

Recently, Cone and Brown (1976) have found that T-cell SIg extraction is highly dependent on detergent concentrations used since they are more firmly bound than their B-cell counterparts. They also determined that murine T-cell SIg had heavy chains of 45,000 daltons which were not disulfide-linked to the light chains, suggesting that this immunoglobulin may not be identical to other classes or subclasses. These studies suggest that a special immunoglobulin-type molecule with strong hydrophobic bonding acts as the SIg for T cells. Perhaps the strongest evidence for at least a portion (V region?) of immunoglobulins being on the surface of T cells is the observation that B and T cells with apparently the same antigen specificity react with the same anti-idiotype antibody (Binz and Wigzell, 1975; Eichmann and Rajewsky, 1975).

It is obvious that without more detailed chemical information about the structure of SIg, particularly amino acid, carbohydrate, and lipid analysis, explanations concerning the mode of attachment of Ig to membranes must be speculative.

2. Fixation to Phagocytes and Lymphocytes—Cytophilic Antibody

In contrast to the surface immunoglobulins discussed in the previous section, immunoglobulins may also bind to the surface of certain cells via a membrane component referred to as a "Fc receptor" (Dickler, 1976). These immunoglobulins are peripheral proteins, and in this and the following sections we shall be discussing the cytophilic properties of different antibody classes for various cell types. We shall refer to these antibodies collectively as "cytophilic," realizing that classically this term was initially reserved for specific types of immunoglobulin which bind to macrophages. The function of the cytophilic antibody is dependent on the cell to which it binds. Immune response cells to which cytophilic antibody may bind include macrophage (Boyden and Sarkin, 1960), monocytes (Huber and Fudenberg, 1968), neutrophils (Messner and Jelinek, 1970), cytotoxic "K" cells (Möller, 1965), B cells (Dickler and Kunkel, 1972; Basten et al., 1972), and activated T cells (Yoshida and Anderson, 1972). Recently, it has become evident that a third population of lymphocytes bearing Fc receptors exists. These "null cells" are neither classical B cells nor classical T cells since they do not form E rosettes or have surface Ig. They may, however, be equivalent to K cells (Abo et al., 1976).

In the case of monocytes, macrophages, neutrophils, and K cells, the cytophilic antibody acts as an opsonin for phagocytosis or is involved in the destruction of a specific target cell by contact lysis. For B cells and activated T cells, the function of the cytophilic antibody is as yet unknown, but it could be involved in the regulation of cellular and humoral immune responses.

Antibodies cytophilic for phagocytes and lymphocytes belong to the IgG class primarily. This has recently been extensively studied by Lawrence et al. (1975). By using ^{125}I-labeled proteins, they were able to study the binding of different classes and subclasses to various cell types. The results are summarized in Figs. 12–14. In the human, IgG1 and IgG3 are cytophilic for monocytes, neutrophils, and lymphocytes. The cytophilic properties of these two classes have previously been reported by Huber and Fudenberg (1968), Messner and Jelinek (1970), and Huber et al. (1971). However these investigators also found that IgG4 was cytophilic for monocytes and IgA1 and IgA2 (especially IgA2) bound to neutrophils. In contrast, IgG2, IgM, IgD, and IgE were found to be noncytophilic. When aggregation of these proteins was accomplished by the use of F(ab')₂ fragments of rabbit anti-human Fab and these aggregates were tested, a considerable increase in binding was seen, and, in addition, IgG2 bound to all cell types. Lymphocytes, but not neutrophils, bound aggregated IgE, but the aggregated IgM and IgD were noncytophilic. This is in agreement with previous results where binding to neutrophils was measured by enzyme release (Spiegelberg et al., 1974).

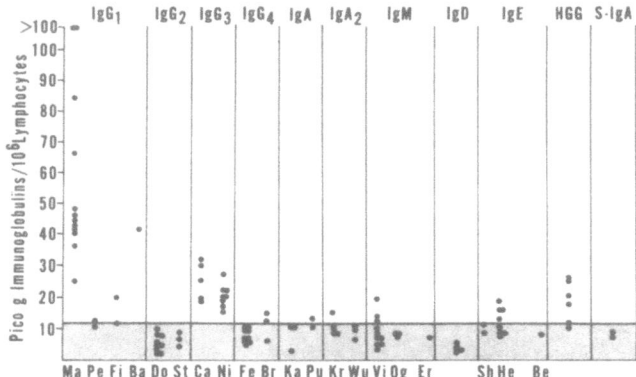

Figure 12. Binding of ¹²⁵I-labeled Ig to human lymphocytes. Each column represents uptake of either HGG, SIgA, or a myeloma protein identified by abbreviation of patient's name, and each point represents the mean of duplicate determinations with various normal lymphocyte preparations. The class of the myeloma protein is indicated on the top of the figure. The shaded area indicates the highest binding of IgG2 proteins below which binding is considered insignificant. Reproduced with permission from Lawrence *et al.* (1975); copyright 1975, Rockefeller University Press.

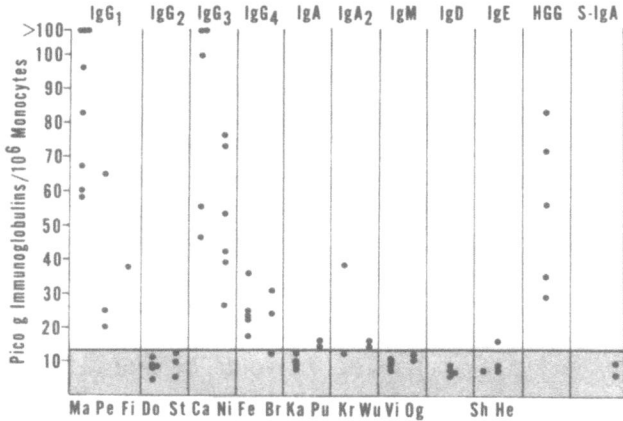

Figure 13. Binding of ¹²⁵I-labeled Ig to human monocytes. Each column represents uptake of either HGG, SIgA, or a myeloma protein identified by abbreviation of patient's name, and each point represents the mean of duplicate determinations with various normal monocyte preparations. The class of myeloma protein is indicated on the top of the figure. The shaded area indicates the highest binding of IgG2 proteins below which binding is considered insignificant. Reproduced with permission from Lawrence *et al.* (1975); copyright 1975, Rockefeller University Press.

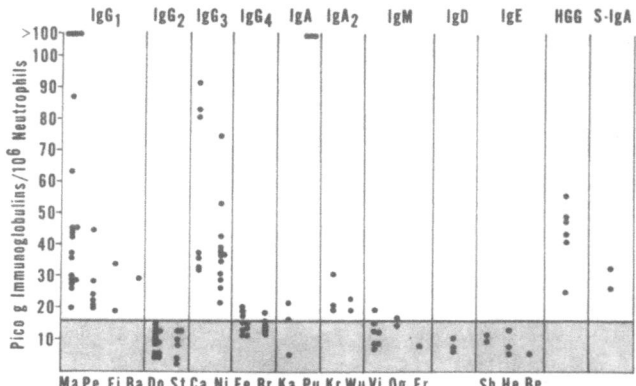

Figure 14.   Binding of ^{125}I-labeled Ig to human neutrophils. Each column represents uptake of either HGG, SIgA, or a myeloma protein identified by abbreviation of patient's name, and each point represents the mean of duplicate determinations with various normal neutrophil preparations. The class of the myeloma protein is indicated on the top of the figure. The shaded area indicates the highest binding of IgG2 proteins below which binding is considered insignificant. Reproduced with permission from Lawrence *et al.* (1975); copyright 1975, Rockefeller University Press.

The binding of IgA to neutrophils was found for both serum and secretory IgA (Lawrence *et al.*, 1975; Spiegelberg *et al.*, 1974), while earlier studies failed to detect the opsonizing properties of IgA (Zipursky *et al.*, 1973; Wilson, 1972). In the study by Lawrence *et al.* (1975), evidence was obtained to indicate that the receptors for IgA and IgG on neutrophils were different, while receptors for the IgG subclasses were the same on all cell types. A recent report indicates that a subpopulation of porcine circulating mononuclear cells bears surface receptors for secretory component (Setcavage *et al.*, 1976). It should be pointed out that the lack of IgA binding to lymphocytes may be due to the use of inappropriate cells for these studies. It would be interesting to investigate whether IgA is cytophilic for cells derived from a secretion, such as colostrum, rather than circulating cells.

The inability of IgM to bind to any cell type in Lawrence's study is surprising in view of previous reports that it was cytophilic in mouse (Lay and Nussenzweig, 1969) and chicken (Webb and Cooper, 1973). One report stated that the 8 S subunit was cytophilic for guinea pig macrophage (Rhodes, 1973), but in the work of Lawrence *et al.* (1975) no binding of the reduced and alkylated pentamer occurred with monocytes or lymphocytes. This could be due to species differences. IgM does appear to be cytophilic for T cells (Moretta *et al.*, 1975; McConnell and

Hurd, 1976) and has been demonstrated to mediate tumor cell cytotoxicity (Lamon *et al.*, 1975*a,b*) and to bind T cells cultured in IgM-free media (Ferrarini *et al.*, 1976). In the latter case, binding occurred through the pentameric $(Fc)_5\mu$.

A recent report has examined the ability of the IgG subclasses to bind to K cells (Spiegelberg *et al.*, 1976). The method used was to coat ^{51}Cr-labeled chicken erythrocytes (CRBC) with rabbit antibody and test the ability of various human subclass myeloma proteins to inhibit lysis in the presence of (human) lymphocytes. The use of rabbit antibody in the test system is justified on the basis that there is little, if any, species specificity involved in binding of immunoglobulin to Fc receptors (Larsson *et al.*, 1973). With this system it was found that the IgG1 and IgG3 subclasses inhibited K-cell-mediated lysis more efficiently (at lower concentration) than IgG2 and IgG4, which often had to be aggregated with BDB to demonstrate activity. However, some proteins of the latter subclasses were shown to be strong inhibitors as well. In other tests, K lymphocytes could be adsorbed onto glass beads coated with IgG1 and IgG3 but not IgG2 and IgG4 even though they were aggregated. The variations in inhibition of cell lysis seen *within* a subclass could not be attributed to known genetic markers or L-chain type. The reason for this is unknown, but it may indicate that small localized sequence differences occur in myeloma proteins which affect their binding affinity. Another possibility may be that the Fab part of the molecule plays an indirect role in cell surface binding as appears to be the case in complement fixation (see Section IIIA1), although there is no evidence for this. Because of the variations between individual molecules, it is important that many samples of a given subclass be tested to obtain a true picture of the biological properties of that subclass.

While subclasses IgG1 and IgG3 were more cytophilic for K cells in the native state, when aggregated by heat or by chemical cross-linking all four subclasses were more consistently cytophilic (MacLennan *et al.*, 1973). This suggests that all four subclasses may potentially participate in antibody-dependent cell-mediated cytotoxicity (ADCC). However, to confirm these observations, experiments with isolated subclass antibodies to known antigens must be carried out. This has recently been done for the IgG2 subclass having antidextran specificity (Larsson *et al.*, 1975). This subclass was shown to be fully active in ADCC in this study. It should also be noted that binding of aggregated Ig and IgG-sensitized RBCs may occur through different mechanisms. Froland *et al.* (1974) have reported that IgG-sensitized RBCs are bound to cells which are neither T nor B cells, whereas heat-aggregated IgG is bound by Ig-positive cells (B cells). Moreover, binding of the heat-aggregated IgG was shown to be mediated by sites on the $F(ab')_2$ as well as Fc' [heat-aggregated F(ab')$_2$ and pFc' from an IgG3 myeloma protein] and would indicate a "nonspecific" binding of heat-aggregated IgG by B lymphocytes as opposed to specific binding through sites on the Fc fragment only. This is supported by the results of Weissmann *et al.* (1974) which show considerable interaction between heat-aggregated immunoglobulins and liposomes. However, Dickler (1974) has shown that heat-aggregated albumin and transferrin do not bind lymphocytes. Moreover, he found that heat-aggregated IgG inhibited the binding of rabbit antibody-antigen complexes. Also, heat-aggregated Ig prevented lysis of specific sensitized target cells, indicating that heat-aggregated Ig and antigen-antibody complexes share the same receptor.

There is a difference between binding by cells of antibody-antigen complexes and binding by unliganded antibody (Warner, 1974). The former is referred to as "opsonic adherence" while the latter is "cytophilia," and the difference between them must be kept in mind when designing or evaluating experiments. Recent work suggests that the same effector cells and the same antibodies are operative in both types of reactions (Imir *et al.*, 1976). The fundamental difference between these two mechanisms is whether or not the antibody binds first to a target cell via its antibody site (opsonic adherence) or to the effector cell via its Fc (cytophilia). Higher antibody concentrations are required for cytophilia than for opsonic adherence (approximately 100 times). In most studies the two tests are used interchangeably and little effort is made by the various workers to differentiate between them, but it is clear, according to this distinction, that studies with native proteins measure true cytophilia while those made with aggregated or altered proteins presumably mimic antigen bound antibody and therefore represent sensitization. The binding of liganded antibody by Fc receptors appears to be a higher energy than binding of antibody alone or of monovalent hapten-antibody complexes (Phillips-Quagliata *et al.*, 1971).

There is a conflict concerning certain characteristics of Fc receptors. Some studies indicate that rabbit macrophage receptors are resistant to proteolytic enzymes (Arend and Mannik, 1973) while some indicate that the receptors of mouse macrophage are destroyed by such enzymes (Unkeless and Eisen, 1975). Other reports suggest varying susceptibility to different proteolytic enzymes (Dickler, 1974). In certain studies showing resistance, increased adherence of soluble complexes could be demonstrated as a result of the proteolysis, and the increased adherence resulted from different mechanisms depending on whether male or female rabbit alveolar macrophages were used (Arend and Mannik, 1973). Other reports suggest that early-response cytophilic antibody binds to a trypsin-sensitive receptor, while the late-response cytophilic antibodies bind to a trypsin-resistant receptor (Askenase and Hayden, 1974; Kossard and Nelson, 1968). Some studies indicate that the macrophage receptor may be sensitive to phospholipase (Warner, 1974; Walker, 1976). Haustein *et al.* (1975) reported that mouse T lymphoma cell lines have a surface protein of 40,000–45,000 molecular weight intimately associated with what these workers have considered to be SIg of T cells and suggest that this may be the Fc receptor. Their argument is supported by the fact that two cell lines which lack this component do not form IgG rosettes. Rask *et al.* (1975) have reported the isolation of a murine B-cell Fc receptor having a molecular weight of 65,000. A putative Fc receptor from a human B cell has been shown to have a 70,000 molecular weight, but, in contrast to the murine B-cell receptor, it becomes 35,000 molecular weight after reduction and alkylation (Wernet, 1976). Neauport-Sautes *et al.* (1975) showed that the binding properties of Fc receptors on mouse activated T cells are very similar to those of an immunoglobulin-binding factor (IBF) produced by these cells. Moreover, under conditions known to cause loss of Fc receptor bearing cells as well as release of bound immunoglobulin from mononuclear cells (Kumagai *et al.*, 1975), increased secretion of IBF occurs. Some workers have associated B-cell Fc receptors with I-region-associated antigens (Ia antigens) present on these cells (Dickler and Sachs, 1974). Recent work, however, has not supported this view (Halloran *et al.*, 1975). It appears therefore that Fc receptors probably do not represent a single protein moiety. The nature of this receptor may indeed be dependent on several factors, including type of cell (e.g., B cell, mastocytoma, T cell, epithelial cells), age of the cell, species of cell and Ig, and subclass of Ig.

While there are uncertainties associated with the properties of the receptor, other facts appear to be clear. Among these are the apparent specificity of certain classes and subclasses for different cell types and the apparent lack of species specificity (Imir *et al.*, 1976). It is also evident that while native monomeric Ig may bind to Fc receptors, polymeric forms have much greater affinity (Phillips-Quagliata *et al.*, 1971). Unkeless and Eisen (1975) have measured the affinity of unaggregated mouse myeloma proteins for mouse macrophages. For mouse IgG2a, a K_a of 1.4×10^8 M^{-1} was measured at 4°C (K_a increases with decreasing temperature, i.e., the reaction is exothermic). This is the highest affinity reported. Guinea pig has a K_a of 1.5×10^6 M^{-1} at 20°C (Leslie and Cohen, 1974*a,b*), and mouse IgG2b has a K_a of 6.8×10^6 M^{-1} at 4°C. The affinity constant for aggregated forms has not been measured. However, the increased binding seen with altered Ig reflects their ability to bind either to multiple receptors or to receptors specific for newly exposed sites (or both). Dorrington has pointed out that this lower affinity for unaltered Ig is advantageous to the organism since the concentration of a specific antigen-antibody complex is sure to be less than that of native Ig and therefore competes favorably for sites on macrophages and other cells (Dorrington, 1976).

A question of importance is whether or not all cytophilic immunoglobulins bind the same receptor on a given cell or whether there are different receptors for different classes, subclasses, and species. The studies of Lawrence *et al.* (1975) clearly indicate that for human IgA and IgG different receptors exist, as previously stated, while for IgG subclasses binding apparently occurs on the same receptor since significant cross-inhibition was observed. In contrast to this, there appear to be separate receptors for mouse IgG2a and IgG2b on an established line of mouse peritoneal (C57BL/6 transformed by SV40 virus) macrophage (Walker, 1976), termed "IG21." A recent study (Unkeless, 1977) shows that two receptors can be differentiated on mouse peritoneal macrophage, one of which is trypsin sensitive and binds IgG2a in either monomeric or liganded form, and another which is trypsin resistant and binds heterologous antibody (rabbit) in antigen-antibody complexes. The uncomplexed heterologous antibody was also found to bind to the trypsin-sensitive receptor, although very weakly. Another recent report (Ghetie *et al.*, 1976) has demonstrated that lymphocytes of mouse, rabbit, and pig bind heterologous native IgG to a much greater extent (i.e., a greater percentage of binding lymphocytes) than native homologous IgG. These studies were performed using staphylococcal protein A conjugated to red cells (ES) and determining the number of rosettes formed with lymphocytes treated with nonantibody IgG. Similar results were obtained with alveolar and peritoneal macrophage. Matre (1976) has reported that pooled IgG of human, rabbit, and guinea pig origin is able to inhibit the binding of EA cells sensitized with rabbit antibody (A) by normal and malignant lymphoreticular tissue. Binding of native heterologous IgG by human and mouse lymphocytes has also been observed by the authors (R. C. McCarthy, J. A. Velosa, N. J. Calvanico, and T. B. Tomasi, unpublished observations). It therefore appears that considerable controversy exists as to whether or not a given Fc receptor may bind more than one type of immunoglobulin. This controversy is due to the large variety of detection systems, species combinations of cells, and antibodies and ligands used by various workers.

There is little doubt that the Fc receptor interacts with sites on the Fc part of the molecule, as has been demonstrated with all species examined (Walker, 1976; Berken and Benacerraf, 1966; Inchley *et al.*, 1970). Carbohydrates may play a variable role in the opsonic properties of rabbit IgG. It has been shown that while rabbit antipneumococcal antibody loses its cytophilic properties by treatment with glycosidases, other bacterial antibodies (e.g., antistaphylococcal) are unaffected (Williams *et al.*, 1973). The significance of these studies must await further experiments with antibodies to several types of antigens.

Yasmeen *et al.* (1973, 1976) have reported that the C_H3 domain of human IgG contains the site responsible for interaction with guinea pig macrophages. It was shown that tanned sheep RBCs coated with the $C_\gamma3$ fragment (see Section IIc), but not the $C_\gamma2$, retained significant rosette-forming capacity (approximately 30% as effective as native IgG on tanned SRBC). In addition, these workers found that the $C_\gamma3$ fragment, when preincubated with macrophage, inhibited the formation of rosettes between guinea pig peritoneal macrophages and IgG-coated SRBC. On a molar basis, the $C_\gamma3$ fragment was twice as effective as the Fc. This is supported by earlier studies by Okafor *et al.* (1974) showing that the pFc' fragment of IgG inhibited rosette formation between human monocytes and anti-D (Rh0) coated human red cells. These results clearly show the involvement of the C_H3 domain. Mild reduction and alkylation of human IgG cause essentially complete loss of its ability to bind monocytes, lymphocytes, and neutrophils (Lawrence *et al.*, 1975). Ciccimarra *et al.* (1975) have reported that a decapeptide from the C_H3 domain was fully capable (90%) of inhibiting rosette formation between monocytes and anti-Rh-coated human erythrocytes at low concentration (0.6 nmol/8 × 10^5 monocytes). The decapeptide, which is obtained from a dialysate of an acid-CNBr treated Fc fragment of pooled human IgG, has the empirical formula Tyr-Ser$_2$-Lys$_2$-Leu-Thr-Val-Asp-Arg. Although the authors point out that the sequence 407–416 of the Eu myeloma protein has this composition, they have not provided molecular weight or sequence data to support their contention. As pointed out by Dorrington, this sequence might be expected to be buried in the interior of the domain on the basis of crystallographic data obtained on other domains (Okafor *et al.*, 1974). However, the high affinity of the fragment could reflect the fact that this peptide is not the site bound on the native molecule but the one exposed by aggregation. It would be interesting to know if this peptide inhibits binding of native IgG.

Ciccimarra *et al.* (1975) have also tested two deleted proteins, "Dob" (Lopes and Steiner, 1973), an IgG1 protein lacking residues 216–229 (Eu numbering) in the hinge region, and an IgG3 protein, "Web" (Grossman *et al.*, 1972), with deletions in the C_H2 region (residues 240–300). Both were equally efficient in binding to monocytes.

These data support a C_H3 binding site. Other workers, however, have not been in agreement with these conclusions. This is particularly true of studies involving species other than man. A recent study by

Alexander *et al.* (1976) on the cytophilic activity of guinea pig IgG2 for homologous peritoneal macrophage implicates the C_H2 region and not the C_H3. Both Fc' and pFc' showed no binding activity, and neither did the Fab and F(ab)$_2$ fragments. Only complete Fc fragments with interchain disulfide bonds intact were cytophilic. Reduction of the interchain disulfide caused almost complete loss of binding even though the fragment remained a noncovalent dimer. Urea-acid denaturation also causes irreversible loss of activity. A fragment intermediate between Fc and Fc' containing only one C_H2 domain (but two C_H3 domains) was also inactive indicating a need for two closely linked C_H2 domains. This work agrees with an earlier report (Kazmierowski *et al.*, 1971) showing that opsonic activity of rabbit IgG was lost by reduction and alkylation of the native molecule. Unfortunately, these workers could not isolate a C_H2 fragment to test directly. Therefore, their data can be interpreted as a requirement for C_H2 alone or a combination of C_H2 and C_H3 domains for full activity. This latter reasoning has been used to explain the loss of activity in the human myleoma "Web" protein (Grossman *et al.*, 1972), which lacks a large part of the C_H2 domain.

Ovary *et al.* (1976) obtained the Facb (plasmin digestion after acid treatment) fragment from rabbit Ig and showed binding to homologous alveolar macrophages. Also, rabbit anti-sheep erythrocyte Facb was equally able to form rosettes with macrophage compared to acid-treated antibody (i.e., acid-treated controls, no plasmin). In addition, the C_H3 fragment obtained by papain digestion (Fc') was completely without inhibitory activity when tested in the same system. On the other hand, neutrophils apparently bind regions on the C_H3 domain. MacLennan *et al.* (1974) have shown that complexes of human serum albumin (HSA) and acid-plasmin digested anti-HSA (Facb anti-HSA–HSA) do not inhibit phagocytosis by neutrophils at concentrations 10 times those of whole antiHSA–HSA complexes required to produce 50% inhibition.

Results from experiments concerned with measuring the binding of rabbit immunoglobulin fragments to cytotoxic K cells in ADCC are in agreement. MacLennan *et al.* (1974) reported that Facb fragments of rabbit antibody (acid-plasmin digestion) lose the ability to lyse target cells when human peripheral blood lymphocytes were used. They did not test Fc'-type fragments. Michaelsen *et al.* (1975) and Wisloff *et al.* (1974*b*) carried out similar experiments with rabbit anti-CRBC and human lymphocytes and found the Facb to be inactive. In addition, pFc' fragments tested for inhibition of the reaction were also inactive (Wisloff *et al.*, 1974*a*), even when heat aggregated. These workers suggest that the absence of noncovalent interaction in the C_H2 domain accounts for the lack of activity in the Facb fragment and that while the actual site of interaction resides in this domain the C_H3 domain is needed to stabilize the proximity of the two C_H2 domains required for binding to K cells. This hypothesis is supported by the finding that mild reduction and alkylation markedly reduce ADCC. It would be interesting in these studies to prepare C_H2 domains chemically cross-linked to test whether such preparations satisfy the necessary structural requirements for binding.

Ramasamy et al. (1975) have carried out studies on the binding of mouse immunoglobulins to lymph node lymphocytes. In this work, mutant proteins of the McPC 21 IgG1 cell line were tested for their ability to inhibit rosette formation. It was found that a mutant lacking only the C_H1 domain was inhibitory while mutants lacking only the C_H3 domains were not. Here again, while this suggests that the C_H3 contains the necessary site, it does not prove it, since mutants without the C_H2 region were not available, and the same arguments can be used to explain these results as were used to explain the ADCC data, i.e., the C_H3 stabilizes the dimeric form of the C_H2 domains.

Attempts have been made to study the active site by chemical modification of amino acid side chains (Messner et al., 1970; Thrasher et al., 1975; Thrasher and Cohen, 1971). No attempts have been made to separate the various products of the modification reactions and to study the individual homogeneous populations of modified proteins. Collectively, however, the results of these studies would appear to implicate an amino group in the cytophilic site. The data of Ciccimarra et al. (1975) suggest that there are two lysine residues in a decapeptide containing the site, but the positions of the modified amino groups have not been ascertained, nor has the effect of these reagents on other side chains and on conformations been studied.

It is difficult to draw firm conclusions regarding the location of the cytophilic site. While most studies suggest the C_H3 domain (for IgM the site appears to be in the last domain also, i.e., the $C_\mu4$ region) (Conradie and Bubb, 1977), there are contradictions not easily explained. The most impressive data are those of Ciccimarra et al. (1975) which implicate residues 407–416 in the site. As pointed out by Dorrington (1976), the only difference in sequence between IgG1 (cytophilic) and IgG4 (relatively noncytophilic) is the replacement of Lys at position 409 in IgG1 with an Arg in IgG4. Most of the contradictory results come from studies involved with nonhuman antibodies such as guinea pig and rabbit. An additional source of confusion may be the cell type for which binding is being investigated. There is no evidence to suggest that the Fc receptors on different cells all have identical specificities. Indeed, a recent report indicates that while binding of native free heterologous IgG is similar with all cell types, the binding of heterologous and homologous antibody-antigen complexes varies with the type of cell (Ghetie *et al.*, 1976). Greater attention should be placed on the system in use, and interchangeable reference to Fc receptors as an all inclusive and single moiety should be avoided. For example, Anderson *et al.* (1975) have reported that human β_2-microglobulin, which shows significant homology to immunoglobulin domains, does not bind to human lymphocytes or neutrophils but does to those of mice and rats. The receptor, however, is different from the Fc receptor specific for immunoglobulins. It is obvious that care is needed in evaluating and comparing results from binding experiments with the immunoglobulins of different species on various cell types.

3. Fixation to Mast Cells—Cytotropic Antibody

An anaphylactic reaction may result from the fixation of certain types of antibodies to basophilic cells in the blood or tissue (mast cells), and the subsequent release from these cells of pharmacological reagents follows the reaction of the surface-fixed antibody with its specific antigen. The released pharmacological agents include histamine, serotonin, slow-reacting substance (SRS-A), eosinophil chemotactic factor (ECF-A), neutrophil chemotactic factor, bradykinin, and prostaglandins. Their effect is to cause vasodilation with leakage of intravascular fluids or to produce smooth muscle constriction, as, for example, in guinea pig bronchi during generalized anaphylaxis. These effects may also be localized to specific organs as in the skin; the passive cutaneous anaphylaxis (PCA) reaction in an example of this phenomenon. It is caused by the injection of the serum from a sensitive animal of the same or another species into the skin of a test animal. After a latent period, antigen is injected intravenously with Evans blue (a protein binding dye). Vascular leakage at the site of antibody fixation is evidenced by the formation of a blue spot (Austen and Brocklehurst, 1961; Ovary *et al.*, 1963; Ishizaka *et al.*, 1970*b*).

The antibodies involved in anaphylactic sensitization are called "cytotropic antibodies." Those able to passively sensitize animals of another species are called "heterocytotropic" while those able to sensitize only members of the same or closely related species are called "homocytotropic." Heterocytotropic antibodies are primarily IgG, while homocytotropic antibodies belong primarily to the IgE class (Ishizaka and Ishizaka, 1966; Johansson, 1967; Vaz and Ovary, 1968). IgG homocytotropic antibodies have been demonstrated in animals such as guinea pig (Amkraut *et al.*, 1973), rat (Bach *et al.*, 1971), and mouse (Vaz and Ovary, 1968). In humans, although there are reports claiming the existence of IgG reagins (Reid, 1970; Parish, 1970; Malley *et al.,* 1974), these antibodies have not as yet been well characterized.

Heterologous sensitization can be demonstrated in a manner similar to the PCA reaction, but instead of using antigen to elicit the release of the pharmacological agents, antibody to the class or subclass of the sensitizing antibody can be used. This technique by which antigen (in this case an antibody acting as an antigen) is injected locally and an antiserum directed against it injected systemically is termed the "reverse passive cutaneous reaction" (RPCA) (Ovary, 1960). Using this method it has been determined that all subclasses of human IgG except IgG2 sensitize heterologous skin (Ovary *et al.,* 1970), in this case the guinea pig. This subclass specificity is different from complement-fixing subclasses (IgG1, 2, 3), which would appear to indicate that the two sites are distinct.

Only one report suggests that subfragments of the Fc can be used to elicit a RPCA reaction. This study (Minta and Painter, 1972) examined the ability of pepsin (pFc') and papain (Fc') subfragments from pooled human IgG and IgG1 myeloma proteins to inhibit the PCA reaction in guinea pigs. Two methods were used to quantitate the results. The first method entailed the usual measurement of the diameter of the blue area resulting from extravasation of the dye. The second method involved the measurement of ^{131}I-labeled serum albumin, which was used in combination with the dye (Udaka *et al.,* 1970). It was found that while both the Fc and its subfragments (F'c) were able to inhibit accumulation of labeled albumin, only Fc reduced the diameter of the blue zone when injected simultaneously with antibody. No differences were noted between papain Fc' and pepsin Fc' activities. Interestingly, however, when tested by RPCA using pFc' specific antisera, the COOH-terminal domain fragment showed no activity in guinea pig, as has been found previously with Fc' fragments of both human IgG (Calvanico and Tomasi, 1971; Frommel and Hong, 1970) and rabbit IgG (Prahl, 1967; Utsumi, 1969). It is difficult to reconcile the results of the blue dye and radiolabeled albumin experiments, since both dye and label presumably are bound to protein. The inability to demonstrate RPCA with the subfragments could not be explained on the basis of loss of reactivity of the antiserum since, with the Fc, RPCA could be demonstrated with the same Fc'-specific antiserum.

There are few data concerning the ability of the amino-terminal half of the Fc fragment of human IgG to elicit PCA reactions, but there are some data available for rabbit IgG. The Facb fragment resulting from acid-plasmin treatment of rabbit antibody (contains C_H2 domains) did not fix to guinea pig skin, suggesting that the C_H2 domain (Stewart *et al.,*

1973; Ovary et al., 1976) is not involved. The investigators have interpreted these findings as an indication that both the C_H2 and C_H3 domains are needed for the PCA reaction, acting conjointly to fix and release histamine from the mast cell, or, alternatively, each carrying the site for a separate function, i.e., fixation by the C_H3 domain with subsequent histamine release a function of the C_H2 domain.

Some amino acid modification studies have been done on rabbit antibody effects on the PCA reaction in guinea pig. Carbamylation of approximately 90% of the available amino groups is needed to obtain a reduction in PCA titer; but the effect appears to be nonspecific since changes in the precipitating ability of antibody can be detected (Cohen et al., 1969). Amidination of 71% of the amino groups and benzylation of 2.3 tryptophan residues/molecule caused no significant loss in PCA titer. These studies suggest that amino groups and tryptophan residues play an insignificant role in the PCA reaction. This is not in agreement with earlier studies which implicated tryptophan (Griffin et al., 1967) and lysine (Ljaljevic et al., 1968) residues. However, in these studies, greater degrees of modification were used to obtain the reduced PCA titer, and indications of change of the native structure of the antibody were present. More recently, it has been shown that fluorescein conjugation of rabbit antibody causes considerable loss of PCA activity in guinea pig even at relatively low fluorescein-to-protein ratios (Thrasher et al., 1975). However, no information concerning possible conformational changes, sites of conjugation, or heterogeneity of conjugation products was reported in these studies. It was stated that antibody activity was intact, but this is not evidence that the Fc part of the molecule had not been altered.

Taken collectively, the data appear to indicate that no single domain is responsible for the PCA activity in IgG antibody in the guinea pig. It would be interesting to carry out mixing experiments with the C_H2 and C_H3 domains to see if the two separated domains can act together to elicit a PCA reaction. If they can, it would be strong evidence that both domains are needed for the receptor site. The modification studies are hard to evaluate, but they do not support an important role for amino groups as in the C'-fixing site.

Homocytotropic antibody, or "reagin" as it is called in humans, is primarily IgE, although an IgG1 homocytotropic antibody has been reported in some species. In contrast to IgE, the IgG1 homocytotropic antibody has a short half-life in skin, a long half-life in plasma, and a low affinity for receptors in the skin (Spiegelberg, 1974). The chemistry and biology of IgE have recently been reviewed by Ishizaka and Ishizaka (1975), and the reader is directed to this reference for an extensive account of this class of immunoglobulins. For our purposes, only a short discussion of the structure of IgE is required. This has partly been covered in Sections IIA and IIC.

IgE has a sedimentation coefficient of 8 S and a molecular weight of 190,000–200,000. The physicochemical properties of the molecule are based on results obtained from the six IgE myeloma patients which have thus far been reported (Ishizaka and Ishizaka, 1975). The ϵ chain (IgE heavy chain) is approximately the same size as the μ chain of IgM and is also composed of five domains (Bennich and Bahr-Lindstrom, 1974). Cleavage of the molecule by papain and pepsin is diagrammed in Fig. 15. It should be noted that papain digestion yields a Fc fragment composed of three domains and that the Fc' fragment represents the C_H2 domain rather than the COOH-terminal domain. Peptic cleavage occurs between constant domains 2 and 3, with concomitant destruction of C_H3 and C_H4, yielding a F(ab')$_2$ fragment having the C_H2 domain, the C_H2 also being present in the Fc fragment obtained from papain digestion (Ishizaka et al., 1970a; Bennich and Johansson, 1971).

The mast cell receptor for IgE appears to be a glycoprotein of approximately 50,000 molecular weight (Kulczycki et al., 1976; Conrad and Froese, 1976). These results are only tentative as it is not known if this represents part of the receptor, a subunit of it or the entire moiety. An antiserum to the native receptor would be helpful, and it appears that one has recently been prepared (Froese, 1976). The receptor has been shown to be sensitive to trypsin, pepsin, and pronase treatment (Gonzalez-Molina and Spiegelberg, 1976; Kulczycki et al., 1976).

Rat and mouse normal and neoplastic cells all contain the receptor (Mendoza and Metzger, 1976) but do not distinguish between rat and mouse IgE. The affinity constants of both rat and mouse mast cells for rat IgE are high (K_a = approximately 10^{10}), but the normal rat mast cell has 40–80 times greater affinity than that of the mouse normal mast cell. Receptors for IgE have also been found on certain human cultured lymphoblastoid cell lines (Gonzalez-Molina and Spiegelberg, 1976) and are specific for human IgE.

The sensitizing activity of IgE antibody is lost by heating to 56°C

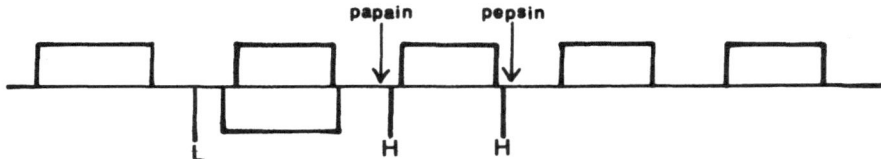

Figure 15.   Positions of cleavage of ϵ chain by pepsin and papain.

(Coca and Gorve, 1925; Loveless, 1940) and by reduction and alkylation (Ishizaka and Ishizaka, 1969; Stanworth *et al.*, 1970), although these treatments do not alter antigen-binding ability. Several studies have shown that the site responsible for skin fixation of IgE is located on the Fc fragment (Ishizaka *et al.*, 1970a; Stanworth *et al.*, 1968). The papain Fc' containing the C_H2 domain does not sensitize, suggesting that the site is on either the C_H3 or the C_H4 domain (or both).

The effect of heating IgE at 56°C has been studied by CD (Dorrington and Bennich, 1973). IgE myeloma proteins from two patients were studied as well as their $F(ab')_2$ and Fc fragments. Both proteins showed irreversible conformational changes on heating to 56°C for 30 min. Some reversible changes were also seen. In contrast to the thermal changes, denaturation by 6 M guanidinium chloride appears to be completely reversible. In addition, 6 M guanidinium chloride is able to reverse the "irreversible" thermal changes. When the fragments were studied, the $F(ab')_2$ (which includes the Fc' or amino-terminal C_H2 domain of the Fc) showed completely reversible thermal changes, while the Fc undergoes irreversible changes similar to those of the intact IgE. These changes are paralleled by irreversible losses of antigenic determinants in the C_H3 and C_H4 domains during heating. These findings support the contention that the heat lability of IgE sensitization results from conformational changes associated with the skin-fixing site in the C_H3 and C_H4 domains and indicate a requirement for three-dimensional integrity of the involved region rather than simply a linear sequence of amino acids. This is supported by studies on the effects of reduction and alkylation of the native molecule (Takatsu *et al.*, 1975). Reduction of IgE with 1 mM dithiothreitol (DTT) cleaves the inter-H-L disulfide bonds but does not affect the reverse PK reaction. Two additional disulfide bonds are lost by treatment with 2 mM DTT, also in the $F(ab')_2$ part of the molecule, and this diminishes affinity for target cells and subsequent PK activity. The Fc fragment from the reduced protein has a greater affinity than the reduced and alkylated protein, indicating that a conformational change in the Fc is associated with reduction in the $F(ab')_2$ and this is reversible after the Fc is cleaved from the molecule. Complete loss of affinity occurs when a fifth disulfide bond is reduced by 10 mM DTT (Takatsu *et al.*, 1975; Stanworth *et al.*, 1970). The fifth bond is most probably the COOH-terminal inter-H-H bond in the C_H2 domain (Bennich *et al.*, 1974), but the two ε chains remain joined by a single inter-H-H disulfide. Clearly, what is needed to further these studies is a method for the preparation of a fragment containing the C_H3 and C_H4 regions as well as a method for isolating each of these domains.

The lack of sufficient material has curtailed chemical studies on the

IgE-binding site. However, one report has appeared of a synthetic pentapeptide with the structure Asp-Ser-Asp-Pro-Arg which is able to inhibit PK tests up to approximately 90% (Hamburger, 1975). This remarkable peptide corresponds to the IgE (ND) sequence located at positions 320–324 in the C_H3 domain. Other peptides were also synthesized but were found to be moderately to minimally active. The addition of Ala to the NH_2-terminal Asp of the inhibitory pentapeptide causes a loss of 30–80% inhibition, and a homologous peptide, Asp-Thr-Glu-Ala-Arg, inhibits up to 80%. In all, five peptides were synthesized based on their uniqueness to the structure of the ϵ chain as compared to those of the γ, α, and μ chains. If these results are consistent, they would implicate a simple linear sequence as the binding site of IgE rather than a conformational site, contrary to the indications of the heating and reduction studies. In this event the thermal and reductive changes observed could be attributed to conformational burying of the binding site in the C_H3 domain.

It should be noted that the obvious approaches to the treatment of allergic diseases resulting from the availability of a peptide that inhibits IgE binding to cells illustrates the type of benefits obtainable from studies of functional sites on antibodies.

4. Placental Transfer

Although the human fetus is able to produce some immunoglobulins as early as 10 weeks, the primary source of immunoglobulins during uterine life is the mother's blood (Van Furth et al., 1965). Thus the first 5 months of postnatal life is marked by the decline of maternal immunoglobulins and the rapid increase of the child's own immunoglobulin levels (Alford, 1971). IgM concentration first reaches adult levels, followed by IgG and then IgA.

The protection afforded the fetus by the mother occurs by transfer of immunoglobulins from the maternal circulation to the fetal circulation across the placental barrier (the chorioallantoic placenta). This is not true of all species of mammals. In some the yolk sac appears to be the major route across which immunoglobulins are transferred (e.g., rabbit, guinea pig, and mouse). In others, such as goats, cows, and sheep, no immunoglobulins are transferred during intrauterine life but are obtained by the neonate from maternal colostrum by absorption across the gut. In some mammals (mouse, rat, dog) both pre- and postnatal transfer occurs (Schlamowitz, 1976).

While postnatal transfer across the gut may be nonselective, as in ungulates (Halliday, 1965), prenatal transfer via the placenta and yolk sac is always specific for the IgG class of antibody (Brambel, 1970). The mechanism of this transfer is unknown, but several theories have been proposed. These have been reviewed by Schlamowitz (1976). They all have in common the requirement of a specific receptor for the transfer of the IgG class of immunoglobulins. This has been found to be true in all species examined (Jones and Waldmann, 1972; Hemmings *et al.*, 1973; Gitlin and Gitlin, 1974; Leslie and Swate, 1972). In humans it has been shown that all four subclasses of IgG (Virella *et al.*, 1972) are transferred, although IgG1 and IgG3 may be somewhat preferred.

Evidence for the presence of specific cell-surface receptors for IgG in the human placenta has been reported (Matre *et al.*, 1975). Sections of human placenta have been shown to bind antibody-coated sheep erythrocytes (EA). While EA prepared with rabbit or guinea pig IgG also binds placental tissue, human IgA- and IgM-coated RBC do not. Inhibition of binding could be demonstrated by monomeric and heat-aggregated IgG equally well. IgD and IgE have not been investigated. Receptors for IgG have also been demonstrated in a similar fashion for mouse cultured yolk sac cells and placentas (Elson *et al.*, 1975). Vesicles prepared from rabbit yolk sac splanchnopleure have been shown to bind fluorescence-labeled rabbit IgG (Schlamowitz *et al.*, 1975). In contrast to mouse yolk sac, which bound heterologous IgG, rabbit yolk sac did not bind bovine labeled IgG. These studies, however, should be repeated with heterologous species other than ungulates which do not undergo prenatal transfer. The nature of the receptor is unknown, but it appears to be associated with the glycocalyx (Sonoda *et al.*, 1973). A recent report indicates that the receptor is sensitive to proteolytic enzymes and resistant to neuraminidase and glycosidases (Hellman *et al.*, 1977).

The specificity of the IgG receptor has been located on the Fc fragment (Gitlin *et al.*, 1964; Matre *et al.*, 1975; McNabb *et al.*, 1976). In a recent study (McNabb *et al.*, 1976) binding of ^{125}I-labeled human IgG to a cell-free suspension of human placental membranes was investigated. It was found that the amount of IgG bound was temperature and pH dependent, optimal conditions being at 37°C and pH 7.4. Binding activity was destroyed by heating the suspension of membrane homogenate to 60°C. IgG1 and IgG3 bound better than IgG2 and IgG4, with IgG2 being the weakest binder. Rabbit IgG was only slightly better than IgG2, and IgA and IgM did not bind at all. These studies also point out the importance of careful interpretation of results since nonspecific binding was a significant factor that had to be corrected for. Also, as pointed out in this report, macrophages, which also have Fc receptors, have been reported in human placentae (Moskalewski *et al.*, 1975). This must also be accounted for when using tissue slices. These workers have calculated 2×10^{15} receptors exist per placenta.

Although binding of the Fc fragment was found to be equal to that of the entire molecule (K_a = 4.6 ± 0.4 × 10^6 M^{-1}), none of its subfragments or the Fab exhibited any binding. Conflicting results were obtained by Matre *et al.* (1975), who found that pFc' fragments inhibited the binding of EA cells by placental tissue sections, although weakly. These results were interpreted as a requirement for the $C_\gamma 2$ region in addition to the $C_\gamma 3$ for full binding activity. In view of the nonspecific binding and macrophage binding reported by McNabb *et al.* (1976), the weak positive results are difficult to interpret. The Facb fragment did not inhibit binding, which indicates little or no activity in the $C_\gamma 2$ domain. Here again it would be interesting to test mixed Facb and pFc' fragments.

The fact that neither $C_\gamma 2$ nor $C_\gamma 3$ alone exhibits binding activity is similar to the results obtained with Ig binding to K cells (Section IIIB2). As discussed previously, it has been shown that neither the $C_\gamma 2$ nor the $C_\gamma 3$ domain exhibits any activity in inhibition of antibody-dependent cytotoxicity. Michaelsen *et al.* (1974) have suggested that this can be due to a requirement for the juxtaposition of the $C_\gamma 2$ domains, a structure maintained not by the noncovalent interactions between themselves but rather by interactions between the two $C_\gamma 3$ domains. Loss of the $C_\gamma 3$ domain would result in the formation of monomeric $C_\gamma 2$, which interacts very weakly. Alternatively, of course, it could simply mean that both domains share in the site. Further work is necessary to differentiate these two alternatives.

Reduction and alkylation of IgG1 to selectively cleave the interchain disulfide bonds completely destroy the ability of the molecule to bind the placental receptor (McNabb *et al.*, 1976). Interestingly, the same treatment of the Fc has almost no effect. This suggests that the native protein devoid of its interchain disulfides is less rigid, allowing the Fab to interfere with the binding site, as has been discussed with regard to complement binding (Section IIIA1). It may be of interest to test isolated Fc fragments from nonbinding IgG2 molecules for binding. An alternative explanation is that the site on the Fc is somewhat different than that on intact IgG. It should be noted that while β_2-microglobulin exhibits complement-binding activity it does not bind placental receptor.

Some preliminary studies have been reported (Schlamowitz, 1976) on the chemical characteristics of the placental receptor. It appears to be protein in nature with little carbohydrate and resists solubilization by several detergents. Further work is needed here.

5. Catabolism of Immunoglobulins

The serum level of antibody is a result of several processes including synthesis, redistribution, and catabolism. Each of these processes is in turn dependent on several factors, most of which are incompletely understood. However, it has become clear by metabolic turnover studies that immunoglobulins are heterogeneous with respect to their lifetimes.

Catabolic rates of immunoglobulins are studied by several methods which usually involve the isolation of a class, or subclass, followed by labeling of the isolated antibodies by radioactive labels and reintroduction of the tracer into the animal. The disappearance qf circulating label is then followed as a function of time. These methods have been reviewed by Waldmann and Strober (1969). The results obtained have shown that the disappearance of labeled immunoglobulin follows a biphasic course (Fig. 16). The first phase is a rapid exponential loss due to equilibration and loss of the label from the intravascular pool. The second phase is a more gradual linear decline which represents the catabolic degradation of the molecule. The half-life ($t_{1/2}$) of immunoglobulins is calculated from the second phase. A more meaningful figure is the fraction of the serum pool catabolized and cleared per day, referred to as the "fractional turnover" rate (FTR). Some figures for immunoglobulins are shown in Table I, along with their respective synthetic rates (Wells, 1976).

Although IgG as a class has the longest survival and lowest catabolic rate of any of the serum proteins, it can be seen that the subclasses do

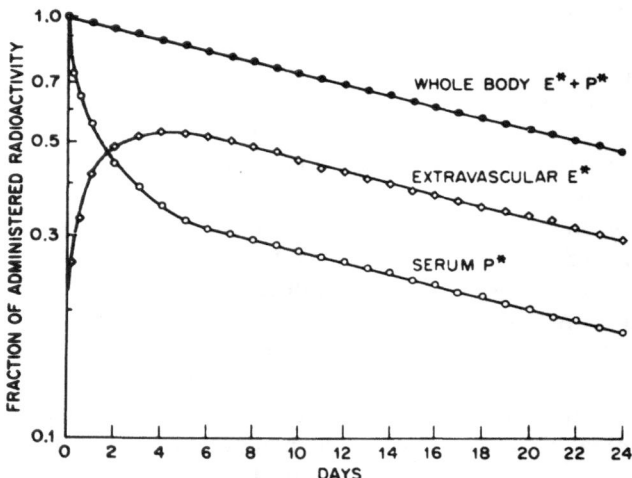

Figure 16.   Semilogarithmic plot of the time course of decline of radioactivity from the whole body, serum, and extravascular pools following intravenous administration of [^{125}I]-IgG. The radioactivity retained in the body (E* + P*) was determined by cumulative subtraction of the radioactivity excreted in the urine from the injected activity. The curve of activity in the extravascular pool (E*) was determined by subtracting the activity in the plasma pool (P*) from that retained in the whole body (E* + P*). Reproduced with permission from Waldmann and Strober (1969); copyright 1969, S. Karger, AG, Basel.

Table V. Site of Effector Functions of Human Immunoglobulins

	C_H2		C_H3		C_H4	
	Facb	C_H2^a	Fc'	C_H3^a	Tryptic 37°C	Tryptic 60°C
Complement fixation (IgG)	+	+	−	−		
Complement fixation (IgM)					+	
Staphylococcal protein A binding			−			
Macrophage binding			−	+		
Monocyte binding			+			
Passive cutaneous anaphylaxis			+			
Placental transfer	−		−			
Catabolic rate		+	−			
IgM binding to T cells						+

^{a} Acid-trypsin digestion.

not have equivalent half-lives, IgG3 being considerably shorter lived (Spiegelberg and Weigle, 1965; Morell *et al.*, 1970). IgM and IgA have similar (from 4 to 6 days) half-lives, and both polymeric and monomeric forms have similar properties (Spiegelberg, 1974). IgD and IgE have the shortest half-lives.

The serum level of IgG regulates its own rate of catabolism (Fahey *et al.*, 1965; Lippincott *et al.*, 1960; Solomon *et al.*, 1963). At high serum levels, the $t_{1/2}$ may fall to a lower limit of approximately 11 days (FTR increases to 185). In the event of low levels of IgG, the survival time may double or triple. This concentration-catabolic effect of IgG is not affected by the concentration of the other immunoglobulins. Furthermore, in contrast to IgG, the half-lives of IgA and IgM are independent of their serum levels (Barth *et al.*, 1964; Strober *et al.*, 1968), while IgE and possibly IgD appear to have the reverse effect, i.e., higher serum levels promote longer survival times (Wells, 1976).

Studies show that the catabolism of IgG depends on the presence of the Fc part of the molecule (Fahey and Robinson, 1963). While the papain Fab and pepsin $F(ab')_2$ are rapidly eliminated from the circulation, the Fc fragment is cleared in a manner similar to that of intact IgG (Spiegelberg and Weigle, 1965). It has also been shown that infusion of Fc fragment accelerates the catabolism of IgG, while infusion of Fab has no effect. Mild reduction and alkylation of the IgG (interchain bonds) lowers the $t_{1/2}$ very little, if at all, and the isolated H chain is similar in half-life to the reduced and alkylated molecule (Cohen and Mannik, 1966; Spiegelberg and Weigle, 1966). The L chains or Bence Jones proteins, in contrast, are rapidly catabolized at a rate approximately 100 times that of the intact molecule (Wochner *et al.*, 1967) and have little effect on the survival of intact IgG. Neuraminidase treatment of IgG also has little effect on its catabolic rate. These studies indicate that the Fc fragment contains a structure or site which determines its survival in the circulation and serves to regulate its own levels. This has therapeutic significance since attempts to use passively administered γ-globulin by preparing F(ab′)₂ fragments (in order to prevent harmful side effects due to aggregates of IgG) must consider the shortened half-life of the F(ab)₂′ compared with IgG. Apparently, milder pepsin treatment reduces the tendency to aggregate IgG without significantly altering the survival (Koblet *et al.*, 1967).

The mechanism and site of catabolism of immunoglobulins are unknown. No single organ has been identified as the major site of immunoglobulin catabolism. The liver, kidney, and gastrointestinal tract all appear to be implicated, but considerable controversy exists (Anderson *et al.*, 1963; Solomon *et al.*, 1964; Cohen *et al.*, 1962). In the case of Bence-Jones or light chains, it is clear that the kidney is the major catabolic organ (Wochner *et al.*, 1967). A recent report (Arend and Silverblatt, 1975) on the metabolic clearance of Fab and Fc fragments in rats shows that the kidney is a major route of clearance and catabolism of both fragments in the early phases of disappearance. Shortly afterward, however, the Fc becomes equilibrated with an unidentified pool and does not undergo glomerular filtration or catabolism in the proximal tubule.

Little is known about the mechanism by which the Fc regulates the survival of the intact molecule. The data suggest the presence of cell receptors which protect the whole molecule or Fc fragment from catabolic degradation. Such receptors could be similar to those postulated for placental transfer, although this anatomical location and cellular nature have not been determined. Current data would suggest a wide dispersal of these putative receptors since no single organ has been shown to be the site of catabolism of the majority of immunoglobulin molecules.

Very little has been done to characterize chemically the catabolic site on the Fc fragment. Some information is available concerning the fate of pFc′ fragments and plasmin subfragments of IgG (Yasmeen *et al.*, 1976). The $C_\gamma 2$ domain has been shown to have a catabolic rate similar to that of IgG and Fc in rabbits, although the initial rapid phase of elimination is much greater. Approximately 80% of the $C_\gamma 2$ fragments are rapidly eliminated while the remaining 20% undergo the more gradual linear catabolism of the second phase from which $t_{1/2}$ is determined. No differences were detected between two pools of $C_\gamma 2$ fragments. Sialic acid had little influence on the catabolic rate, which is of interest in view of the role of sialic acid in controlling catabolism of many serum glyco-proteins. In contrast to the gradual degradation of the $C_\gamma 2$ domain, ex-periments with pFc' ($C_\gamma 3$) and Fab showed that these fragments have little similarity to the intact molecule since both were rapidly eliminated. It was also found that β_2-microglobulin is rapidly catabolized. These studies would tend to localize the catabolic site to the $C_\gamma 2$ region.

6. Other Cells

Platelets from all mammals studied bind antigen-antibody complexes and aggregated immunoglobulins, with the subsequent release of vaso-active amines (Mueller-Eckhardt and Lüscher, 1968a,b). Only the IgG class reacts with these cells, including all four subclasses (Pfueller and Lüscher, 1972; Henson and Spiegelberg, 1973). It has been shown that the site of interaction is on the Fc fragment and that binding of comple-ment by the Fc apparently prevents this interaction. Reduction of the IgG with 0.02 M DTT and subsequent alkylation result in some loss of activity which varies with the subclass, IgG4 being most affected.

Binding of nonantibody IgG to red blood cells has been observed with both D-positive and D-negative cells (Boursnell et al., 1953). The binding is not, however, specific for the Fc part of the molecule, as both Fab and Fc bind equally (Grob et al., 1967). Albumin competes for this binding, indicating that there is little specificity involved. IgM has also been found to bind to these surfaces (Frommel et al., 1967). The binding appears to be preferential for denatured or aggregated immunoglobulins, but nonaggregated immunoglobulin will also bind, the extent being de-pendent on the immunoglobulin concentration. It is interesting that these nonspecifically bound immunoglobulins are not available for reaction with anti-Fc antisera. The nature and physiological significance of this binding are unknown. However, it has been reported that the bound IgG may play a role in the survival and functioning of the red blood cell (Fidalgo et al., 1967a,b). The characteristic biconcave shape of erythro-cytes is lost on removal of these bound immunoglobulins at high ionic strength (Lahiri et al., 1970).

IV. Conclusions

Immunology has progressed to a new era. Immunochemists and immunobiologists initially took separate paths and have now returned, with the focal point being the cell. While the immunochemists were laying the structural framework of immunology, the immunobiologists were concerned with the mechanisms of regulation of the immune response from the whole organism to the single cell. Now both disciplines are interdependent and seek the molecular mechanisms for cellular phenomena. This chapter is an effort to review the progress made in one aspect of this: how the antibody molecule carries out its functions.

Certain biological properties can be localized to a given Fc domain, and in some cases to a limited subregion of that domain, e.g., complement fixation, catabolic rate, and reagin binding. Others have not been localized to a single domain, e.g., placental transfer and heterocytotropic antibody binding, and there are others which appear to be a function of different domains depending on the experimental systems used, i.e., antibody cytophilic for phagocytic and lymphoid cells. In general, the findings support the domain theory (Edelman, 1970), which states that each of these regions evolved for specific functions. The clearest evidence is the complement fixation studies that localized the site in the $C_\gamma2$ region of IgG and the $C_\mu4$ region of IgM. The domain theory suggests that the $C_\gamma2$ region may have evolved from the $C_\mu4$ region on the basis of this common function, although the regions do not appear exceptionally homologous in sequence (Low et al., 1976). The maximum homology is between the $C_\mu4$ and $C_\alpha3$ domains (approximately 50%) and is least between the $C_\mu3$ and $C_\alpha2$ domains (approximately 19%). Overall, therefore, homology appears to have little predictive value regarding function. This is supported by findings suggesting that effector functions are often associated with a short stretch of amino acid sequence.

It appears that the presently available data on placental transfer and heterocytotropic antibody binding argue against domain theory in its strictest interpretation; e.g. a given function localized to one domain. However, it should be stressed that processes other than simple binding are being measured in these assays and both domains may be required for separate stages of the event. Alternatively, the site may be localized to a single domain, but stabilization of this domain may be required by another domain. This cooperation between domains may be necessary for certain effector functions. Table V summarizes the data on localization of the effector functions discussed in this chapter.

Modification of protein side chains has not been extensively employed in studies of functional sites, and, where it has been used, little has been done to characterize the nature of the products by either chemical or physical methods. This approach, used in its fullest capacity to delineate the complete antigenic structures of sperm whale myoglobin (Atassi, 1975) and lysozyme (Atassi et al., 1976a,b; Lee and Atassi, 1977a,b; Atassi and Lee, 1978a,b; Atassi, 1978), could be of great value in localizing more precisely the functional sites on antibodies. While fragmentation has provided significant information, it is limited in its usefulness, and selective modification of amino acids could extend these findings considerably. Ultimately, the goal will be to sequence and synthesize the active site of the various effector functions.

ACKNOWLEDGMENTS

The authors with to thank their colleagues Drs. W. Anderson, R. Keller, J. Velosa, D. McKean, and Z. Atassi, who read the manuscript and made helpful suggestions. We also wish to acknowledge the considerable secretarial skills of Ms. P. Mahone, T. Lee, and J. Jones.

V. References

Abney, E. R., and Parkhouse, R. M. E., 1974, *Nature (London)* **252**:600.
Abney, E. R., Hunter, I. R., and Parkhouse, R. M. E., 1976, *Nature (London)* **259**:404.
Abo, T., Yamaguchi, T., Shimizu, F., and Kumagai, K., 1976, *J. Immunol.* **117**:1781.
Adlersberg, J. B., Franklin, E. C., and Frangione, B., 1975, *Proc. Natl. Acad Sci. USA* **72**:723.
Alexander, M. D., Leslie, R. G. Q., and Cohen, S., 1976, *Eur. J. Immunol.* **6**:101.
Alford, C. A., 1971, *Pediatr. Clin. N. Am.* **18**:99.
Allan, R., and Isliker, H., 1974a, *Immunochemistry* **11**:175.
Allan, R., and Isliker, H., 1974b, *Immunochemistry* **11**:243.
Amiraian, K., and Leikhim, E. J., 1961, *Proc. Soc. Exp. Biol. Med.* **108**:454.
Amkraut, A., Malley, A., and Begley, D., 1973, *Int. Arch. Allergy* **44**:369.
Amzel, L. M., Poljak, R. J., Saul, F., Varga, J. M., and Richards, F. F., 1974, *Proc. Natl. Acad. Sci. USA* **71**:1427.
Anderson, C. L., Kubo, R. T., and Grey, H. M., 1975, *J. Immunol.* **114**:997.
Anderson, S. B., Glenert, J., and Wallevik, K., 1963, *J. Clin. Invest.* **42**:1873.
Arend, W. P. and Mannik, M., 1973, *J. Immunol.* **110**:1455.
Arend, W. P., and Silverblatt, F. J., 1975, *Clin. Exp. Immunol.* **22**:502.
Arroyave, C. M., Vallota, E. H., and Müller-Eberhard, H. J., 1974, *J. Immunol.* **113**:764.
Ashman, R. F., and Metzger, H., 1971, *Immunochemistry* **8**:643.
Ashman, R. F., Kaplan, A. P., and Metzger, H., 1971, *Immunochemistry* **8**:627.
Askenase, P. W., and Hayden, B. J., 1974, *Immunology* **27**:563.
Atassi, M. Z., 1975, *Immunochemistry* **12**:423.
Atassi, M. Z., 1978, in: *Immunobiology of Proteins and Peptides* (M. Z. Atassi and A. B. Stavitsky, Eds.), Vol. 1, pp. 41–100, Plenum, New York.
Atassi, M. Z., and Lee, C.-L., 1978a, *Biochem. J.* **171**:419.
Atassi, M. Z., and Lee, C.-L., 1978b, *Biochem. J.* **171**:429.
Atassi, M. Z., Koketsu, J., and Habeeb, A. F. S. A., 1976a, *Biochim. Biophys. Acta* **420**:358.
Atassi, M. Z., Lee, C.-L., and Pai, R.-C., 1976b, *Biochim. Biophys. Acta* **427**:745.
Augener, W., and Grey, H. M., 1970, *J. Immunol.* **105**:1024.

Augener, W., Grey, H. M., Cooper, N. R., and Müller-Eberhard, H. J., 1971, *Immunochemistry* **8**:1011.

Austen, K. F., and Brocklehurst, W. E., 1961, *J. Exp. Med.* **113**:521.

Bach, M. K., Bloch, K. J., and Austen, K. F., 1971, *J. Exp. Med.* **133**:772.

Barth, W. F., Wochner, R. D., Waldmann, T. A., and Fahey, J. L., 1964, *J. Clin. Invest.* **43**:1036.

Basten, A., Miller, J. F. A. P., Sprent, J., and Pye, J., 1972, *J. Exp. Med.* **135**:610.

Baur, S., Schenkein, I., and Uhr, J. W., 1972, *J. Immunol.* **108**:748.

Beale, D., and Feinstein, A., 1969, *Biochem. J.* **112**:187.

Bennich, H., and Johansson, S. G. O., 1971, *Adv. Immunol.* **13**:1.

Bennich, H., and Turner, M. W., 1969, *Biochim. Biophys. Acta* **175**:388.

Bennich, H., and von Bahr-Lindstrom, H., 1974, *Progr. Immunol.* **1**:49.

Bennich, H., Ishizaka, K., Johansson, S. G. O., Rowe, D. S., Stanworth, D. R., and Terry, W. D., 1968, *Immunology* **15**:323.

Berken, A., and Benacerraf, B., 1966, *J. Exp. Med.* **123**:119.

Bernier, G. M., Tominaga, K., Easley, C. W., and Putnam, F. W., 1965, *Biochemistry* **4**:2072.

Biewenga, J., and Feltkamp, T. E. W., 1975, *Clin. Chim. Acta* **58**:239.

Biewenga, J., and Thijs, L. G., 1970, *Clin. Chim. Acta* **27**:293.

Bigelow, C. C., Smith, B. R., and Dorrington, K. J., 1974, *Biochemistry* **13**:4602.

Bing, D. H., 1971, *J. Immunol.* **107**:1243.

Binz, H., and Wigzell, H., 1975, *J. Exp. Med.* **142**:197.

Bjork, I., and Lindh, E., 1974, *Eur. J. Biochem.* **45**:135.

Bjork, I., and Tanford, C., 1971*a*, *Biochemistry* **10**:1280.

Bjork, I., and Tanford, C., 1971*b*, *Biochemistry* **10**:1289.

Bjork, I., Karlsson, F. A., and Berggard, I., 1971, *Proc. Natl. Acad. Sci. USA* **68**:1707.

Bjork, I., Petersson, B.-A, and Sjoquist, J., 1972, *Eur. J. Biochem.* **29**:579.

Boackle, R. J., Pruitt, K. M., and Mestecky, J., 1974, *Immunochemistry* **11**:543.

Borsos, T., and Rapp, H. J., 1963, *J. Immunol.* **91**:851.

Borsos, T., and Rapp, H. J., 1965, *Science* **150**:505.

Boursnell, J. C., Coombs, R. R. A., and Rigk, V., 1953, *Biochem. J.* **55**:745.

Boyden, S. V., and Sarkin, E., 1960, *Immunology* **3**:272.

Brambel, F. W. R., 1970, *Frontiers of Biology*, Vol. 18, North-Holland, Amsterdam.

Brandtzaeg, P., 1973, *Scand. J. Immunol.* **2**:441.

Brandtzaeg, P., 1976, *Scand. J. Immunol.* **5**:411.

Brown, J. C., and Koshland, M. E., 1975, *Proc. Natl. Acad. Sci. USA* **72**:5111.

Burnet, F. M., 1959, *The Clonal Selection Theory of Acquired Immunity*, Vanderbilt University Press, Nashville, Tenn.

Burritt, M. F., Calvanico, N. J., Mehta, S., and Tomasi, T. B., 1977, *J. Immunol.* **118**:723.

Calvanico, N. J., and Tomasi, T. B., 1971, *Arch. Biochem. Biophys.* **144**:269.

Calvanico, N. J., and Tomasi, T. B., 1976, *Immunochemistry* **13**:203.

Capaldi, R. A., and Vanderkooi, G., 1972, *Proc. Natl. Acad. Sci. USA* **69**:930.

Capra, J. D., and Kindt, T. J., 1975, *Immunogenetics* **1**:417.

Cathou, R. E., and Dorrington, K. J., 1975, in: *Biologic Macromolecule Series*, Vol. 7: *Subunits in Biological Systems*, Part C (S.N. Timasheff and G. D. Fasman, eds.), p. 91, Dekker, New York.

Cathou, R. E., and Haber, E., 1967, *Biochemistry* **6**:513.

Cathou, R. E., and O'Konski, C. T., 1970, *J. Mol. Biol.* **48**:125.

Cathou, R. E., Kulczycki, A., and Haber, E., 1968, *Biochemistry* **7**:3958.

Chavin, S. I., and Holliman, A., 1975, *Biochem. J.* **152**:267.

Chen, J. P., Reichlin, M., and Tomasi, T. B., 1969, *Biochemistry* **8:**2246.

Chesebro, B., Bloth, B., and Svehag, S. E., 1968, *J. Exp. Med.* **127:**399.

Choi, Y. S., 1976, *Biochemistry* **15:**1037.

Ciccimarra, F., Rosen, F. S., and Merler, E., 1975, *Proc. Natl. Acad. Sci. USA* **72:**2081.

Cioli, D., and Baglioni, C., 1968, *J. Exp. Med.* **128:**517.

Coca, A. F., and Grove, E. F., 1925, *J. Immunol.* **10:**445.

Cochrane, C. G., 1967, *Arthritis Rheum.* **10:**392.

Cohen, G. L., and Mannik, M., 1966, *J. Immunol.* **96:**683.

Cohen, S., 1968, *J. Immunol.* **100:**407.

Cohen, S., and Becker, E. L., 1968*a*, *J. Immunol.* **100:**403.

Cohen, S., and Becker, E. L., 1968*b*, *J. Immunol.* **100:**395.

Cohen, S., Gordon. A. H., and Matthews, C., 1962, *Biochem. J.* **82:**197.

Cohen, S., Feinman, L., and Becker, E, 1969, *J. Immunol.* **103:**387.

Colman, P. M., Fehlhammer, H., Epp, O., Bode, H., Schiffer, M., Lattman, E. E., Jones, T. A., and Palm, W., 1974, *FEBS Lett.* **44:**194.

Colman, P. M., Deisenhofer, J., Huber, R., and Palm, W., 1976, *J. Mol. Biol.* **100:**257.

Colomb, M., and Porter, R. R., 1975, *Biochem. J.* **145:**177.

Cone, R. E., and Brown, W. C. 1976, *Immunochemistry* **13:**571.

Connell, G. E., and Painter, R. H., 1966, *Can. J. Biochem.* **44:**371.

Connell, G. E., and Porter, R. R., 1971, *Biochem. J.* **123:**33P.

Conrad, D. H., and Froese, A., 1976, *J. Immunol.* **116:**319.

Conradie, J. D., and Bubb, M. O., 1977, *Nature (London)* **265:**5590.

Constantopoulos, A., Najjar, V. A., Wish, J. B., Necheles, T. H., and Stolbach, L. L., 1973, *Am. J. Dis. Child.* **125:**663.

Cunniff, R. V., and Stollar, B. D., 1968, *J. Immunol.* **100:**7.

Cunniff, R. V. H., Cole, H. H., and Stollar, B. D., 1968, *J. Immunol* **101:**695.

Cunningham, B. A., and Berggard, I., 1974, *Transplant. Rev.* **21:**3.

Dammacco, F., Franklin, E. C., and Frangione, B., 1972, *J. Immunol.* **109:**565.

Danes, B. S., Litwin, S. D., Hutteroth, T. H., Cleve, H., and Bearn, A. G., 1973, *J. Exp. Med.* **137:**1538.

Davies, D. R., Sarma, R. V., Labaw, L. W., Silverton, E., Segal, D., and Terry, W. D., 1971, *Ann. N.Y. Acad. Sci.* **190:**122.

Davies, D. R., Padlan, E. A., and Segal, D. M., 1975, *Annu. Rev. Biochem.* **44:**639.

Deisenhofer, J., Colman, P. M., Huber, R., Haupt, H., and Schivick, G., 1976*a*, *Hoppe-Seyler's Z. Physiol. Chem.* **357:**435.

Deisenhofer, J., Colman, P. M., Epp, O., and Huber, R., 1976*b*, *Hoppe-Seyler's Z. Physiol. Chem.* **357:**1421.

Della Corte, E., and Parkhouse, R. M. E., 1973, *Biochem. J.* **136:**597.

Deutsch, H. F., Stiehm, E. R., and Morton, J. I., 1961, *J. Biol. Chem.* **236:**2216.

Dickler, H. B., 1974, *J. Exp. Med.* **140:**508.

Dickler, H. B., 1976, *Adv. Immunol.* **24:**167.

Dickler, H. B., and Kunkel, H. G., 1972, *J. Exp. Med.* **136:**191.

Dickler, H. B., and Sachs, D. H., 1974, *J. Exp. Med.* **140:**779.

Dorrington, K. J., 1976, *Immunol. Commun.* **5:**263.

Dorrington, K. J., and Bennich, H., 1973, *J. Biol. Chem.* **248:**8378.

Dorrington, K. J., and Kortan, C., 1974, *Biochem. Biophys. Res. Commun.* **56:**529.

Dorrington, K. J., and Smith, B. R., 1972, *Biochim. Biophys. Acta* **263:**70.

Dorrington, K. J., and Tanford C., 1968, *J. Biol. Chem.* **243:**4745.

Dorrington, K. J., Bennich, H., and Turner, M. W., 1972, *Biochem. Biophys. Res. Commun.* **47:**512.

Dossett, J. H., Kronvall, G., Williams, R. C., and Quie, P. G., 1969, *J. Immunol.* **103**:1405.
Dourmashkin, R. R., Virella, G., and Parkhouse, R. M. E., 1971, *J. Mol. Biol.* **56**:207.
Dreyer, W. J., and Bennett, J. C., 1965, *Proc. Natl. Acad. Sci. USA* **54**:864.
Edelman, G. M., 1970, *Biochemistry* **9**:3197.
Edelman, G. M., and Gally, J. A., 1964, *Proc. Natl. Acad. Sci. USA* **51**:846.
Edelman, G. M., Cunningham, B. A., Gall, W. E., Gottlieb, P. D., Rutishauser, U., and
  Waxdal, M. J., 1969, *Proc. Natl. Acad. Sci. USA* **63**:78.
Edmundson, A. B., Schiffer, M., Wood, M. K., Hardman, K. D., Ely, K. R., and Ain-
  sworth, C. F., 1971, *Cold Spring Harbor Symp. Quant. Biol.* **36**:427.
Edmundson, A. B., Schiffer, M., Ely, K. R., and Wood, M. K., 1972, *Biochemistry*
  11:1822.
Edmundson, A. B., Ely, K. R., Girling, R. L., Abola, E. E., Schiffer, M., Westholm, F.
  A., Fausch, M. D., and Deutsch, H. F., 1974, *Biochemistry* **13**:3816.
Eichmann, K., and Rajewsky, K., 1975, *Eur. J. Immunol.* **5**:661.
Ellerson, J. R., Yasmeen, D., Painter, R. H., and Dorrington, K. J., 1972, *FEBS Lett.*
  24:318.
Ellerson, J. R., Yasmeen, D., Painter, R. H., and Dorrington, K. J., 1976, *J. Immunol.*
  116:510.
Elson, J., Jenkinson, E. J., and Billington, W. D., 1975, *Nature (London)* **255**:412.
Engelman, D. M., and Morowitz, H. J., 1968, *Biochim. Biophys. Acta* **150**:385.
Epp, O., Palm, W., Fehlhammer, H., Ruhlman, A., Ztergemann, W., Schwager, P., and
  Huber, R., 1972, *J. Mol. Biol.* **69**:315.
Epp, O., Colman, P., Fehlhammer, H., Bode, H., Schiffer, M., Huber, R., and Palm, W.,
  1974, *Eur. J. Biochem.* **45**:513.
Epp, O., Lattman, E. E., Schiffer, M., Huber, R., and Palm, W., 1975, *Biochemistry*
  14:4943.
Eskeland, T., and Brandtzaeg, P., 1974, *Immunochemistry* **11**:161.
Fahey, J. L., 1963, *J. Immunol.* **90**:576.
Fahey, J. L., and Robinson, A. G., 1963, *J. Exp. Med.* **118**:845.
Fahey, J. L., Barth, W. F., and Law, L. W., 1965, *J. Natl. Cancer Inst.* **35**:663.
Fauci, A. S., Frank, M. M., and Johnson, J. S., 1970, *J. Immunol.* **105**:215.
Feinstein, A., and Munn, E. A., 1969, *Nature (London)* **224**:1307.
Feinstein, A., Munn, E. A., and Richardson, N. E., 1971, *Ann. N.Y. Acad. Sci.* **190**:104.
Ferrarini, M., Moretta, L., Mingari, M. C., Tonda, P., and Pernis, B., 1976, *Eur. J.
  Immunol.* **6**:520.
Fidalgo, B. V., Najjar, V. A., Zukoski, C. F., and Katayama, Y., 1967a, *Proc. Natl. Acad.
  Sci. USA* **57**:665.
Fidalgo, B. V., Katayama, Y., and Najjar, V. A., 1967b, *Biochemistry* **6**:3378.
Finkelman, F. D., van Boxel, J. A., Asofsky, R., and Paul, W. E., 1976, *J. Immunol.*
  116:1173.
Forsgren, A., 1969, *Acta Pathol. Microbiol. Scand.* **75**:481.
Forsgren, A., 1970, *Infect. Immun.* **2**:672.
Forsgren, A., and Sjoquist, J., 1966, *J. Immunol.* **97**:822.
Forsgren, A., and Sjoquist, J., 1969, *Acta Pathol. Microbiol. Scand.* **75**:466.
Forsgren, A., Nordström, K., Phillipson, L., and Sjoquist, J., 1971, *J. Bacteriol.* **107**:245.
Frangione, B., and Franklin, E. C., 1972, *FEBS Lett.* **20**:321.
Frangione, B., and Wolfenstein-Todel, C., 1972, *Proc. Natl. Acad. Sci. USA* **69**:3673.
Frangione, B., Prelli, F., and Franklin, E. C., 1967, *Immunochemistry* **4**:95.
Frank, M. M., Gaither, T., Adkinson, F., Terry, W. D., and May, J. E., 1976, *J. Immunol.*
  116:1733.

Franklin, E. C., 1960, *J. Clin. Invest.* **39**:1933.
Franklin, E. C., and Frangione, B., 1968, *Biochemistry* **7**:4203.
Fraser, K. J., Poulsen, K., and Haber, E., 1972, *Biochemistry* **11**:4974.
Fridman, W. H., and Golstein, P., 1974, *Cell. Immunol.* **11**:442.
Friedhandler, L., Berk, J. E., and Wong, D., 1974, *Clin. Chem.* **20**:22.
Froese, A., 1976, *Immunol. Commun.* **5**:437.
Froland, S. S., Natvig, J. B., and Michaelsen, T. E., 1974, *Scand. J. Immunol.* **3**:375.
Frommel, D., and Hong, R., 1970, *Biochim. Biophys. Acta* **200**:113.
Frommel, D., Grob, P. J., Masouredis, S. P., and Isliker, H. C., 1967, *Immunology* **13**:501.
Frommhagen, L. H., and Fudenberg, H. H., 1962, *J. Immunol.* **89**:336.
Fu, S. M., and Kunkel, H. G., 1974, *J. Exp. Med.* **140**:895.
Fu, S. M., Winchester, R. J., and Kunkel, H. G., 1975, *J. Immunol.* **114**:250.
Füst, G., Csecsi-Nagy, M., Medgyesi, G. A., Kulics, J., and Gergely, J., 1976, *Immunochemistry* **13**:793.
Gall, W. E., and D'Eustachio, P., 1972, *Biochemistry* **11**:4621.
Gally, J. A., 1973, in: *The Antigens*, Vol. I, p. 161.
Gally, J. A., and Edelman, G. M., 1972, *Annu. Rev. Genet.* **6**:1.
Genco, R. J., Plaut, A. G., and Moellering, R. C., 1975, *J. Infect. Dis.* **131**:517.
Gergely, J., Fudenberg, H. H., and Van Loghem, E., 1970, *Immunochemistry* **7**:1.
Ghetie, V., Moraru, I., Sulica, A., Gherman, M., and Sjoquist, J., 1976, *Rev. Roum. Biochem.* **13**:263.
Ghose, A. C., 1971, *Biochem. Biophys. Res. Commun.* **45**:1144.
Ghose, A. C., and Jirgensons, B., 1971, *Biochim. Biophys. Acta* **251**:14.
Gitlin, J. D., and Gitlin, D., 1974, *J. Clin. Invest.* **54**:1155.
Gitlin, D., Kumate, J., Urrusti, J., and Morales, C., 1964, *J. Clin. Invest.* **43**:1938.
Glueck, H. I., and Hong, R. J., 1965, *Clin. Invest.* **44**:1866.
Goding, J. W., Warr, G. W., and Warner, N. L., 1976, *Proc. Natl. Acad. Sci. USA* **73**:1305.
Gonzalez-Molina, A., and Spiegelberg, H. L., 1976, *J. Immunol.* **117**:1838.
Goodman, J. W., 1963, *Science* **139**:1292.
Götze, O., and Müller-Eberhard, H. J., 1971, *J. Exp. Med.* **134**:90s.
Gray, W. R., Dreyer, W. J., and Hood, L., 1967, *Science* **155**:465.
Green, N. M., 1969, *Adv. Immunol.* **11**:1.
Grey, H. M., and Abel, C. A., 1967, *Immunochemistry* **4**:315.
Grey, H. M., Sher, A., and Shalitin, N., 1970, *J. Immunol.* **105**:75.
Grey, H. M., Kubo, R. T., and Cerottini, J. C., 1972, *J. Exp. Med.* **136**:1323.
Grey, H. M., Kubo, R. T., Colon, S. M., Poulik, M. D., Cresswell, P., Springer, T., Turner, M., and Strominger, J. L., 1973, *J. Exp. Med.* **138**:1608.
Griffin, D., Tachibana, D. K., Nelson, B., and Rosenberg, L. T., 1967, *Immunochemistry* **4**:23.
Griffiths, R. W., and Gleich, G. J., 1972, *J. Biol. Chem.* **247**:4543.
Grob, P. J., Frommel, D., Isliker, H. C., and Masouredis, S. P., 1967, *Immunology* **13**:489.
Grossberg, A. L., Markus, G., and Pressman, D., 1965, *Proc. Natl. Acad. Sci. USA* **54**:942.
Grossman, J., Abraham, G. N., Leddy, J. P., and Condemi, J. L., 1972, *Ann. Intern. Med.* **77**:395.
Grov, A., 1967, *Acta Pathol. Microbiol. Scand.* **69**:567.
Grov, A., 1975, *Acta Pathol. Microbiol. Scand.* **83**:173.
Grov, A., Myklestad, B., and Oeding, P., 1964, *Acta Pathol. Microbiol. Scand.* **61**:588.
Grubb, R., 1956, *Acta Pathol. Microbiol. Scand.* **39**:195.
Guidotti, G., 1972, *Annu. Rev. Biochem.* **41**:731.
Gustafson, G. T., Sjoquist, J., and Stalenheim, G., 1967, *J. Immunol.* **98**:1178.

Gustafson, G. T., Stalenheim, G., Forsgren, A., and Sjoquist, J., 1968, *J. Immunol.* **100**:530.

Haber, E., and Stone, M., 1967, *Biochemistry* **6**:1974.

Halliday, R., 1965, *J. Immunol.* **95**:510.

Halloran, P., Schirrmacher, V., and David, C. S., 1975, *Immunogenetics* **2**:349.

Halpern, M. S., and Koshland, M. E., 1970, *Nature (London)* **228**:1276.

Halpern, M. S., and Koshland, M. E., 1973, *J. Immunol.* **111**:1653.

Hamburger, R., 1975, *Science* **189**:389.

Hammerling, U., Mack, C., and Pickel, H. G., 1976a, *Immunochemistry* **13**:525.

Hammerling, U., Pickel, H. G., Mack, C., and Masters, D., 1976b, *Immunochemistry* **13**:533.

Hanly, W. C., Lichter, E. A., Dray, S., and Knight, K. L., 1973, *Biochemistry* **12**:733.

Hansen, H. R., van Kley, H., and Knight, W. A., 1972, *Am. J. Med.* **52**:712.

Harboe, M., and Folling, I., 1974, *Scand. J. Immunol.* **3**:471.

Haustein, D., and Goding, J. W., 1975, *Biochem. Biophys. Res. Commun.* **65**:483.

Haustein, D., Marchalonis, J. J., and Harris, A. W., 1975, *Biochemistry* **14**:1826.

Heimer, R., and Schnoll, S. H., 1968, *J. Immunol.* **100**:231.

Heimer, R., Schnoll, S. H., and Primock, A., 1967, *Biochemistry* **6**:127.

Hemmings, W. A., Jones, R. E., and Williams, E. W., 1973, *Immunology* **25**:645.

Henney, C. S., and Ishizaka, K., 1968, *J. Immunol.* **100**:718.

Henney, C. S., and Stanworth, D. R., 1966, *Nature (London)* **210**:1071.

Henney, C. S., Stanworth, D. R., and Gill, P. G. H., 1965, *Nature (London)* **205**:1079.

Henney, C. S., Welscher, H. D., Terry, W. D., and Rowe, D. S., 1969, *Immunochemistry* **6**:445.

Henson, P. M., and Spiegelberg, H. L., 1973, *J. Clin. Invest.* **52**:1282.

Heremans, J. F., 1960, *Les Globulines Seriques du Systeme Gamma*, Arscia, Brussels, and Masson, Paris.

Hester, R. B., Mole, J. E., and Schrohenloher, R. E., 1975, *J. Immunol.* **114**:486.

Higuchi, Y., Honda, M., and Hayashi, H., 1975, *Cell. Immunol.* **15**:100.

Hillman, K., Schlamowitz, M., and Shaw, A. R., 1977, *J. Immunol.* **118**:782.

Hinrichs, W. A., and Smyth, D. G., 1970, *Immunology* **18**:769.

Hjelm, H., Sjodahl, J., and Sjoquist, J., 1975, *Eur. J. Biochem.* **57**:395.

Hochman, J., Inbar, D., and Givol, D., 1973, *Biochemistry* **12**:1130.

Holowka, D. A., Stasberg, A. D., Kimball, J. W., Haber, E., and Cathou, R. E., 1972, *Proc. Natl. Acad. Sci. USA* **69**:3379.

Horton, H. R., and Koshland, D. E., 1965, *J. Am. Chem. Soc.* **87**:1126.

Hsiao, S., and Putnam, F. W., 1961, *J. Biol. Chem.* **236**:122.

Huber, H., and Fudenberg, H. H., 1968, *Int. Arch. Allergy Appl. Immunol.* **34**:18.

Huber, H., Douglas, S. D., Nubacher, J., Kochwa, S., and Rosenfield, R. E., 1971, *Nature (London)* **229**:419.

Hurst, M. M., Volanakis, R. B., Hester, R. B., Stroud, R. M., and Bennett, J. C., 1974, *J. Exp. Med.* **140**:1117.

Hurst, M. M., Volanakis, J. E., Stroud, R. M., and Bennett, J. C., 1975, *J. Exp. Med.* **142**:1322.

Huston, J. S., Bjork, I., and Tanford, C., 1972, *Biochemistry* **11**:4256.

Hyslop, N. E., Dourmashkin, R. R., Green, N. M., and Porter, R. R., 1970, *J. Exp. Med.* **131**:783.

Ikeda, K., Hamaguchi, K., and Migita, S., 1968, *J. Biochem. (Tokyo)* **63**:654.

Imahori, K., 1963, *Biopolymers* **1**:563.

Imahori, K., and Momoi, H., 1962, *Arch. Biochem. Biophys.* **97**:236.

Imir, T., Saksela, E., and Makela, O., 1976, *J. Immunol.* **117**:1938.

Inbar, D., Hochman, J., and Givol, D., 1972, *Proc. Natl. Acad. Sci. USA* **69**:2659.

Inchley, C., Grey, H. M., and Uhr, J. W., 1970, *J. Immunol.* **105**:362.

Inman, F. P., and Hazen, S. R., 1968, *J. Biol. Chem.* **243**:5598.

Irimajiri, S., Franklin, E. C., and Frangione, B., 1968, *Immunochemistry* **5**:383.

Isenman, D. E., Dorrington, K. J., and Painter, R. H., 1975a, *J. Immunol.* **114**:1726.

Isenman, D. E., Painter, R. H., and Dorrington, K. J., 1975b, *Proc. Natl. Acad. Sci. USA* **72**:548.

Isenman, D. E., Ellerson, J. R., Painter, R. H., and Dorrington, K. J., 1977, *Biochemistry* **15**:233.

Ishizaka, K., 1973, in: *The Antigens,* Vol. I (M. Sela, ed.), p. 479, Academic Press, New York.

Ishizaka, K., and Ishizaka, T., 1960, *J. Immunol.* **85**:163.

Ishizaka, K., and Ishizaka, T., 1966, *J. Allergy* **37**:169.

Ishizaka, K., and Ishizaka, T., 1969, *J. Immunol.* **102**:69.

Ishizaka, K., Ishizaka, T., and Sugahara, T., 1962, *J. Immunol.* **88**:690.

Ishizaka, K., Ishizaka, T., Salmon, S., and Fudenberg, H., 1967, *J. Immunol.* **99**:82.

Ishizaka, K., Ishizaka, T., and Lee, E. H., 1970a, *Immunochemistry* **7**:687.

Ishizaka, K., Tomioka, H., and Ishizaka, T., 1970b, *J. Immunol.* **105**:1459.

Ishizaka, T., and Ishizaka, K., 1975, *Progr. Allergy* **19**:60.

Ishizaka, T., Ishizaka, K., and Borsos, T., 1961, *J. Immunol.* **87**:433.

Ishizaka, T., Tada, T., and Ishizaka, K., 1968, *J. Immunol.* **100**:1145.

Ishizaka, T., Sean, C. M., and Ishizaka, K., 1972, *J. Immunol.* **108**:848.

Isliker, H., Allan, R., Boesman, M., Hensser, C., and Knobel, H., 1974, *Adv. Biosci.* **12**:270.

Ito, K., Wicher, K., Arbesman, C. E., 1971, *Int. Arch. Allergy Appl. Immunol.* **41**:477.

Jaton, J.-C., Huser, H., Blatt, Y., and Pecht, I., 1975a, *Biochemistry* **14**:5308.

Jaton, J.-C., Huser, H., Braun, D. G., Schlessinger, J., Pecht, I., and Givol, D., 1975b, *Biochemistry* **14**:5312.

Jaton, J.-C., Huser, H., Riesen, W. F., Schlessinger, J., and Givol, D., 1976, *J. Immunol.* **116**:1363.

Jeffries, R., Weston, P. D., Stanworth, D. R., and Clamp, J. R., 1968, *Nature (London)* **219**:646.

Jensen, K., 1958, *Acta Pathol. Microbiol. Scand.* **44**:421.

Jirgensons, B., 1961, *Arch. Biochem. Biophys.* **94**:59.

Jirgensons, B., 1965, *J. Biol. Chem.* **240**:1064.

Johansson, S. G. O., 1967, *Lancet* **2**:951.

Johnson, B. J., and Thames, K. E., 1976, *J. Immunol.* **117**:1491.

Johnson, P. M., Scopes, P. M., Tracey, B. M., and Watkins, J., 1974, *Immunology* **27**:27.

Johnson, P. M., Howard, A., and Scopes, P. M., 1975, *FEBS Lett.* **49**:310.

Jones, E. A., and Waldmann, T. A., 1972, *J. Clin. Invest.* **51**:2916.

Kabat, E. A., and Wu, T. T., 1972, *Proc. Natl. Acad. Sci. USA* **69**:960.

Kakimoto, K., and Onoue, K., 1974, *J. Immunol.* **112**:1373.

Kang, Y.-S., Calvanico, N. J., and Tomasi, T. B., 1974, *J. Immunol.* **112**:162.

Kaplan, M. H., and Volanakis, J. E., 1974, *J. Immunol.* **112**:2135.

Karlsson, F. A., Peterson, P. A., and Berggard, I., 1969, *Proc. Natl. Acad. Sci. USA* **64**:1257.

Karlsson, F. A., Peterson, P. A., and Berggard, I., 1972, *J. Biol. Chem.* **247**:1065.

Katz, D. H., and Benacerraf, B., 1972, *Adv. Immunol.* **15**:1.

Kauzman, W., 1959, *Adv. Protein Chem.* **14**:1.

Kazmierowski, J. A., Nisonoff, A., Quie, P. G., and Williams, R. C., 1971, *J. Immunol.* **106**:605.

Kehoe, J. M., and Capra, J. D., 1971, *Proc. Natl. Acad. Sci. USA* **68**:2019.

Kehoe, J. M., and Fougereau, M., 1969, *Nature (London)* **224**:1212.

Kehoe, J. M., Bourgois, A., Capra, J. D., and Fougereau, M., 1974, *Biochemistry* **13**:2499.

Kellander, J., 1963, *Acta Soc. Med. Upsal.* **68**:230.

Kennel, S. J., and Lerner, R. A., 1973, *J. Mol. Biol.* **76**:485.

Kincaid, H. L., and Jirgensons, B., 1972, *Biochim. Biophys. Acta* **271**:23.

Kindmark, C. O., 1969, *Scand. J. Clin. Lab. Invest.* **24**:49.

Kishimoto, T., Onoue, K., and Yamamura, Y., 1968, *J. Immunol.* **100**:1032.

Koblet, H., Barandun, S., and Diggelmann, H., 1967, *Vox Sang.* **13**:93.

Kochwa, S., Terry, W. D., Capra, J. D., and Yand, N. L., 1971, *Ann. N.Y. Acad. Sci.* **190**:49.

Konno, T., and Hirai, H., 1975, *Immunochemistry* **12**:773.

Kossard, S., and Nelson, D. S., 1968, *Aust. J. Exp. Biol. Med. Sci.* **46**:63.

Kratzin, H., Altevogt, P., Ruban, E., Kortt, A., Staroscik, K., and Hilschmann, N., 1975, *Z. Physiol. Chem.* **356**:1337.

Kronvall, G., 1967, *Acta Pathol. Microbiol. Scand.* **69**:619.

Kronvall, G., and Frommel, D., 1970, *Immunochemistry* **7**:124.

Kronvall, G., and Gewurz, H., 1970, *Clin. Exp. Immunol.* **7**:211.

Kronvall, G., and Williams, R. C., 1969, *J. Immunol.* **103**:828.

Kronvall, G., and Williams, R. C., 1971 *Immunochemistry* **8**:577.

Kronvall, G., Grey, H., and Williams, R. C., 1970a, *J. Immunol.* **105**:1116.

Kronvall, G., Quie, P. G., and Williams, R. C., 1970b, *J. Immunol.* **104**:273.

Kronvall, G., Seal, U. S., Finstad, J., and Williams, R. C., 1970c, *J. Immunol.* **104**:140.

Kronvall, G., Dossett, J. H., Quie, P. G., and Williams, R. C., 1971, *Infect. Immun.* **3**:10.

Kronvall, G., Seal, U. S., Svensson, S., and Williams, R. C., 1974, *Acta Pathol. Microbiol. Scand.* **82**:12.

Kulczycki, A., Jr., McNearney, T. A., and Parker, C. W., 1976, *J. Immunol.* **117**:661.

Kumagai, K., Abo, T., Sekizawa, T., and Sasaki, M., 1975, *J. Immunol.* **115**:982.

Labaw, L. W., and Davies, D. R., 1971, *J. Biol. Chem.* **246**:3760.

Labib, R. W., Calvanico, N. J., and Tomasi, T. B., 1976, *J. Biol. Chem.* **251**:1969.

Labib, R. W., Calvanico, N. J., and Tomasi, T. B., 1978, *Biochim. Biophys. Acta* **526**:547.

Lahiri, A. K., Mitchell, W. M., and Najjar, V. A., 1970, *J. Biol. Chem.* **245**:3906.

Lamon, E. W., Whitten, H. D., Lidin, B., and Fudenberg, H. H., 1975a, *J. Exp. Med.* **142**:542.

Lamon, E. W., Whitten, H. D., Skurzak, H. M., Andersson, B., and Lidin, B., 1975b, *J. Immunol.* **115**:1288.

Larsson, A., Perlmann, P., and Natvig, J. B., 1973, *Immunology* **25**:675.

Larsson, A., Pierri-Salsano, S., Ohlander, C., Natvig, J. B., and Perlmann, P., 1975, *Scand. J. Immunol.* **4**:241.

Laurell, C.-B., and Thulin, E., 1975, *J. Exp. Med.* **141**:453.

Lawrence, D. A., Weigle, W. O., and Spiegelberg, H. L., 1975, *J. Clin. Invest.* **55**:368.

Lay, W. H., and Nussenzweig, V., 1969, *J. Immunol.* **102**:1172.

Lee, C.-L., and Atassi, M. Z., 1977a, *Biochem. J.* **167**:571.

Lee, C.-L., and Atassi, M. Z., 1977b, *Biochim. Biophys. Acta* **495**:354.

Leslie, G. A. and Swate, T. E., 1972, *J. Immunol.* **109**:47.

Leslie, R. G. Q., and Cohen, S., 1974a, *Immunology* **27**:577.

Leslie, R. G. Q., and Cohen, S., 1974b, *Immunology* **27**:589.

Lewis, L. A., and Page, I. H., 1965, *Am. J. Med.* **38**:286.

Liberti, P. A., Stylas, W. A., and Maurer, P. H., 1972a, Biochemistry 11:3312.

Liberti, P. A., Stylos, W. A., Maurer, P. H., and Callahan, H. J., 1972b, Biochemistry 11:3321.

Lind, I., 1974, Scand. J. Immunol. 3:689.

Lind, I., and Mansa, B., 1974, Scand. J. Immunol. 3:147.

Lind, I., Harboe, M., and Folling, I., 1975, Scand. J. Immunol. 4:843.

Lindh, E., 1975, J. Immunol. 114:284.

Lindh, E., and Bjork, I., 1976, Eur. J. Biochem. 62:271.

Lippincott, S. W., Korman, S., Fong, C., Stickley, E., Wolins, W., and Hughes, W. L., 1960, J. Clin. Invest. 39:565.

Liu, Y.-S. V., Low, T. L. K., Infante, A., and Putnam, F. W., 1976, Science 193:1017.

Ljaljevic, M., Ljaljevic, J., and Parker, C. W., 1968, J. Immunol. 100:1051.

Löfkvist, T., 1966, Int. Arch. Allergy 29:240.

Löfkvist, T., and Sjoquist, J., 1962, Acta Pathol. Microbiol. Scand. 56:295.

Lopes, A. D., and Steiner, L. A., 1973, Fed. Proc. 32:1003.

Loveless, M. H., 1940, J. Immunol. 38:25.

Low, T. L. K., Liu, Y.-S. V., and Putnam, F. W., 1976, Science 191:390.

Mach, J. P., 1970, Nature (London) 228:1278.

MacKenzie, M. R., Creevy, N., and Heh, M., 1971, J. Immunol. 106:65.

MacLennan, I. C. M., Howard, A., Gotch, F. M., and Quie, P. G., 1973, Immunology 25:459.

MacLennan, I. C. M., Connell, G. E., and Gotch, F. M., 1974, Immunology 26:303.

Mage, R., Lieberman, R., Potter, M., and Terry, W., 1973, in: The Antigens, Vol. I (M. Sella, ed.), p. 300, Academic Press, New York.

Malley, A., Baecher, L., Porter, G., and Gerding, R., 1974, Int. Arch. Allergy Appl. Immunol. 47:194.

Mannik, M., 1967, J. Immunol. 99:899.

Marchalonis, J. J., 1975, Science 190:20.

Martin, R. R., Crowder, J. G., and White, A., 1967, J. Immunol. 99:269.

Matre, R., 1976, Scand. J. Immunol. 5:963.

Matre, R., Tonder, O., and Endresen, C., 1975, Scand. J. Immunol. 4:741.

Matthews, N., Stewart, G., and Stanworth, D. R., 1971, Immunochemistry 8:973.

Mayer, M. M., 1961, in: Experimental Immunochemistry (E. A. Kabat and M. M. Mayer, eds.), p. 133, Thomas, Springfield, Ill.

McConnell, I., and Hurd, C. M., 1976, Immunology 30:835.

McNabb, T., Koh, T. Y., Dorrington, K. J., and Painter, R. H., 1976, J. Immunol. 117:882.

Medgyesi, G. A., Csecsi-Nagy, M., Gorini, G., Puskas, E., Gergely, J., Sajgo, M., and Czvppon, A., 1973, Immunochemistry 10:509.

Mehta, S. K., Plaut, A. G., Calvanico, N. J., and Tomasi, T. B., 1974, J. Immunol. 113:289.

Melcher, U., and Uhr, J. W., 1976, J. Immunol. 116:409.

Melcher, U., Vitetta, E. S., McWilliams, M., Lamm, M. E., Phillips-Quagliata, J. M., and Uhr, J. W., 1974, J. Exp. Med. 140:1427.

Melcher, U., Eidels, L., and Uhr, J. W., 1975, Nature (London) 258:434.

Melchers, F., and Knopf, R. M., 1967, Cold Spring Harbor Symp. Quant. Biol. 32:255.

Mendoza, G. R., and Metzger, H., 1976, J. Immunol. 117:1573.

Messner, R. P., and Jelinek, J., 1970, J. Clin. Invest. 49:2165.

Messner, R. P., Parker, C. W., and Williams, R. C., 1970, J. Immunol. 104:238.

Mestecky, J., Zikan, J., and Butler, W. T., 1971, Science 171:1163.

Mestecky, J., Schrohenloher, R. E., Kulhavy, R., Wright, G. P., and Tomana, M., 1974, *Proc. Natl. Acad. Sci. USA* **71**:544.

Metzger, H., 1970, *Adv. Immunol.* **12**:57.

Metzger, H., 1974, *Adv. Immunol.* **18**:169.

Michaelsen, T. E., and Natvig, J. B., 1971, *Immunochemistry* **8**:235.

Michaelsen, T. E., and Natvig, J. B., 1972, *Scand. J. Immunol.* **1**:255.

Michaelsen, T. E., and Natvig, J. B., 1974a, *J. Biol. Chem.* **249**:2778.

Michaelsen, T. E., and Natvig, J. B., 1974b, *Scand. J. Immunol.* **3**:865.

Michaelsen, T. E., Natvig, J. B., and Sletten, K., 1974, *Scand. J. Immunol.* **3**:491.

Michaelsen, T. E., Wisloff, F., and Natvig, J. B., 1975, *Scand. J. Immunol.* **4**:71.

Mihaesco, C., and Seligmann, M., 1968a, *J. Exp. Med.* **127**:431.

Mihaesco, C., and Seligmann, M., 1968b, *Immunochemistry* **5**:457.

Miller, F., and Metzger, H. J., 1965, *J. Biol. Chem.* **240**:4740.

Miller, F., and Metzger, H., 1966, *J. Biol. Chem.* **241**:1732.

Milstein, C., 1967, *Nature (London)* **216**:330.

Minta, J. O., and Painter, R. H., 1972, *Immunochemistry* **9**:1041.

Mole, J., Bhown, A. S., and Bennett, J. C., 1977, *Biochemistry* **16**:3507.

Möller, E., 1965, *Science* **147**:873.

Morell, A., Terry, W. D., and Waldmann, T. A., 1970, *J. Clin. Invest.* **49**:673.

Moretta, L., Ferrarini, M., Durante, M. L., and Mingari, M. C., 1975, *Eur. J. Immunol.* **5**:565.

Mortensen, R. F., Osmand, A. P., Lint, T. F., and Gewurz, H., 1976, *J. Immunol.* **117**:774.

Moskalewski, S., Ptak, W., and Czannik, Z., 1975, *Biol. Neonate* **26**:268.

Mueller-Eckhardt, C. L., and Lüscher, E. F., 1968a, *Thromb. Diath. Haemorrh.* **20**:155.

Mueller-Eckhardt, C. L., and Lüscher, E. F., 1968b, *Thromb. Diath. Haemorrh.* **20**:168.

Müller-Eberhard, H. J., 1975, *Annu. Rev. Biochem.* **44**:697.

Munn, E. A., Feinstein, A., and Munro, A. J., 1971, *Nature (London)* **231**:527.

Murray, E. S., O'Connor, J. M., and Gaon, J. B., 1965, *Proc. Soc. Exp. Biol. Med.* **119**:291.

Natvig, J. B., Turner, M. W., and Michaelsen, T. E., 1971, *Ann. N.Y. Acad. Sci.* **190**:150.

Natvig, J. B., Gaarder, P. I., and Turner, M. W., 1972, *Clin. Exp. Immunol.* **12**:177.

Neauport-Sautes, C., Dupuis, D., and Fridman, W. H., 1975, *Eur. J. Immunol.* **5**:849.

Nisonoff, A., Wissler, F. C., and Lipman, L. N., 1960, *Science* **132**:1770.

Noelken, M. E., Nelson, C. A., Buckley, C. E., and Tanford, C., 1965, *J. Biol. Chem.* **240**:218.

Oeding, P. and Hankenes, G., 1963, *Acta Pathol. Microbiol. Scand.* **57**:438.

Ohta, Y., Gill, T. J., III, and Leung, C. S., 1970, *Biochemistry* **9**:2708.

Okafor, G. O., and Turner, M. W., 1974, *Scand. J. Immunol.* **3**:181.

Okafor, G. O., Turner, M. W., and Hay, F. C., 1974, *Nature (London)* **248**:228.

Onoue, K., Kishimoto, T., and Yamamura, Y., 1968, *J. Immunol.* **100**:238.

Osler, A. G., Oliveira, B., Shin, H. S., and Sandberg, A. L., 1969, *J. Immunol.* **102**:269.

Osterland, C. K., Harboe, M., and Kunkel, H. G., 1963, *Vox Sang.* **8**:133.

Ovary, Z., 1960, *Immunology* **3**:19.

Ovary, Z., Benacerraf, B., and Bloch, K. J., 1963, *J. Exp. Med.* **117**:951.

Ovary, Z., Kunkel, H. G., and Joslin, F. G., 1970, *J. Immunol.* **105**:1103.

Ovary, Z., Saluk, P. H., Ouijada, L., and Lamm, M. E., 1976, *J. Immunol.* **116**:1265.

Padlan, E. A., Segal, D. M., Spande, T., Davies, D. R., Rudikoff, S., and Potter, M., 1973, *Nature (London) New Biol.* **245**:165.

Painter, R. H., Yasmeen, D., Assimeh, S. N., and Poulik, M. D., 1974, *Immunol. Commun.* **3**:19.

Palm, W. H., 1970, *FEBS Lett.* **10**:46.

Parish, W. E., 1970, *Lancet* **2**:591.

Parr, D. M., Connell, G. E., Kells, D. I. C., and Hoffmann, T., 1976a, *Biochem. J.* **155**:31.

Parr, D. M., Hoffmann, T., and Connell, G. E., 1976b, *Biochem. J.* **157**:535.

Pernis, B., Forni, L., and Amante, L., 1970, *J. Exp. Med.* **132**:1001.

Perry, M. B., and M:lstein, C., 1970, *Nature (London)* **228**:934.

Pfueller, S. L., and Lüscher, E. F., 1972, *J. Immunol.* **109**:517.

Phillips-Quagliata, J. M., Levine, B. B., Quagliata, F., and Uhr, J. W., 1971, *J. Exp. Med.* **133**:589.

Pilz, I., Puchwein, G., Kratky, O., Herbst, M., Haager, O., Gall, W. E., and Edelman, G. M., 1970, *Biochemistry* **9**:211.

Plaut, A. G., and Tomasi, T. B., 1970, *Proc. Natl. Acad. Sci. USA* **65**:318.

Plaut, A. G., Cohen, S., and Tomasi, T. B., 1972, *Science* **176**:55.

Plaut, A. G., Wistar, R., and Capra, J. D., 1974a, *J. Clin. Invest.* **54**:1295.

Plaut, A. G., Genco, R. J., and Tomasi, T. B., 1974b, *J. Immunol.* **113**:289.

Plaut, A. G., Gilbert, J. V., Artenstein, M. S., and Capra, J. D., 1975, *Science* **190**:1103.

Poljak, R. J., 1975a, *Adv. Immunol.* **21**:1.

Poljak, R. J., 1975b, *Nature (London)* **256**:373.

Poljak, R. J., Amzel, L. M., Avey, H. P., Chen, B. L., Phızackerley, R. P., and Saul, F., 1973, *Proc. Natl. Acad. Sci. USA* **70**:3305.

Poljak, R. J., Amzel, L. M., Chen, B. L., Phizackerley, R. P., and Saul, F., 1974, *Proc. Natl. Acad. Sci. USA* **71**:3440.

Porter, R. R., 1959, *Biochem. J.* **73**:119.

Porter, R. R., 1973, *Science* **180**:713.

Poulik, M. D., 1966, *Nature (London)* **210**:133.

Prahl, J. W., 1967, *Biochem. J.* **104**:647.

Putnam, F. W., Florent, G., Paul, C., Shinoda, T., and Shimizu, A., 1973, *Science* **182**:287.

Rabellino, E., Colon, S., Grey, H. M., and Unanue, E. R., 1971, *J. Exp. Med.* **133**:156.

Raff, M. C., Sternberg, M., and Taylor, R. B., 1970, *Nature (London)* **225**:553.

Ramasamy, R., Secher, D. S., and Adetugbo, K., 1975, *Nature (London)* **253**:656.

Rask, L., Klareskog, L., Ostberg, L., and Peterson, P. A., 1975, *Nature (London)* **257**:231.

Reid, K. B. M., 1971, *Immunology* **20**:649.

Reid, K. B. M., Lowe, D. M., and Porter, R. R., 1972, *Biochem. J.* **130**:749.

Reid, R. T., 1970, *J. Immunol.* **104**:935.

Rhodes, J., 1973, *Nature (London)* **243**:527.

Richardson, J., Richardson, D. C., Thomas, K. A., Silverton, E. W., and Davies, D. R., 1976, *J. Mol. Biol.* **102**:221.

Richardson, S. H., Hultin, H. O., and Green, D. E., 1963, *Proc. Natl. Acad. Sci. USA* **50**:821.

Riesen, W. F., Huser, H., and Skvaril, F., 1976, *FEBS Lett.* **61**:243.

Robert, S., and Grabar, P., 1957, *Ann. Inst. Pasteur* **92**:56.

Ropartz, C., Lenoir, J., Aurel, R., Hemet, Y., and Breteau, G., 1958, *Rev. Hematol.* **13**:511.

Rose, G. D., Winters, R. H., and Wetlaufer, D. B., 1976, *FEBS Lett.* **63**:10.

Ross, D. L., and Jirgensons, B., 1968, *J. Biol. Chem.* **243**:2829.

Rowe, D. S., Dolder, F., and Welscher, H. D., 1969, *Immunochemistry* **6**:437.

Rowe, D. S., Hug, K., Forni, L., and Pernis, B., 1973, *J. Exp. Med.* **138**:965.

Rudikoff, S., Potter, M., Segal, D. M., Padlan, E. A., and Davies, D. R., 1972, *Proc. Natl. Acad. Sci. USA* **69**:3689.

Salsano, F., Froland, S. S., Natvig, J. B., and Michaelsen, T. E., 1974, *Scand. J. Immunol.* **3**:841.

Sandberg, A. L., Oliveira, B., and Osler, A. G., 1971, *J. Immunol.* **106**:282.

Sarkar, P. K., and Doty, P., 1966, *Proc. Natl. Acad. Sci. USA* **55**:981.

Sarma, R. V., and Zaloga, G., 1975, *J. Mol. Biol.* **98**:479.

Sarma, R. V., Silverton, E. W., Davies, D. R., and Terry, W. D., 1971, *J. Biol. Chem.* **246**:3753.

Schiffer, M., Hardman, K. D., Wood, M. K., Edmundson, A. B., Hook, M. E., and Ely, K. R., 1970, *J. Biol. Chem.* **245**:728.

Schiffer, M., Girling, R. L., Ely, K. R., and Edmundson, A. B., 1973, *Biochemistry* **12**:4620.

Schlamowitz, M., 1976, *Immun. Commun.* **5**:481.

Schlamowitz, M., Hillman, K., Lechtiger, B., and Abearn, M. J., 1975, *J. Immunol.* **115**:296.

Schlessinger, J., Steinberg, I. Z., Givol, D., Hochman, J., and Pecht, I., 1975, *Proc. Natl. Acad. Sci. USA* **72**:2775.

Schrohenloher, R., 1963, *Arch. Biochim. Biophys.* **101**:456.

Schur, P. H., and Becker, E. L., 1963, *J. Exp. Med.* **118**:891.

Schur, P. H., and Christian, G. D., 1964, *J. Exp. Med.* **120**:531.

Segal, D. M., Padlan, E. A., Cohen, G. H., Rudikoff, S., Potter, M., and Davies, D. R., 1974, *Proc. Natl. Acad. Sci. USA* **71**:4298.

Segrest, J. P., and Feldman, R. J., 1974, *J. Mol. Biol.* **87**:853.

Segrest, J. P., Kahane, I., Jackson, R. L., and Marchesi, V. T., 1973, *Arch. Biochem. Biophys.* **155**:167.

Seon, B.-K., and Pressman, D., 1975, *Immunochemistry* **12**:333.

Setcavage, T. M., Rothlein, R., Muscoplat, C. C., and Kim, Y. B., 1976, *Cell. Immunol.* **27**:47.

Shelton, E., Yonemasu, K., and Stroud, R. M., 1972, *Proc. Natl. Acad. Sci. USA* **69**:65.

Shimizu, A., Watanabe, S., Yamamura, Y., and Putnam, F. W., 1974, *Immunochemistry* **11**:719.

Shuster, J., 1971, *Immunochemistry* **8**:405.

Siegel, J., Rent, R., and Gewurz, H., 1974, *J. Exp. Med.* **140**:631.

Singer, S. J., 1971, in: *Structure and Function of Biological Membranes* (L. I. Rothfield, ed.), p. 145, Academic Press, New York.

Singer, S. J., 1974, *Adv. Immunol.* **19**:1.

Singer, S. J., and Nicolson, G. L., 1972, *Science* **175**:720.

Sjodahl, J., 1976, *FEBS Lett.* **67**:62.

Sjoholm, I., 1975a, *Eur. J. Biochem.* **51**:55.

Sjoholm, I., 1975b, *FEBS Lett.* **52**:53.

Sjoholm, I., and Ljungdahl, M., 1973, *Immunochemistry* **10**:287.

Sjoholm, I., and Sjodin, T., 1974, *Eur. J. Biochem.* **47**:491.

Sjoholm, I., Ekenas, A.-K., and Sjoquist, J., 1972, *Eur. J. Biochem.* **29**:455.

Sjoholm, I., Bjerken, A., and Sjoquist, J., 1973, *J. Immunol.* **110**:1562.

Sjoquist, J., and Stalenheim, G., 1969, *J. Immunol.* **103**:467.

Sjoquist, J., Meloun, B., and Hjelm, H., 1972a, *Eur. J. Biochem.* **29**:572.

Sjoquist, J., Movitz, J., Johnsson, I.-B., and Hjelm, H., 1972b, *Eur. J. Biochem.* **30**:190.

Sledge, C. R., and Bing, D. H., 1973, *J. Biol. Chem.* **248**:2818.

Smith, B. R., and Dorrington, K. J., 1972, *Biochem. Biophys. Res. Commun.* **46**:1061.

Smith, G. P., Hood, L., and Fitch, W. M., 1971, *Annu. Rev. Biochem.* **40**:969.

Solomon, A., Waldmann, T. A., and Fahey, J., 1963, *J. Lab. Clin. Med.* **62**:1.

Solomon, A., Waldmann, T. A., Fahey, J. L., and MacFarlane, A. S., 1964, *J. Clin. Invest.* **48**:103.

Sonoda, S., Shigematsu, T., and Schlamowitz, M., 1973, *J. Immunol.* **110**:1682.

Spiegelberg, H. L., 1974, *Adv. Immunol.* **19**:259.

Spiegelberg, H. L., and Weigle, W. O., 1965, *J. Exp. Med.* **121**:323.
Spiegelberg, H. L., and Weigle, W. O., 1966, *J. Immunol.* **95**:1034.
Spiegelberg, H. L., Prahl, J. W., and Grey, H. M., 1970, *Biochemistry* **9**:2115.
Spiegelberg, H. L., Lawrence, D. A., and Henson, P. M., 1974, *Adv. Exp. Med. Biol.* **45**:67.
Spiegelberg, H. L., Perlmann, H., and Perlmann, P., 1976, *J. Immunol.* **116**:1464.
Springer, T. A., and Strominger, J. L., 1976, *Proc. Natl. Acad. Sci. USA* **73**:2481.
Stalenheim, G., and Castensson, S., 1971, *FEBS Lett.* **14**:79.
Stalenheim, G., and Sjoquist, J., 1970, *J. Immunol.* **105**:944.
Stanworth, D. R., Humphrey, J. H., Bennich, H., and Johansson, S. G. O., 1968, *Lancet* **2**:17.
Stanworth, D. R., Housley, J., Bennich, H., and Johansson, S. G. O., 1970, *Immunochemistry* **7**:321.
Steinberg, A., 1962, *Progr. Med. Genet.* **2**:1.
Steiner, L. A., and Lowey, S., 1966, *J. Biol. Chem.* **241**:231.
Stevenson, G. T., and Dorrington, K. J., 1970, *Biochem. J.* **118**:703.
Stewart, G. A., and Stanworth, D. R., 1975, *Immunochemistry* **12**:713.
Stewart, G. A., Smith, A. K., and Stanworth, D. R., 1973, *Immunochemistry* **10**:755.
Stobo, J. D., and Tomasi, T. B., 1967, *J. Clin. Invest.* **46**:1329.
Stone, M. J., and Metzger, H. J., 1968, *J. Biol. Chem.* **243**:5977.
Strober, W., Wochner, R. D., Barlow, M. H., McFarlin, D. E., and Waldmann, T. A., 1968, *J. Clin. Invest.* **47**:1905.
Svehag, S. E., and Bloth, B., 1970, *Science* **168**:847.
Swenson, R. M., and Kern, M., 1967, *J. Biol. Chem.* **242**:3242.
Takakazu, A., Shimizu, A., and Yamamura, Y., 1976, *Immunochemistry* **13**:461.
Takatsu, K., Ishizaka, T., and Ishizaka, K., 1975, *J. Immunol.* **114**:1838.
Tanford, C., 1973, in: *The Hydrophobic Effect: Formation of Micelles and Biological Membranes*, Wiley, New York.
Taranta, A., and Franklin, E. C., 1961, *Science* **134**:1981.
Terry, W. D., Matthews, W., and Davies, D. R., 1968, *Nature (London)* **220**:239.
Thrasher, S. G., and Cohen, S., 1971, *J. Immunol.* **107**:672.
Thrasher, S. G., Bigazzi, P. E., Yoshida, T., and Cohen, S., 1975, *J. Immunol.* **114**:762.
Titani, K., Whitley, E., and Putnam, F. W., 1966, *Science* **152**:1513.
Titani, K., Wikler, M., and Putnam, F. W., 1967, *Science* **155**:828.
Todd, C. W., 1972, *Fed. Proc.* **31**:188.
Tomana, M., Niedermeier, W., and Skvaril, F., 1974, *Immunochemistry* **11**:337.
Tomasi, T. B., 1973, *Proc. Natl. Acad. Sci. USA* **70**:3410.
Tomasi, T. B., and Bienenstock, J., 1968, *Adv. Immunol.* **9**:1.
Tomasi, T. B., and Czerwinski, D. S., 1976, *Scand. J. Immunol.* **5**:647.
Tomasi, T. B., and Grey, H. M., 1972, *Progr. Allergy* **16**:81.
Tomasi, T. B., and Hauptman, S. P., 1974a, *J. Immunol.* **112**:2274.
Tomasi, T. B., and Hauptman, S., 1974b, in: *The Immunoglobulin A System* (J. Mestecky and A. R. Lawton, eds.), p. 111, Plenum, New York.
Turner, M. W., and Bennich, H., 1968, *Biochem. J.* **107**:171.
Turner, M. W., and Berggard, I., 1969, *Nature (London)* **224**:912.
Turner, M. W., and Rowe, D. S., 1966, *Nature (London)* **210**:130.
Turner, M. W., Martensson, L., Natvig, J. B., and Bennich, H., 1969a, *Nature (London)* **221**:1166.
Turner, M. W., Stanworth, D. R., Normansell, D. E., and Bennich, H. H., 1969b, *Biochim. Biophys. Acta* **188**:265.
Turner, M. W., Bennich, H. H., and Natvig, J. B., 1970a, *Nature (London)* **255**:853.

Turner, M. W., Bennich, H. H., and Natvig, J. B., 1970*b*, *Clin. Exp. Immunol.* 7:603.

Turner, M. W., Bennich, H. H., and Natvig, J. B., 1970*c*, *Clin. Exp. Immunol.* 7:627.

Udaka, K., Takeuchi, Y., and Movat, H. Z., 1970, *Proc. Soc. Exp. Biol. Med.* 133:1384.

Underdown, B. J., and Dorrington, K. J., 1974, *J. Immunol.* 112:949.

Unkeless, J. C., 1977, *J. Exp. Med.* 145:931.

Unkeless, J. C., and Eisen, H. N., 1975, *J. Exp. Med.* 142:1520.

Utsumi, S., 1969, *Biochem. J.* 112:343.

Utsumi, S., and Karush, F., 1965, *Biochemistry* 4:1766.

Vaerman, J. P., Fudenberg, H. H., Vaerman, C., and Mandy, W. J., 1965, *Immunochemistry* 2:263.

Valentine, R. C., and Green, N. M., 1967, *J. Mol. Biol.* 27:615.

Van Furth, R., Schint, H. R., and Hymans, W., 1965, *J. Exp. Med.* 122:1173.

Van Loghem, E., Wang, A. C., and Shuster, J., 1973, *Vox Sang.* 24:481.

Vaz, N. M., and Ovary, Z., 1968, *J. Immunol.* 100:1014.

Virella, G., and Parkhouse, R. M. E., 1971, *Immunochemistry* 8:243.

Virella, G., Amelia Silveira Nunes, M., and Tamagnini, G., 1972, *Clin. Exp. Immunol.* 10:475.

Vitetta, E. S., and Uhr, J. W., 1975, *Science* 189:964.

Vitetta, E. S., Baur, S., and Uhr, J. W., 1971, *J. Exp. Med.* 134:242.

Vitetta, E. S., Bianco, C., Nussenzweig, V., and Uhr, J. W., 1972, *J. Exp. Med.* 136:81.

Waldmann, T. A., and Strober, W., 1969, *Progr. Allergy* 13:1.

Walker, W. S., 1976, *J. Immunol.* 116:911.

Waller, M., 1967, *Immunology* 13:623.

Warner, N. L., 1974, *Adv. Immunol.* 19:67.

Webb, S. R., and Cooper, M. D., 1973, *J. Immunol.* 111:275.

Weicker, J., and Underdown, B. J., 1975, *J. Immunol.* 114:1337.

Weissman, G., Brand, A., and Franklin, E. C., 1974, *J. Clin. Invest.* 53:536.

Wells, J. V., 1976, in: *Basic and Clinical Immunology* (H. H. Fudenberg, D. P. Stites, J. L. Caldwell, J. V. Wells, eds.), p. 195, Lange Medical Publications, Los Altos, Calif.

Welter, O., 1972, *Clin. Chim. Acta* 36:284.

Werner, T. C., Bunting, J. R., and Cathou, R. E., 1972, *Proc. Natl. Acad. Sci. USA* 69:795.

Wernet, P., 1976, *Transplant. Rev.* 30:271.

Wernet, P., Feizi, T., and Kunkel, H. G., 1972, *J. Exp. Med.* 136:650.

Wetlaufer, D., Kwok, E., Anderson, W. L., and Johnson, E. R., 1974, *Biochem. Biophys. Res. Commun.* 56:380.

Wiedermann, G., Miescher, P. A., and Franklin, E. C., 1963, *Proc. Soc. Exp. Biol. Med.* 113:609.

Williams, R. C., Osterland, C. K., Marghertia, S., Tokuda, S., and Messner, R. P., 1973, *J. Immunol.* 111:1690.

Wilson, D., 1972, *J. Immunol.* 108:726.

Wilson, I. D., and Williams, R. C., 1969, *J. Clin. Invest.* 48:2409.

Winkler, M., and Doty, P., 1961, *Biochim. Biophys. Acta* 54:448.

Wirtz, G. H., 1965, *Immunochemistry* 2:95.

Wisloff, F., Froland, S. S., and Michaelsen, T. E., 1974*a*, *Int. Arch. Allergy* 47:139.

Wisloff, F., Michaelsen, T. E., and Froland, S. S., 1974*b*, *Scand. J. Immunol.* 3:29.

Wochner, R. D., Strober, W., and Waldmann, T. A., 1967, *J. Exp. Med.* 126:207.

Wolcott, M., Freeman, D. G., Schrohenloher, R. E., Hammack, W., and Bennett, J. C., 1975, *Immunochemistry* 12:685.

Woodward, D. O., and Munkres, K. D., 1966, *Proc. Natl. Acad. Sci. USA* 55:827.

Wu, T. T., and Kabat, E. A., 1970, *J. Exp. Med.* 132:211.

Yasmeen, D., Ellerson, J. R., Dorrington, K. J., and Painter, R. H., 1973, *J. Immunol.* **110**:1706.

Yasmeen, D., Ellerson, J. R., Dorrington, K. J., and Painter, R. H., 1976, *J. Immunol.* **116**:518.

Yguerabide, J., Epstein, H. F., and Stryer, L., 1970, *J. Mol. Biol.* **51**:573.

Yonemasu, K., and Stroud, R. M., 1972, *Immunochemistry* **9**:545.

Yoshida, A., Mudd, S., and Lenhart, N. A., 1963, *J. Immunol.* **91**:777.

Yoshida, T. O., and Andersson, B., 1972, *Scand. J. Immunol.* **1**:401.

Zegers, B. J. M., Van Der Sluis, J. J., and Ballieux, R. E., 1974, *Biochim. Biophys. Acta* **351**:261.

Zegers, B. J. M., Ballieux, R. E., and Van Loghem, E., 1975, *Scand. J. Immunol.* **4**:161.

Zimmerman, B., and Grey, H. M., 1972, *Biochemistry* **11**:78.

Zipursky, A., Brown, E. J., and Bienenstock, J., 1973, *Proc. Soc. Exp. Biol. Med.* **142**:181.

2

Antigenic Features of Immunoglobulins

J. Michael Kehoe and Rochelle Seide-Kehoe

I. Introduction

In addition to carrying out the diverse functions of the humoral immune system, the family of proteins collectively referred to as "immunoglobulins" possesses important antigenic features. These proteins, in other words, are themselves immunogenic, as would be expected of such large and complex molecules. Detailed study of the precise nature of the antigenic features of immunoglobulins has provided important insights into the organization and complexity of the various members of this protein family, knowledge of how their synthesis is genetically controlled, and information showing how immunological reactions involving immunoglobulins as target molecules can contribute to a number of disease states. It is the purpose of this chapter to provide an overview of what is currently known about these various antigenic properties of immunoglobulins. The chapter by Calvanico and Tomasi in this volume provides relevant information regarding the elements of immunoglobulin structure.

II. Basic Features of Antigenic Determinants

The fundamental nature of antigenic determinants has been clearly described by Sela (1969). For the purpose of the following discussion,

J. Michael Kehoe and Rochelle Seide-Kehoe · Department of Microbiology and Immunology, Northeastern Ohio Universities College of Medicine, Rootstown, Ohio 44272. J. M. K. was supported by an Established Investigator Award from the American Heart Association, by the New York Heart Association, and by NIH Grant AI-09810.

which concerns protein determinants exclusively, only a few basic points need be reemphasized. Antigenic determinants are the subcomponents of a larger intact entity (e.g., a globular protein) that are *individually recognized* by a responding animal. Sela (1969) subcategorized these determinants as *"conformational,"* the uniqueness of which is due to their three-dimensional structure, and *"sequential,"* whose specificity is dependent purely on the linear arrangement of their constituents (e.g., the linear array of amino acids in proteins). It thus follows that the identity of a given determinant is ultimately related, in both instances, to the primary structure of the area concerned. Consequently, it is feasible to search for correlates of particular antigenic determinants, which were defined initially by serological methods, in terms of primary structure. An understanding of the complete antigenic character of a given protein requires both knowledge of the primary structure of the protein and detailed information concerning the tertiary structure of the molecule as determined by X-ray diffraction analysis. In such cases, it is conceivable, at least in theory, to construct a comprehensive antigenic "map" including all of the antigenic determinants characteristic of the molecule in question. Such an ideal state of affairs has been approximated in only a few cases and, as shall become clear, certainly not yet for immunoglobulins.

III. Constant Region Determinants

A. Heavy-Chain Isotypic Determinants

The extreme complexity of the immunoglobulins has been known for many years. The precise basis for this complexity has become much clearer recently because of the extensive structural studies, especially involving amino acid sequence analysis, that have been performed on homogeneous immunoglobulins. For the most part, these proteins have been isolated as paraproteins from the sera of human patients or animals having some form of lymphoid malignancy. However, prior to these elegant chemical studies, much progress was made in understanding some of the reasons for the heterogeneity of antibody molecules through purely immunological studies. The techniques used in this work depended on the presence within the protein of a number of specific antigenic determinants which defined such a particular subcategory of immunoglobulin proteins. Such determinants are characteristic of antibody classes and subclasses in *all* normal individuals of a given species, and are mainly, although not exclusively, associated with the Fc segment of the protein. All are included in the constant region of the heavy chains. These antigenic determinants are referred to as "isotypic" determinants and are detected, in the main, using heterologous antisera produced in a species different from the one serving as the source of the immunoglobulin. An excellent example of the analytical use of isotypic determinants to subcategorize immunoglobulins is the original definition of the four human IgG subclasses by Grey and Kunkel (1964). These workers prepared heterologous antisera to human IgG myeloma proteins in monkeys. Appropriate adsorption of these antisera followed by agar gel precipitin tests allowed the demonstration of the four *subclasses,* now termed "IgG1," "IgG2," "IgG3," and "IgG4."

The antigenic distinctions among *classes* of immunoglobulins are even more pronounced. For example, a general idea of fundamental differences between the IgM and IgG classes can be observed when any attempt (filtration chromatography or analytical ultracentrifugation) is made to physically separate them. However, an even more clear distinction is possible utilizing heterologous antisera that contain specificities directed against isotypic determinants characteristic of the two classes. In such a case, the structure of the isotypic determinants is so divergent between the two classes that no cross-reactivity is discernible. This, in fact, serves to define the class difference of the two groups of proteins.

It seems clear that the existence of distinct isotypic determinants is due to specific conformational features of the constant region of the heavy chains of immunoglobulins. Unlike for some other protein systems, however, such as myoglobin (Atassi, 1975) and lysozyme (Atassi *et al.,* 1976; Lee and Atassi, 1977*a,b*; Atassi and Lee, 1978*a,b*; Atassi, 1978), the location of the various determinants has not been precisely mapped and correlated with particular structural features.

It is also known that some isotypic determinants are common to *all* members of a given class (e.g., IgG) while others are peculiar to individual subclasses (e.g., human IgG1 or IgG3). Still other isotypic determinants are present in more than one subclass but not in *all* subclasses characteristic of a particular class. For example, the human IgG1, IgG2, and IgG3 subclasses share a common determinant correlated with the presence of a proline residue at position 445 of the heavy chain (Eu numbering, C_H3 domain; see Fig. 1). The IgG4 subclass lacks this determinant and has a leucine residue at position 445 (Natvig and Kunkel, 1973).

Known sequences of the Fc segments of proteins representative of the various human IgG subclasses are displayed in Fig. 1. As emphasized previously, information regarding the precise location of specific heavy-chain determinants, be they class, subclass, or allotype specific, is regrettably sparse. They are to be found, however, in large measure, in the

```
        210             215             220             225             230
IgG1 Lys-Val-Asp-Lys-Lys-Val-Glu-Pro-Lys-Ser-Cys-Asp-Lys-Thr-His-Thr-Cys-Pro-Pro-Cys-Pro-Ala-
IgG2 _____Thr_____Arg_____Cys_____[        ]Val-Glu_____
IgG3 Thr-Pro-His)Arg-Cys-Pro_____Thr-Pro-Pro-Pro_____Arg_____
IgG4 _____Arg_____Ser_____Tyr-Gly-[        ]Pro-Pro_____

        235             240             245             250
IgG1 Pro-Glu-Leu-Leu-Gly-Gly-Pro-Ser-Val-Phe-Leu-Phe-Pro-Pro-Lys-Pro-Lys-Asp-Thr-Leu-Met-Ile-
IgG2 ____Pro-Val-Ala [    ]_____
IgG3 _____
IgG4 Ser_____Phe_____

        255             260             265             270             275
IgG1 Ser-Arg-Thr-Pro-Glu-Val-Thr-Cys-Val-Val-Val-Asp-Val-Ser-His-Glu-Asp-Pro-Gln-Val-Lys-Phe-
IgG2 _____Glx-Asx_____Glx_____Glx____
IgG3 _____Glx_____Glx____
IgG4 _____Gln_____(_____Glx_____)

        280             285             290             295
IgG1 Asn-Trp-Tyr-Val-Asp-Gly-Val-Gln-Val-His-Asn-Ala-Lys-Thr-Lys-Pro-Arg-Glu-Gln-Gln-Tyr-Asx-
IgG2 Asx_____Asx_____Glx_____Asx_____
IgG3 Lys_____(Glu_____)_____Glx-Glx-Glx-Phe____
IgG4 _____Glu_____Glu_____Phe____

        300             305             310             315
IgG1 Ser-Thr-Tyr-Arg-Val-Val-Ser-Val-Leu-Thr-Val-Leu-His-Gln-Asn-Trp-Leu-Asp-Gly-Lys-Glu-Tyr-
IgG2
IgG3 _____Phe_____Glx(Asx_____Asx____)_____
IgG4 _____(_____Glx-Asx_____)_____

        320             325             330             335             340
IgG1 Lys-Cys-Lys-Val-Ser-Asn-Lys-Ala-Leu-Pro-Ala-Pro-Ile-Glu-Lys-Thr-Ile-Ser-Lys-Ala-Lys-Gly-
IgG2
IgG3 _____Thr_____
IgG4 _____Gly_____Ser-Ser_____
```

Figure 1.   Available amino acid sequences for the four human IgG subclasses. Numbering system is that of the IgG1 protein shown, Eu (Edelman et al., 1969). The IgG2 sequence is from Wang and Fudenberg (1972), the IgG3 sequence from Wolfenstein-Todel et al. (1976) and Michaelsen et al. (1977), and the IgG4 sequence from Pink et al. (1970). Intersubclass comparisons show primary structure differences of less than 10%, so all antigenic determinant distinctions seen must be accommodated within this degree of covalent structure difference. Structural correlates for the common determinants (i.e., IgG class-specific determinants) should be both more numerous and easier to specifically identify than others (e.g., subclass-specific or allotype-related determinants).

segments of the polypeptide chain shown in Fig. 1. As originally noted by Pink et al. (1970), human subclasses differ by 10% or less in primary sequence in this region on the basis of work completed to date. Thus the subclass-specific determinants (e.g., IgG1 vs. IgG4) result from very modest differences in primary structure. Very likely, detailed crystallo-

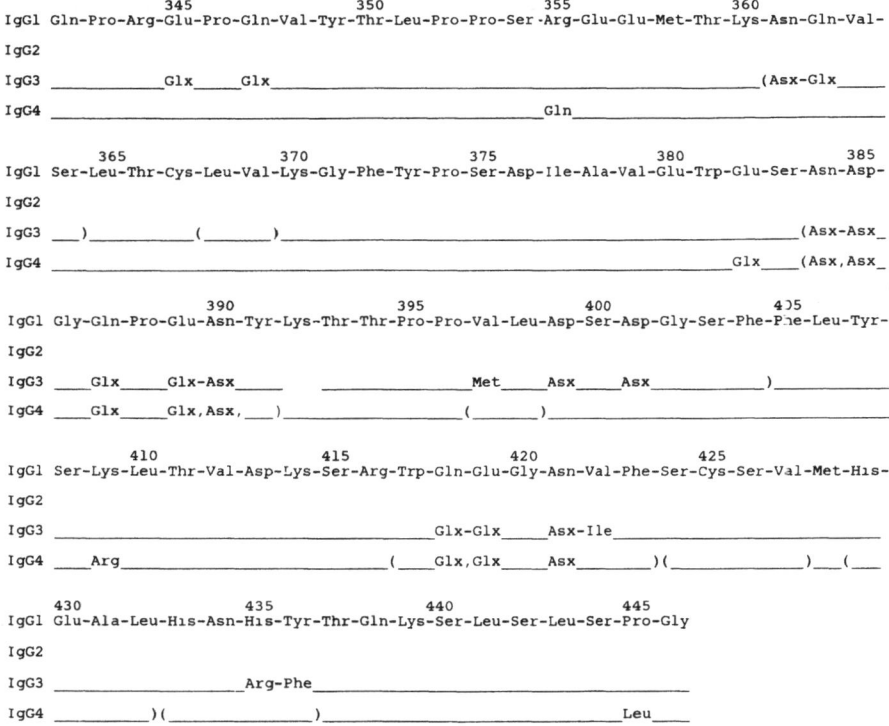

Figure 1 (*continued*)

graphic analyses of Fc structure, such as that being reported by Deisenhofer and Huber and their associates (Deisenhofer *et al.*, 1976; Huber *et al.*, 1976), as well as the preparation of synthetic peptide analogues, will indicate the segments that are of greatest significance with respect to the expression of the various antigenic determinants characteristic of this region of immunoglobulins.

B. Light-Chain Isotypic Determinants

The λ light chains have been shown to express a number of antigenic determinants which also reflect isotypic differences (Fett and Deutsch, 1975). Two distinct antigenic types of human λ chains, termed Oz⁺ and Oz⁻, were originally thought to be allotypic markers (see below) but were later shown by genetic analyses to be isotypic in nature. *Both* types of chain are thus found in all normal individuals. The structural correlate for the Oz^+ and Oz^- distinction is associated with position 193 (Mcg numbering) of the λ chain, which contains lysine in Oz^+ proteins and arginine in Oz^- proteins (Table I). Another isotypic variant, termed "Kern," has been associated with position 156, where $Kern^+$ proteins have a glycine residue and $Kern^-$ proteins a serine. The antigenic differences shown by serological analyses appear to be fully explained by these small differences in primary structure. The determinants, in these cases, have consequently been very precisely mapped, especially when information on the three-dimensional structure of human λ proteins is taken into account (Shiffer et al., 1973).

Still another λ chain variant has been described by Fett and Deutsch (1975) totally on the basis of the primary structure of a λ chain termed "Mcg" and related proteins. This variant is correlated with differences in *three* positions of the Mcg λ constant region, as compared with other λ proteins. Mcg^+ variants have asparagine at position 116, threonine at position 118, and lysine at position 167. Mcg^- proteins, on the other hand, have alanine, serine, and threonine at these respective positions (Table I).

Very recently, Solomon (1977) has shown that the distinct antigenic determinants characteristic of the two variants can both be detected serologically by appropriate antisera. The determinants involved in the Mcg isotype are complex since their expression is dependent on the presence of *both* the variable and constant domains of the λ chain, in spite of the fact that the primary structure correlates are entirely in the constant region, as established by the studies of Fett and Deutsch (1975). Very likely, as proposed by Solomon, the amino-terminal segment of the variable domain participates in the expression of the determinant associated with the Mcg variants.

Table I. λ-Chain Isotypic Variants[a]

Isotypic variant	Position[b]	Residue found
Oz^+		Lys
Oz^-	193	Arg
$Kern^+$		Gly
$Kern^-$	156	Ser
Mcg^+		Asp/Thr/Lys
Mcg^-	116/118/167	Ala/Ser/Thr

[a] The identity and location of important λ-chain isotypic variants. See text for further discussion and references.
[b] Mcg numbering.

C. Nonisotypic Light-Chain Constant Region Determinants

Immunoglobulin light chains also contain other important antigenic determinants in the constant segments. Early studies of the urinary Bence-Jones proteins that commonly accompany multiple myeloma and related neoplastic disorders involving the lymphoid system showed that two main types of human light chains exist, which were termed "κ" and "λ." These protein types are readily distinguished by heterologous antisera, which can recognize antigenic determinants present in the constant region of the respective chains. The precise nature and location of most of these determinants are also presently unclear, however, even though the details of the covalent structure of the polypeptide segments involved have been known for some time. The resolution of this question will also require careful determinant mapping studies, a project which should be aided enormously by the availability of high-resolution X-ray diffraction models of human light chains (Schiffer *et al.*, 1973). To the authors' knowledge, there have been no reports to date of the existence of antigenic determinants common to both κ and λ chains.

McLaughlin and Solomon (1973) described an interesting "hidden" antigenic determinant in the constant region of a human kappa Bence-Jones protein. This determinant was not detectable in the intact polypeptide chain but could be revealed either by cleaving the chain between the variable and constant domains or by unfolding in denaturing solvents such as urea. Here again, the details of the three-dimensional structure of the intact protein would seem to define the reactivity of a given determinant.

An idea of the complexities associated with light-chain determinants is clear from the difficulties that are occasionally encountered in adsorbing antisera that contain anti-light-chain specificities. For example, Prendergast *et al.* (1966), using IgA proteins, observed that anti-κ-chain specificities elicited by the injection of one protein were not always removed by adsorption with a different κ protein. It would appear that there can be modulation of certain κ-specific determinants by the interaction of the light chain with the heavy chain. This kind of phenomenon has been observed in a number of different systems and must always be taken into account in the interpretation of data based on the recognition of antigenic determinants in any proteins of complex quaternary structure.

An undoubtedly related phenomenon has been seen with respect to the influence of interchain disulfide bonds on the detection of light-chain-specific and other types of immunoglobulin determinants. It is occasionally observed that the simple reduction of an immunoglobulin, by the inclusion of a mercaptan reductant in the buffer, will facilitate the detection of light-chain or other determinants. An important overall principle regarding the antigenic determinants of immunoglobulins, and other proteins, thus emerges: such determinants can be modulated by a number of different factors, including, but not restricted to, the conformation of neighboring local regions of the polypeptide chain and the disposition of critical disulfide bonds. Specific procedures may be required to fully reveal many of these determinants.

IV. Allotypic Markers

Allotypes are serologically detected genetic markers present on some, but not all, immunoglobulin molecules in a given species. In most cases, they are under the control of allelic genes, and as such are analogous to many other known protein polymorphisms. As opposed to isotypic and some idiotypic determinants, these markers are detected by alloantisera, i.e., sera raised in the *same* species. There are some immunoglobulin genetic markers described in the mouse and rabbit that are not antigenic and are detected by exclusively chemical methods, but discussion of these is beyond the scope of this chapter (Edelman and Gottlieb, 1970; Thunberg *et al.*, 1973; Mole, 1976).

Allotypic markers have been of great importance in helping to understand the structure of immunoglobulins and the genetic regulation of immunoglobulin synthesis. For example, the study of allotypic markers contributed to the notion that a single polypeptide chain may be encoded by two genes (Todd, 1963) and that the structural genes for heavy and light chains are unlinked (Dubiski *et al.*, 1962).

By far the greatest number of different allotypic markers have been found in man. Allotypes have also been found in a number of other species, however, including the rabbit, mouse, rat, cow, and chicken. For this chapter, we will be concerned mainly with structural correlates of human and rabbit allotypes. The general subject of allotypes is extremely well described in several excellent reviews (Mage *et al.*, 1973; Natvig and Kunkel, 1973; Kindt, 1975; Kunkel and Kindt, 1975), and the reader is directed to these for additional information.

Antigenic markers (allotypes) of immunoglobulin molecules were almost simultaneously reported for human and rabbit antibodies. Oudin (1956) observed that rabbit antibodies themselves elicited precipitating antibodies when they were injected into certain other rabbits. Oudin named the phenomenon "allotypy" and the antigenic determinants on the immunoglobulin molecules were called "allotypes." At the same time, Grubb (1956) reported that some sera from patients with rheumatoid arthritis which contain rheumatoid factors (see below) would specifically agglutinate human red blood cells (RBC) coated with certain incomplete antihuman RBC antibodies. These agglutination reactions could be inhibited by sera from particular individuals whose immunoglobulins presumably had the same antigenic determinants as the molecules coated on the RBC. Those rheumatoid factors that agglutinate antibody-coated RBC are called "Raggs" and may be directed against more than one specificity. Other, more specific agglutinators have been found in normal sera. Some of these agglutinating activities, which are called "Snaggs" (serum normal agglutinators), arise as a result of maternal-fetal incompatibilities, whereas some may be induced as a result of frequent transfusions. It is not necessary to use incomplete antibodies to coat RBC to detect allotypic specificities; indicator immunoglobulins can be passively adsorbed onto RBCs by the use of a bifunctional reagent, such as chromium chloride, bis-diazotized benzidine, or glutaraldehyde.

The very sensitive hemagglutination inhibition system is most often used to detect human and certain rabbit allotypes since most antisera are not of very high titer or affinity. In the rabbit, certain antiallotype sera (e.g., those sera directed against the group a and b allotypes) are relatively higher in precipitin titer.

Most rabbit allotypes are qualitatively determined by interfacial (ring) precipitation or by precipitation in gels using appropriate antisera. Quantitative measurements of rabbit allotypes can be made by the use of very sensitive radiobinding assays (Gottlieb et al., 1975).

The differences in the titer of antiallotype antibody produced reflect the particular antigenic determinants involved. The allotypic determinants of human immunoglobulins are small, often single amino acid interchanges in proteins of the same subclass. Amino acids involved in the determinant may be considerably removed from one another in the linear sequence in those instances when more than one amino acid is important, however. Examples are the group a and b allotypic determinants of rabbits which involve multiple amino acid differences scattered along the chain (Kindt, 1975).

Gutman et al. (1975) have classified allotypes into two categories on the basis of determinant complexity. Simple allotypes are those whose different forms are determined by single amino acid differences, while complex allotypes are those that differ at multiple positions in the polypeptide chain. As more structural and X-ray diffraction data have become available for immunoglobulins, it has become apparent that amino acids far removed in the linear sequence could be correlated with allotypy and were, in fact, in close approximation in the tertiary structure. The juxtaposition of these distinct residues gives rise to the specific conformational determinants characteristic of the allotype.

With the exception of group a allotypes in the rabbit and a single report of a human heavy chain determinant (Wang *et al.*, 1978; see below), all of the serologically identifiable allotypic markers so far described are localizable to the constant regions of immunoglobulin polypeptide chains. In man the Gm markers are found on IgG heavy chains, the Am marker is found on heavy chains from the IgA2 subclass, and the Km(InV) markers are found on κ light chains. The newly proposed nomenclature for presenting human immunoglobulin allotypes will be used here (WHO, 1976). The currently recommended and previous designations for allotypic determinants as well as their localization to a specific polypeptide chain are presented in Table IIA.

As yet, allotypic markers on human λ light chains and the heavy

Table IIA. Recommended Nomenclature for Human Allotypes[a]

Location	Chain	Previous designation		Current designation	
		Alphameric	Numeric	Alphameric	Numeric
IgG1	γ_1	Gm(a)	Gm(1)	G1m(a)	G1m(1)
		(x)	(2)	(x)	(2)
		(b^w), (b2), (f)	(3)(4)	(f)	(3)
		(z)	(17)	(z)	(17)
IgG2	γ_2	Gm(n)	Gm(23)	G2m(n)	G2m(23)
IgG3	γ_3	Gm(bβ), (b0)	Gm(11)	G3m(b0)	G3m(11)
		(b), (b1), (bγ)	(5)(12)	(b1)	(5)
		(b3), (Bet)	(13)(25)	(b3)	(13)
		(b4)	(14)	(b4)	(14)
		(bα), (b5)	(10)	(b5)	(10)
		Gm-like, (c), (c3)	(6)	(c3)	(6)
		Gm-like, (c), (c5)	(24)	(c5)	(24)
		(g)	(21)	(g)	(21)
		(s)	(15)	(s)	(15)
		(t)	(16)	(t)	(16)
		(Pa)		(u)	(26)
		(Ray)		(v)	(27)
IgA2	α_2	Am(1)	Am$_2$	A2m(1)	A2m(1)
				A2m(2)	A2m(2)
k chain	κ	InV, Inv(1)	Inv(1)	Km(1)	Km(1)
		(a)	(2)	(2)	(2)
		(b)	(3)	(3)	(3)

[a] Nomenclature as proposed by WHO and reported in *J. Immunol.* **117**:1056 (1976).

chains of IgA1, IgD, and IgE have not been found. On the other hand, allotypic determinants on the heavy chain from murine "IgD-like" proteins and rabbit λ light chains as well as allotypes of heavy chains from rabbit IgM and IgA have been described (Kunkel and Kindt, 1975; Goding et al., 1976).

A. Allotypes of Human Immunoglobulins

1. Light Chains: The Km Markers

There are three Km antigenic types of human κ light chains designated as "Km(1)," "Km(2)," and "Km(3)," formerly referred to as "Inv(1)," "Inv(2)," and "Inv(3)" (see Table IIA). It has been shown that the inheritance of these markers is determined by three Km alleles, termed $Km^{1,2}$, Km^1, and Km^3 (Ropartz et al., 1964). In most whites (98%), the Km(1) and Km(2) markers are found together. These are inherited through the $Km^{1,2}$ allele. A small proportion (2%) of the white population carries only the Km(1) antigen and therefore the rare Km^1 allele So far, there have been no individuals described who carry only the Km(2) marker.

Sequence analysis carried out mainly on κ chains of the Km(1,2) type or Km(3) type has allowed the correlation of certain amino acid residues with antigenic activity. The Km(1,2) antigen is associated with a leucine at position 191 of κ chains, while Km(3) is associated with a valine at that position (Milstein, 1966). Recently, it was shown that Km(1) is also associated with a leucine at position 191 and furthermore that the Km markers are additionally associated with an amino acid interchange at position 153 of κ chains (Milstein et al., 1974). In Km(1,2) and Km(3) chains, an alanine is present at position 153, whereas Km(1) chains have a valine in this position. Comparison of the location of these residues in κ chains to X-ray crystallographic data available for the homologous regions of human λ chains indicates that these two positions are exposed on the surface of the molecule and are located in close spatial proximity, no more than 8–10 A apart (Poljak et al., 1974). It is now thought that antiserum to Km(2) recognizes the leucine at position 191 but also includes position 153. Replacement of alanine by valine at position 153 probably hinders the binding of anti-Km(2) to its antigenic determinant. Furthermore, the antiserum to Km(1) recognizes only position 191 and is not inhibited by the amino acid interchange at position 153 (Milstein et al., 1974).

2. Heavy Chains

a. Variable Region Markers. A most interesting heavy-chain variable region genetic marker has recently been described by Wang *et al.* (1978). This is the first report of a human variable region allotypic marker. The determinant, termed "Hv(1)," was discovered when an antiserum elicited in rabbits to an IgM protein (McE) was found to react with a number of monoclonal immunoglobulins of various classes (IgG, IgA, IgM). Experiments using a variety of individual polypeptide chains and proteolytic fragments of immunoglobulins showed that this determinant was localized in the variable region of the heavy chain. Genetic and population studies suggested that the marker was transmitted as an autosomal dominant trait, although some alternative genetic mechanisms could not be formally excluded.

In view of the unique character of this marker, it will be of considerable interest to examine further its distribution in human populations and, in addition, to see if additional, comparable determinants can be found.

b. Gm Markers. Gm allotypic markers are located in the constant regions of IgG heavy chains. Some serological specificities require the presence of light chains, however, to assume the proper quaternary structure necessary for antigenic expression (Natvig and Kunkel, 1973), a point alluded to earlier in this chapter.

Elegant studies by Natvig and Turner (1971), utilizing different enzyme digestion schemes, localized several of the different allotypic specificities within different homology regions of the subclasses where they are found. Constant region heavy-chain markers were assigned to the C_H1 homology region if they were detected on Fab fragments. Markers were assigned to the C_H2 region if allotype test systems were inhibited by the intact Fc fragment, but not by the pFc' fragment. Other antigens were assigned to the C_H3 homology regions when the test systems could be inhibited by both Fc and pFc' fragments. By these methods, various subclass and allotypic markers have been localized to one or another of the homology regions (see Table III).

G1m(f) and (z) are found in the C_H1 homology region of IgG1 molecules, while G1m(a), G1m(x), and nG1m(a) (nonmarkers will be discussed further below) are found in the C_H3 homology region of IgG1. Likewise, G2m(n) and G3m(g) and (b1) have been localized to the C_H2 homology regions of IgG_2 and IgG_3 heavy chains, respectively. Furthermore, amino acid interchanges presumably responsible for different allotypic differences have been found. For example, in IgG1 heavy chains carrying the G1m(a) allotype, the tetrapeptide Arg-*Asp*-Glu-*Leu* is found in positions

355–358 (Eu numbering, Fig. 1). Heavy chains carrying the antithetical marker nGlm(a) have a sequence Arg-*Glu*-Glu-*Met* in this region. Thus these markers are associated with two amino acid interchanges, an Asp to Glu interchange at position 356 and a Leu to Met interchange at position 358. Glm(f) and (z) are associated with an arginine to lysine interchange, respectively, at position 214 (see Table III).

Although allotypic determinants have been localized to immunoglobulin fragments and subfragments and in some instances are associated with specific amino acid interchanges, certain allotypic markers require the integrity of the immunoglobulin quaternary structure for their antigenic expression. This is particularly true for the Glm(f) and (z) markers on the IgG Fd fragment and the Km markers of Cκ domains. Heterologous mixing of heavy and light chains has shown, however, that the markers are specifically on one chain or the other but are expressed only in combination with each other (Litwin and Kunkel, 1967). Furthermore, tertiary structure integrity is necessary for the expression of Glm(a) and nGlm(a). The antigenic integrity of these determinants is intact in a complete pFc' fragment but is lost on further enzymatic degradation of the fragment (Natvig and Turner, 1971).

Population studies have shown that various allotypic markers are inherited as a result of particular gene complexes (Natvig and Kunkel, 1968, 1973). For example, in whites, Glm(a) and (z) are found on the same IgG molecule, whereas Glm(a) and (f) are not found together. However, in orientals Glm(a) and (f) have been found together. The glm(x) marker, when it is present, is always associated with the Glm(a) marker. Also, the presence of the Glm(a) and (z) markers is associated with the expression of the G3m(g) marker in whites. These associations have proved very informative, not only for elucidating the genetic linkage relationship of immunoglobulins in various populations but also for identifying hybrid immunoglobulin molecules that have provided useful information on the order and number of IgG heavy-chain constant region genes (Kunkel *et al.*, 1969; Natvig and Kunkel, 1974).

     c. Am Markers.   Am markers are found on the heavy chains of the IgA2 subclass, most of which lack the heavy-chain–light-chain disulfide bond. There are two variants of these markers known as "A2m(1)" and "A2m(2)." The A2m(1) marker is found in IgA2 molecules lacking the heavy-chain–light-chain disulfide bridge, whereas the A2m(2) marker is found in those IgA2 molecules that have the interchain disulfide bridge. Chemical analysis has shown that the peptide around the interchain disulfide bridge in both IgA1 and A2m(2) IgA2 proteins is the same (Mihaesco *et al.*, 1971).

     d. Isoallotypes (Nonmarkers).   Isoallotypes (formerly known as "nonmarkers") are markers that behave as allotypes within one IgG subclass but are always present in one or more of the other subclasses, therefore behaving as though they were isotypes (Table IIB). These markers were originally described for myeloma proteins and can be serologically detected in normal proteins by the use of antisera raised in animals and specifically adsorbed; they are not recognized by alloantisera. For example, Glm(a) and nG1m(a) are allotypes of IgG1 for which specific amino acid interchanges have been determined (see above and Table III). However, the antigenic determinant of NG1m(a), and its associated sequence stretch, is always found in IgG2 and IgG3 proteins. A similar sequence appears in IgG4 proteins, but the determinant is not antigenic. There must be some unique orientation of this segment of the IgG4 chain (buried in solvent?) that precludes its full antigenic expression. Isoallotypic markers related to other allotypes have also been found (Table IIA).

There are two markers of IgG4 that behave as allelic variants of each other (and are therefore mutually exclusive) in this subclass but are present in all the other subclasses. The nG4m(a) marker is present in some IgG4 molecules and in all IgG1 and IgG3 molecules, whereas the nG4m(b) antigen is present in IgG2 proteins and in IgG4 proteins that lack nG4m(a). No IgG4 protein has been found that has both markers. These antigens can be used as genetic markers for IgG4 only after its Fc fragments have been isolated from normal serum. The nG4m(a) marker is associated with a leucine at position 309 of the heavy chain of IgG4 proteins, whereas the nG4m(b) marker is associated with a deletion at this position (Table III).

Table IIB.   Recommended Nomenclature for
             Human Isoallotypes[a]

Previous designation	Current designation	
	Alphameric	Numeric
non-a	nG1m(a)	nG1m(1)
nG1m(z)	nG1m(z)	nG1m(17)
non-b0	nG3m(b0)	nG3m(11)
non-b1	nG3m(b1)	nG3m(5)
non-g	nG3m(g)	nG3m(21)
4a	nG4m(a)	nG4m(a)
4b	nG4m(b)	nG4m(b)
nA2m(2)	nA2m(2)	nA2m(2)

[a] Nomenclature as proposed by WHO and reported in J. Immunol. 117:1056 (1976).

Table III. Localization of Certain Human Allotypic Markers[a]

Antigen	Chain	Homology region	Position	Amino acid found
Glm(a)	γ_1	C_H3	355–358	Arg-*Asp*-Glu-*Leu*
nGlm(a)	$\gamma_{1,2,3}$	C_H3	355–358	Arg-*Glu*-Glu-*Met*
Glm(f)	γ_1	C_H1	214	Arg
Glm(z)	γ_1	C_H1	214	Lys
Glm(g)	γ_3	C_H2	296	Tyr
nG3m(g)	$\gamma_{2,3}$	C_H2	296	Phe
G3m(b0)	γ_3	C_H3	436	Phe
nG3m(b0)	$\gamma_{1,2,3}$	C_H3	436	Tyr
nG4m(a)	γ_4	C_H2	309	Val-Leu-His
nG4m(b)	γ_4	C_H2	309	Val-(—)-His
Km(1)	κ	C_κ	153 . . . 191	*Val* . . . *Leu*
Km(1, 2)	κ	C_κ	153 . . . 191	Ala . . . *Leu*
Km(3)	κ	C_κ	153 . . . 191	Ala . . . *Val*

[a] Localization of certain human allotypic markers. Refer to Fig. 1 for linear location within the heavy-chain constant region of the various IgG subclasses.

Thus considerable progress has been made in identifying, characterizing, and locating the antigenic determinants associated with a number of human allotypic markers. These determinants are often quite complex with contributions from amino acids that are widely removed from one another in the linear sequence. This is therefore still another area where the details of the tertiary, or quaternary, structure of the immunoglobulin are crucial to the expression of a given function.

B. Allotypes of Rabbit Imunoglobulins

Allotypic determinants have been described for most of the different rabbit immunoglobulin chains (Kindt, 1975). Allotypes are present in the *variable* region of all heavy chains (groups a, x, and y). Other allotypic determinants have been localized to the constant region of γ heavy chains (groups d and e), α_1 heavy chains (group f), α_2 heavy chains (group g), and μ heavy chains (groups n and ms). Furthermore, allotypes have been described for κ (group b) and λ (group c) light chains and for the secretory component (group t) of IgA. These allotypic specificities and their location are summarized in Table IV.

Although many different allotypic groups are known in the rabbit, structural data on what constitutes the antigenic determinants are available (and, in most instances, only partially) only for the allotypes of groups a, b, d, e, f, g, and a negative (x and y).

Table IV. Allotypic Specificities of Rabbit Immunoglobulins[a]

Allotype group	Specificities	Location	References
a	1, 2, 3	Heavy chain, variable region	Oudin (1956, 1960), Todd (1963), Stemke (1964)
x	32		Kim and Dray (1972, 1973)
y	33		Kim and Dray (1972, 1973)
d	11, 12	γ chain, constant region	Mandy and Todd (1968, 1969, 1970)
e	13, 14		Dubiski (1969a,b)
	A8, A10	γ chain, constant region (a1 molecules only)	Hamers and Hamers-Casterman (1965)
f	69, 70, 71, 72, 73	α_1 chain, constant region	Conway et al. (1969a), Hanly et al. (1973)
g	74, 75, 76, 77	α_2 chain, constant region	Conway et al. (1969b), Hanly et al. (1973)
n	81, 82	μ chain, constant region	Gilman-Sachs and Dray (1972)
ms	1, 2, 3, 4, 5, 6		Kelus and Pernis (1971)
b	4, 5, 6, 9	κ light chains	Oudin (1960), Stemke (1964), Dubiski and Muller (1967)
c	7, 21	λ light chains	Mage et al. (1968)
t	61, 62	Secretory component	Knight et al. (1974)

[a] Intramolecular localization of rabbit allotypic determinants. See text and Fig. 2 for more detailed description.

1. Group d and e Allotypes

Group d markers are simple allotypes associated with a Met (d11) to Thr (d12) interchange at position 225 in the hinge region of rabbit γ chains (Prahl et al., 1969). The sequence of positions 220–230 of d11 heavy chains is Thr-Cys-Ser-Lys-Pro-Met-Cys-Pro-Pro-Pro-Glu. The only difference found in d12 chains is the Thr at position 225. It has recently been shown (McBurnette and Mandy, 1974) that a small hinge region peptide, containing Met-225, isolated from a γ chain carrying the d11 allotype, quantitatively reacted with antisera directed against the d11 allotype, thereby confirming the correlation of the Met at position 225 with antigenic activity.

Group e allotypes have been correlated with a Thr (e14) to Ala (e15) interchange at position 309 of rabbit γ chains (Appella et al., 1971). This difference was the only one found among tryptic peptides from the Fc region of e14 and e15 heavy chains.

2. Group f and g Allotypes

The f and g markers are complex allotypes composed of multiple amino acid residues located in the constant region of rabbit secretory IgA (SIgA) heavy chains (Conway *et al.*, 1969*a,b*; Hanly *et al.*, 1973). Two subclasses of rabbit SIgA termed "SIgA-f" and "SIgA-g" have been found based on their susceptibility to proteolytic cleavage (Hanly *et al.*, 1973; Knight *et al.*, 1973; Tseng and Knight, 1975). The SIgA-f subclass, which is resistant to papain and trypsin cleavage, carries the f allotypic specificities (see Table IV). The SIgA-g subclass, which carries the g determinants, can be cleaved by both papain and trypsin to yield $Fc_{2\alpha}$ and $F(ab)_{2\alpha}$ fragments.

Malek and Knight (1977) have recently shown that if SIgA was mildly reduced and alkylated prior to papain digestion, the SIgA-f molecules could be cleaved. Using this method in conjunction with quantitative radioprecipitation by specific antisera directed against f allotypic determinants, they were able to show that many of the relevant antigenic determinants were located in the $Fc_{2\alpha}$ fragment of the SIgA-f molecule.

Previous immunochemical and serological studies on the papain-sensitive SIgA-g subclass had shown that some of the g allotypic determinants were localized to the Fc region while other g determinants were found on the Fd region of the alpha heavy chain (Knight *et al.*, 1973). In a recent study, Malek *et al.* (1978) found an allotype-related Cys to Ser interchange at position 311 when they compared sequences of heavy-chain fragments from g75 and g76 molecules. Furthermore, they found evidence for an "extra" intradomain disulfide bridge in the $C_{\alpha}2$ domain of g74 heavy chains. The relationship of this finding to the nature of the specific allotypic determinant is not yet known.

3. Group a Allotypes

Rabbits are unique in that they possess allotypic specificities in the variable portion of their heavy chains (Todd, 1963). The group a markers are complex allotypes (Gutman *et al.*, 1975) correlated with multiple amino acid interchanges. Mole *et al.* (1975) have shown that the group a allotypes are totally localizable within the variable region by isolating the intact variable regions from rabbit IgG heavy chains and demonstrating that these fragments quantitatively react with allotype-specific antisera.

In early studies to determine the structural basis for allotypic specificities, Wilkinson (1969*a,b*) isolated amino-terminal peptides from IgG and IgA molecules with defined allotypes. He was able to find differences in amino acid sequence in the peptides isolated from chains with different allotypes and concluded that structural correlates for the various group a markers did exist.

Further sequence analysis by Mole *et al.* (1971) of pooled IgG heavy chains of either allotype a1 or a3 delineated additional areas for potential allotypic correlations (Todd, 1972). These were compared with the sequence of a homogeneous antibody of allotype a2 (Fleischman, 1971). These studies showed, when corrected for hypervariable sequences and group a negative molecules, that amino acid interchanges occurring at positions 4, 7, 9, 11, 12, 15, and 16 could be correlated with group a allotypes. In addition substitutions at positions 80–85 from the amino-terminal end of the heavy chain could also be associated with allotypic differences.

Subsequent studies (Jaton *et al.*, 1973) showed that not all of the differences in this region (positions 80–85) were allotype related. However, these investigators showed that interchanges at positions 84 and 85 were definite allotypic correlates. Allotype a1 molecules were shown to have a Thr-Glu sequence in this region, a2 molecules an Ala-Glu, and a3 molecules an Ala-Ala sequence.

Corrections of sequence alignment may actually move these last allotypic correlates to positions 85–86 (Johnstone and Mole, 1977). Also, it was shown by Mole (1975) that variations in these two residues are the basis for a chemically defined variable region genetic marker. Additional allotype-related sequences occur in the region composed of positions 60–75 (Kindt and Mole, 1974). All amino acid substitutions that have been described as allotypic correlates occur in the variable region framework residues (see below). A composite summary of available sequence data correlating particular amino acid substitutions with group a allotypes is given in Fig. 2.

Although group a allotypic correlates are quite distant from one another along the polypeptide chain, examination of X-ray crystallographic data (Poljak *et al.*, 1973) has shown that certain positions, such as 15–17 and 84–85, are in close proximity in the folded polypeptide chain. This appears analogous to the situation described above for the Km markers of human κ chains where widely spaced amino acid residues can contribute to the relevant antigenic determinant.

It is still not totally clear exactly how the specific amino acid substitutions that correlate with group a allotypes are related to the antigenic determinants involved (Todd, 1972). Especially pertinent are the indications that a given allotype may be composed of numerous subspecificities. For example, Kindt *et al.* (1973) showed that homogeneous anticarbo-

Allotype	Ig	Designation	Antigen	4	7	9	11	12	14	15	16	64	66	69	70	73	84	85
				Glu	Gly	Arg	Val	Thr	Gly	Thr	Pro	Gly	Phe	Ser	Lys	Thr	Thr	Glu
a1		3381	S3	—	—	—	—	—	—	—	—	—	—	—	—	—	—	—
		3374	S3	—	—	—	—	—	—	—	—	—	—	—	—	—	—	—
		120	M. lyso.	—	—	—	—	—	—	—	—	—	—	—	—	—	—	—
		Pool IgG	—	—	—	—	—	—	—	—	—	—	—	—	—	—	—	—
		3T 72	S3	—	—	—	—	—	—	Gly	Ser	—	—	—	—	—	—	—
		BS-5	S3	—	—	—	—	—	Thr	Pro	Gly	—	—	—	—	—	—	—
a2		K 25	S3	Lys	Glu	Gly	Phe	Lys	Thr	Asp	Thr	Ser	Ser	Thr	Arg	Asx	Ala	Gln
		BS-1	S3	Lys	Glu	Gly	Phe	Lys	Thr	Asp	Thr	Ser	Ser	Thr	Arg	Asx	Ala	Glx
		2690	strep C	Lys	Glu	Gly	Phe	Lys	Thr	Asp	Thr	Ser	Ser	Thr	Arg		Ala	Ala
		Pool IgG	—	Lys	Glu	Gly	Phe	Lys	Thr	Asp	Thr		Ser	Thr	Arg			
a3		Pool IgG	—	—	—	Asp	—	Lys	—	Ala	Ser	—	—	—	—		Ala	Ala
a neg.		Pool IgG				Gly		Gln	Glu	Gly	Ser							
		3547	strep A	Val		Gly		Gln		Gly	Ser	Asn	Arg	Ile	Ser	Asn	Ser	Leu

Figure 2.   Rabbit group a allotype structural correlates. Allotype-associated differences in the V_H region exclusive of hypervariable regions are shown. The proteins were prepared either from pools of IgG or from homogeneous antibodies raised against bacterial polysaccharides. Specific references are as follows: the a1 S3 antibodies 3381, 3374, 3T72 (Margolies et al., 1977); a1 S3 antibody BS-5 (Jaton, 1975); a1 micrococcal antibody 120 (van Haegaerden and Strosberg, 1976); a1 pool (Mole, 1976); a2 antibodies K25 and BS-1 (Jaton, 1975, 1976); a2 antibody 2690 streptococcal C antibody (Fleischman, 1973); a2 pool (Mole, 1976); a3 pool (Mole et al., 1971); a-negative pool (Johnstone and Mole, 1977); a-negative streptococcal A antibody 3547 (Johnstone et al., 1978). Reproduced with permission and slight modification from Margolies et al. (1977).

hydrate antibodies bearing the a3 allotype could not totally inhibit the reaction between pooled a3 IgG and anti a3 antisera. Various homogeneous proteins carried somewhat different, but additive, subspecificities. Subspecificities within the a1 allotype have also been reported (Horng *et al.*, 1976). Recently, a serological and structural investigation of a homogeneous antibody which carried the a1 specificity, but was antigenically deficient to pooled IgG, has shown that positions 15 and 16 are probably involved in the a1 allotypic determinant (Margolies *et al.*, 1977). This antibody had the sequence Gly-Ser instead of Thr-Pro which is seen in pooled IgG and several other antibodies (see Fig. 2). Additional detailed structural and serological analysis of this sort should begin to reveal the exact determinants that compose group a allotypes.

4. Group x and y Allotypes

The x and y allotypes are additional variable region markers that are encoded by two separate genes, which are linked to, but distinct from, the gene(s) coding for group a allotypes (Kim and Dray, 1972). Very little information is available on the amino acid correlates of these determinants. They are present on antibodies lacking group a allotypes and are consequently included in that category termed "a-negative" molecules.

Although structural correlates of the x and y allotypes are not yet known, some general comparisons between those heavy chains lacking group a allotypes (group a-negative) and those carrying them (group a-positive) have been made. These types of chains may represent different subgroups (see below) in the rabbit. Sequence studies have shown that group a-positive molecules have a pGlu-Ser-Val or pGlu-Ser-Leu sequence at their amino-terminal end whereas group a-negative molecules have a pGlu-Glu-Gln sequence (Prahl *et al.*, 1973). More recent studies (Johnstone and Mole, 1977; Johnstone *et al.*, 1978) have shown that group a-negative molecules show nearly 80% sequence homology with the human V_HIII subgroup (Capra and Kehoe, 1975) while group a-positive molecules are most homologous to the V_HII subgroup (Mole, 1975; Jaton, 1975). In light of these findings, it would be of interest to see whether the antisera that have been prepared against subgroups of human immunoglobulins (Forre *et al.*, 1976) would react with the appropriate category of rabbit molecules. This similarity may well be relevant to the difficulties that have been observed in eliciting the production of antisera in rabbits that bear specificities for human subgroups.

5. Group b Allotypes

The group b determinants are complex allotypes found on rabbit κ chains. It is generally accepted that these determinants consist of multiple amino acid residues in the constant region of the molecule, although some sequence variation at the amino-terminal segment may be involved (Waterfield *et al.*, 1973). It has been shown, however, that homogeneous anticarbohydrate antibodies carrying the b4 determinant can have identical serological reactivity even though they possess significant amino-terminal sequence differences (Kindt *et al.*, 1972).

Differences in carboxyl-terminal peptides (positions 210–214) have been correlated with group b allotypes (Frangione, 1969; Appella *et al.*, 1969). Light chains with the b4 allotype have the sequence *Asn*-Arg-*Gly*-*Asp*-Cys here, while b5 molecules have a *Ser*-Arg-*Lys*-*Asx*-Cys sequence, and b6 molecules a *Ser*-Arg-*Lys*-*Ser*-Cys sequence in this region. The italicized residues are where b5 and b6 molecules differ from b4. The b4 molecules differ from human κ chains only at position 213, where the human molecule has a *Glu*. The b9 molecule is identical to b4 chains in this region (Goodfleisch, 1975).

Complete or nearly complete amino acid sequence data are available for several b4 light chains (Chen *et al.*, 1974; Margolies *et al.*, 1974; Appella *et al.*, 1973; Jaton, 1974). The reported sequences are identical in the constant region, with the exception of position 174 which is an Asn in one chain (Chen *et al.*, 1974) and either Val or Leu in others (Appella *et al.*, 1973; Strosberg *et al.*, 1972). It is presently unclear whether this position is actually involved in the b4 antigenic determinant. Recently, an inherited variant of the b4 allotype with amino acid substitutions at positions 121 and 124 has been reported (Sogn and Kindt, 1976). Most b4 light chains have Ala at position 121 and Glu at position 124, whereas the variant chain has a Ser at 121 and Leu at 124. These substitutions appeared not to alter the antigenicity of the b4 light chain; however, it has been seen more recently that some b4 antisera will detect antigenic differences between normal b4 chains and the variant b4 chain (T. J. Kindt, personal communication).

Variations in sequence among molecules carrying the b4, b5, and b9 allotypes have been seen in the region around the Cys at position 171. This residue participates in the interdomain disulfide bridge that is found in most rabbit light chains (Poulsen *et al.*, 1972). The b4 chain sequence from position 163–171 is Lys-Thr-Pro-Glu-Asn-Ser-Ala-Asp-Cys. The b5 molecule differs from the b4 only by an Asp substitution at position 169. The b9 molecule, however, differs from the others by four substitutions: a Thr at position 163 and a Ser-Pro-Glu sequence at positions 167–169. The constant region sequence of a b9 molecule that has recently been determined (Goodfleisch, 1975; Farnsworth *et al.*, 1976) differs from that of b4 molecules by about 35% of its total sequence. This has made it difficult to ascertain which of the multiple amino acid substitutions in the constant region of rabbit κ light chains are actually involved in the allotype antigenic determinants. Still more structural data on chains of different allotypes will be needed to fully resolve this question.

Since most rabbit κ chains have been identified either by amino acid sequence analysis or by their reactivity with anti-b-specific allotype sera, it is not known whether purely κ-specific determinants (distinct from allotype-specific determinants) exist in these chains. To the authors' knowledge, there has never been a report of a reaction between any κ-specific antiserum and rabbit light chains. Very likely, it has not yet been looked for seriously.

V. Variable Region Determinants

A. Light-Chain Variable Region Determinants

Light-chain variable region determinants for immunoglobulin κ chains are among the most precisely localized antigenic determinants, in large measure because of the work of Solomon and his associates.

Through the use of heterologous antisera, these workers were able to define three distinct antigenically active regions of human κ chains (e.g., see McLaughlin and Solomon, 1972). Correlation of the results of κ-chain amino acid sequences obtained in a number of laboratories with the antigenic analyses allowed the localization of these three antigenic determinants close to residues 9, 45, and 95. The supposition that the relevant areas of the κ light chain would be located on the surface in the three-dimensional structure of the molecule was confirmed when X-ray crystallographic data for immunoglobulin light chains became available (Schiffer et al., 1973; Poljak et al., 1973).

The utility of these light-chain antisera developed by Solomon and McLaughlin was emphasized by the demonstration that their specificity for κ-chain subgroups could be used to determine the subgroup assignment ($V_{\kappa}I$, $V_{\kappa}II$, $V_{\kappa}III$, $V_{\kappa}IV$) of unknown human κ chains. The fine specificity of some of the sera was such that accurate *predictions* could be made of which amino acids would be found at certain positions of unsequenced κ chains. Thus the potential for the use of antigenic determinants for establishing much detailed information about immunoglobulins is very high. Unfortunately, to date, it has not been possible to achieve the level of precision characteristic of the κ system in all other areas of interest. However, Tischendorf et al. (1970) have been able to identify a subgroup-specific antigenic marker on λ light chains.

B. Heavy-Chain Variable Region Determinants

1. Subgroup-Specific Determinants

It has proven enormously difficult to produce anti-heavy-chain antisera that are capable of distinguishing among the three main heavy-chain subgroups that have been defined by amino acid sequence analysis. Nevertheless, some recent success in this effort has been reported. It is likely that the unusual difficulty in generating antisera with these kinds of specificities is a consequence of some fundamental structural feature of the specific area of the molecule concerned. It may well be related to some aspect of immunological tolerance reflecting a widespread state of true tolerance among the immunized animals to the putative subgroup-specific determinants. If formally established, such a situation would clearly reflect some essential characteristics of the immune response in general which could have important implications regarding the nature of its regulation and control. Alternatively, the determinants in question may simply be hidden or clustered within the interior of the variable region domain of the antibody molecule and thus be unavailable to the potentially responsive cells of the animal that has been immunized with this protein. Additional comparative X-ray diffraction studies may well provide data relevant to this question.

In spite of the difficulties, Forre et al. (1976) succeeded in producing antisera specific for the V_HI, V_HII, and V_HIII subgroups, as these categories have been identified in man. The antisera did not show precipitating activity in agar gel diffusion assays but did show these specific reactivities in hemagglutination or hemagglutination-inhibition assays. The principles used in successfully producing these subgroup-specific reagents were those that have proven useful in many other immunological systems: a heterologous species (generally the rabbit) is injected with a representative protein (e.g., a human V_HIII myeloma protein). Unwanted specificities, such as those characteristic of a given subclass or light chain, are then removed by adsorption with appropriate proteins which *lack* the desired specificity (e.g., specificity of the V_HIII subgroup) but do possess the undesired specificities. The aim, often difficult to reach, is to end up with a reagent unique for a given antigenic characteristic. This aim is exactly what Forre et al. (1976) have achieved with respect to human heavy-chain subgroup-specific reagents.

The exact position of the responsible subgroup-associated antigenic determinants within the heavy-chain variable domain is not yet clear. It seems obvious that they are not likely to be associated with the hypervariable regions (see below). Very probably they do involve, at least partially, those "subgroup-specific" amino acids (Capra and Kehoe, 1975) that are used to categorize the heavy-chain subgroups on the basis of amino acid sequence analysis. Additional studies will also be required here to more closely define the relevant determinants.

A serological marker categorizing a V_H subgroup in murine heavy chains has also recently been reported by Bosma *et al.* (1977). The determinants in question were shown to be present on several different murine myeloma proteins which did not share a ligand-binding specificity. The authors concluded that the determinants they detected were located in the framework regions of the murine heavy-chain variable domain, but a more precise localization will have to await studies using purified murine V_H region peptides, or other approaches.

The identification of heavy-chain subgroup-specific antigenic determinants provides an enormously important investigative tool that should aid studies in a number of areas. For example, the availability of a sensitive, subgroup-specific reagent will allow a more specific analysis of a number of cell-membrane-associated proteins, including true immunoglobulins or closely related molecules. In other words, a serological approach, ideally when the exact identity of the antigenic determinants in question is known, will make many additional contributions to bridging the gap between immunochemistry and other areas of immunobiology.

2. Idiotypic Determinants

a. Discovery. Idiotypic antigenic determinants are also localizable to the variable region of the immunoglobulin molecule. The term "idiotypy" was first proposed by Oudin (1966) following his observation that antiantibodies could be produced against certain antibody proteins present in the serum of rabbits that had been inoculated with bacteria of the genus *Salmonella*. The significant correlate was that the specificity of the antiantibodies could be related to the specificity of the antibodies that were being used as an immunogen. Subsequent studies localized the relevant antigenic determinants first to the Fab segment and then to the variable regions of the immunoglobulin molecule. In retrospect, it is now clear that the observations previously made by Slater *et al.* (1955) pertain to the same phenomenon. They noted that one could generate in a heterologous species (rabbit) antisera to human myeloma proteins which, after adsorption with an appropriate complement of other immunoglobulins, would retain specificity unique for the homologous protein that had been used to immunize the rabbit. Slater *et al.* (1955) thus inferred that such immunoglobulins contained what they named "individual antigenic specificities" to emphasize their singular character. Williams and

Kunkel (1963) and later Williams *et al.* (1968) detected individual antigenic specificities in induced antibodies such as cold agglutinins. The important correlate here was, once again, the association of a particular antibody activity (e.g., the anti-red blood cell specificity characteristic of cold agglutinins) with particular individual antigenic specificities. It is now clear that both "individual antigenic specificity" and "idiotypy" are reflective of the same structural attributes of the immunoglobulin molecule. Accordingly, the term "idiotypy" is now generally used to describe this antigenic feature of antibodies.

    b. Localization of Idiotypic Determinants.   Support for the idea that the idiotypic determinants were present in the Fab region of the immunoglobulin molecule was obtained by Grey *et al.* (1965) in additional studies on the individual antigenic specificity of human myeloma proteins. However, definitive proof of the localization of these determinants to the variable region was not obtained until Wells *et al.* (1973) showed that the F_V fragment (associated light- and heavy-chain variable regions) of the murine myeloma protein McPC 315 contained the idiotypic determinants characteristic of the intact protein.

    An association between the antibody-combining site and idiotypic determinants then seemed a realistic possibility. Brient and Nisonoff (1970) clearly showed that this could be true by finding that a hapten specific for a given antibody could inhibit the reaction between the antibody and its anti-idiotypic antibody by more than 60%. This is what Weigert *et al.* (1974) have termed a "ligand-modifiable" idiotype. Nevertheless, the relationship is not absolute since in some instances idiotypic determinants are shared by antibody molecules that do not have the same binding specificities. There are clearly common determinants that border, or are very near, the antigen-binding cleft, which are bona fide idiotypes. Additional discussion relative to the details of the antigen-binding cleft of antibodies is included in the chapter by Weininger and Richards in this volume.

    The mapping of idiotypic determinants within the immunoglobulin molecule is more advanced than that of a number of the other serologically detected antigenic determinants possessed by this protein family. This has proven true because of the close association between idiotypic determinants and the hypervariable segments of the immunoglobulin variable regions determined by amino acid sequence analysis (Capra and Kehoe, 1975). It was possible to show, for example, that two human anti-γ-globulin antibodies which were known to share idiotypic determinants have very similar or identical hypervariable regions in their heavy (Capra and Kehoe, 1974) and light (Klapper and Capra, 1976) chains. The framework segments of these chains showed a number of sequence differences, the light chains, in fact, even belonging to a different subgroup.

Possibly even more supportive of a strong association between idiotypy and hypervariable regions are the elegant results of the collaboration between Nisonoff and his associates and Capra and his associates on certain antiphenylarsonate antibodies induced in A/J mice (Capra *et al.*, 1977). These antibodies, shown to possess a particular cross-reactive idiotype, can be isolated in pools from individual or small groups of mice in sufficient quantity for amino acid sequence analysis (Tung and Nisonoff, 1975). It is important to emphasize that the relevant structural studies were carried out only on that subpopulation of antiphenylarsonate antibodies that share the cross-reactive idiotype. The crucial observation, when the sequence of the complete variable region of the light chains of such antibodies was determined (Capra *et al.*, 1977), was that, although heterogeneity was apparent in the framework segments of the chain (at least two distinct light chains are included), the *three hypervariable regions showed a homogeneous sequence*. These clear data for a population of molecules specifically selected for a unique idiotype argue strongly for the association of idiotypic antigenic specificity with the structure of the hypervariable regions of antibody molecules.

Feizi *et al.* (1977) have described a heavy-chain variable region marker (V_HMar) that was detected using an antiserum raised against human IgM cold agglutinins. Evidence was presented that the relevant determinant was associable with cross-reactive idiotypes characteristic of the cold agglutinins. It was of particular interest that this antigen is found in both normal pooled IgG and some unselected myeloma paraproteins.

The full expression of an idiotypic determinant is generally dependent on the presence of both the heavy and light chains of an immunoglobulin (e.g., see Carson and Weigert, 1973; Laskin *et al.*, 1977). There are occasional examples, however, where a single chain can be shown to bear a given determinant.

In addition to their intrinsic interest, idiotypic determinants have proven, and are continuing to prove, of great value in analyzing genetic aspects of the control of antibody synthesis, a topic that is beyond the scope of this chapter.

VI. Interspecies Antigenic Determinants

One of the main contributions of the comparative, interspecies approach to the study of antibodies has been the demonstration that the fundamental structural organization of these molecules is remarkably similar across a wide segment of the phylogenetic spectrum. This leads then to the question of the extent of identity of antigenic determinants among various species. These patterns have not been studied in great detail, but some information is available concerning class-specific (heavy-chain constant region) determinants in higher mammals. In one study involving a comparison of myeloma proteins from man and the cat (Kehoe *et al.*, 1972), a panel of ten rabbit antisera specific for human IgG proteins was tested for reactivity with three separate IgG myeloma proteins isolated from cats. Only one of these antisera showed a positive reaction with all three cat IgG proteins. Thus, even for two relatively closely related mammals, there is not extensive antigenic cross-reaction between immunoglobulins of the same class. While it is conceivable that additional studies of this kind of cross-reactivity could reveal additional positive reactions of interest, all indications at present suggest that identities are seen only among very closely related species. The mutational changes that occur in this region of the immunogloblin molecule seem to obliterate relatively quickly the identity of individual, class-specific determinants. Studies of the primary structure of the Fc region of IgG molecules from different species (e.g., see Kehoe *et al.*, 1974) have shown that interspecies variation runs about 40% for this region of the immunoglobulin molecule.

It would be of extreme interest to determine whether any interspecies *idiotypic* cross-reactions could be observed. Could there be, for example, a cross-reaction between idiotypic determinants on an antibody of given specificity (say, antidinitrophenol) produced in a second species. To the authors' knowledge, no reports of such cross-reactivity have yet appeared. However, the basic unity observed in the construction of the antibody-combining-site structure, at least among mammalian species, would suggest that such interspecies cross-reactivity is a very real theoretical possibility.

VII. Other Significant Immunoglobulin Determinants

A. Rheumatoid Factor Determinants

It is well known that a number of antibodies with combining-site specificities directed against antigenic determinants present on *other* immunoglobulins appear during certain diseases. Rheumatoid arthritis is a classical example, where such antiantibodies are important contributors to the pathogenesis of the disease. As indicated previously, the capacity of such rheumatoid serum agglutinators (Raggs) to specifically agglutinate only certain immunoglobulins led Grubb to an early realization of the presence of human allotypic markers. Thus some of the antigenic determinants with which rheumatoid factors interact are the same as those identifiable as allotypic markers. However, the reactivities are not exclusively associated with allotypic determinants since some other rheumatoid factors have been shown to interact with isotypic determinants. One of the best-characterized sites with which rheumatoid factors can interact is termed "Ga" (Gaarder and Natvig, 1970). This determinant is present on human IgG1, IgG2, and IgG4 proteins but is absent on IgG3 proteins. Here again, a detailed mapping of the specific determinants involved has not yet been attained. Most are associated with the Fc region, however, and more refined mapping may be possible now that detailed X-ray diffraction data for this region are becoming available (Deisenhofer *et al.*, 1976; Silverton *et al.*, 1977). Serological analyses (Williams and Lawrence, 1966; Natvig, 1970) have indicated that some of these anti-γ-globulin antibodies have specificity for "hidden" IgG sublcass-specific determinants. Such determinants should also be more localizable with the available three-dimensional structure information concerning the Fc region.

B. J-Chain Determinants

The polymeric immunoglobulins IgM and IgA from a number of species have been shown to contain a third polypeptide chain (besides light and heavy chains) termed "J chain" (Halpern and Koshland, 1970). This polypeptide, which plays an important role in the assembly of the monomeric subunits of IgM and IgA to the polymeric form, is an integral part of the covalent structure of these molecules, being attached to the Fc region of the immunoglobulin molecule (Mestecky *et al.*, 1974). One might thus anticipate that J-chain-associated antigenic determinants would be readily demonstrable in such proteins, especially given the relatively high molecular weight (15,000 d) characteristic of this polypeptide. In fact, this is not the case, since it has proven enormously difficult to raise J-chain-specific antisera, even with the use of vigorous immunizing procedures and careful absorption methods. Evidently the conformational disposition of this chain within the intact polymeric immunoglobulin is such that only a very few J-chain determinants are exposed

```
           5                  10                  15                  20
PCA-Glu-Asp-Glu-Arg-Ile-Val-Leu-Val-Asp-Asn-Lys-CMC-Lys-CMC-Ala-Arg-Ile-Thr-Ser-Arg-Ser-Ser-
      25                  30                  35                  40                  45
Glu-Asp-Pro-Asn-Glu-Asp-Glu-Ile-Val-Arg-Ile-Ile-Val-Pro-Leu-Asp-Asn-Arg-Glu-Asn-Ile-Ser-Asp-
         50                  55                  60                  65
Pro-Thr-Ser-Pro-Leu-Arg-Thr-Arg-Phe-Val-Tyr-His-Leu-Ser-Asp-Leu-CMC-Lys Lys  CMC-Asp-Pro-Thr-
                                                                         Gln
   70                  75                  80                  85                  90
Glu-Val-Glu-Leu-Asp-Asn-Gln-Ile-Val-Thr-Ala-Thr-Gln-CMC-Asx-Ile-CMC-Asp-Glu-Asn(Ser)Ala(Ser)
         95                  100                 105                 110                 115
Glu(Arg)Thr-Tyr-Asp-Arg-Asn-Lys-CMC-Tyr-Thr-Ala-Val-Val-Pro-Leu-Val-Tyr-Gly-Gly-Glu-Thr-Lys-
                120                 125                 129
Met-Val-Glx-Thr-Ala-Leu-Thr-Pro-Asx-Ala-CMC-Tyr-Pro-Asx
```

Figure 3. Complete covalent structure of human J chain as determined by Mole *et al.*
(1977) (reprinted with permission). Such a globular protein should possess numerous potent
antigenic determinants. The relative difficulty of producing anti-J-chain antisera may well
be related to the details of its quaternary association with polymeric immunoglobulins.

(see below). More precise knowledge of this intramolecular orientation
could be of great value in understanding the details of J-chain function.
Alternatively, it is possible that there are sufficient structural similarities
among the J-chain molecules characteristic of the various species so that,
in effect, the different species are immunologically tolerant to the J-chain
molecules of other species and consequently fail to mount an immune
response against this component of the polymeric immunoglobulins. J-
chain-associated antigenic determinants have consequently not been an
important aspect of the immunological analysis of immunoglobulins. Recently, the entire primary structure of the human protein has been determined (Mole *et al.*, 1977). This structure is reproduced in Fig. 3. It is
apparent that such a polypeptide should possess many prominent antigenic determinants. The difficulty in detecting these when J chain is in
association with immunoglobulin thus again suggests that the quaternary
associations involved may lead to extensive masking of the potentially
reactive J-chain determinants that are a part of its native structure.

C. Secretory Piece Determinants

The secretory IgA molecules characteristic of the body secretions
such as saliva, tears, and milk contain a fourth polypeptide component
termed "secretory piece." In contradistinction to the situation with J
chain, secretory component has prominent antigenic determinants which
are displayed in the intact secretory IgA molecule. In fact, the presence
of these determinants was very important in elucidating the unique char-

acter of this secretory immunoglobulin (Tomasi *et al.*, 1965). Although, once again, the precise location of the relevant antigenic determinants on the secretory piece molecule has not been determined, it seems clear from the relative ease of generating strong precipitating antisera that a number of these determinants must be prominently displayed on the surface of the secretory piece, even when it is associated with the IgA molecule. The fact that antisera raised against secretory IgA (and appropriately absorbed of all immunoglobulin-specific antibodies) will react strongly with "free" secretory piece (e.g., from an agammaglobulinemic individual) suggests that at least several prominent antigenic determinants are in the same conformational state in both the bound and free forms of secretory piece. As noted below, however, some exceptions to this pattern have been observed.

Studies of Brandtzaeg (1974, 1976) have suggested a close interaction between the binding of both J chain and secretory component with IgA and IgM proteins. This interaction, which assumes a conformational change in the polymeric immunoglobulin subsequent to J-chain binding and hence a change in its antigenic characteristics, leads, in this hypothesis, to the acquisition of a heightened binding capacity for secretory component. In this conception the firm binding of secretory component to a polymeric immunoglobulin is dependent on its prior union with J chain. One piece of evidence offered by Brandtzaeg (1974, 1976) for this interpretation is that anti-J-chain antibody will markedly inhibit the union of secretory component with IgM or IgA. This is, of course, far from formal proof of this dependence because one might be simply seeing a steric hindrance phenomenon that has nothing to do with the natural route of binding of these distinct polypeptides.

Other experiments of Brandtzaeg (1971, 1977) have identified a specific secretory component antigenic determinant, termed the "I determinant," which is characteristic of "free" secretory piece. Its specificity for the unbound polypeptide is shown by its inaccessibility, or masking, when human secretory component is bound tightly to IgA. This property has been usefully exploited by Brandtzaeg to monitor the degree of binding of secretory component to immunoglobulin. This approach, for example, allowed the demonstration of a much tighter binding of secretory component to IgA than to IgM molecules (Brandtzaeg, 1977). Thus, even though the precise location and molecular characteristics of this determinant are unknown, it has considerable analytical significance. The presence of an additional secretory component determinant, termed "determinant A," was also demonstrated by Brandtzaeg (1977). In contradistinction to the findings with the I determinant, determinant A was not useful as a guide to the quaternary associations of secretory component with the immunoglobulins. Much additional structural information concerning secretory piece is required to map these determinants in greater detail.

As indicated in Table IV, allotype-specific antigenic determinants on rabbit secretory piece have been described by Knight *et al.* (1974). These markers have been shown to be unlinked to those associated with the other polypeptide chains found in rabbit immunoglobulins that were discussed previously.

VIII. Summary and Conclusions

Immunoglobulins are themselves strongly immunogenic proteins. The antigenic determinants involved have been very important in the immunological analyses that have contributed so much to our current understanding of immunoglobulin structure. This has been especially true with respect to the delineation of the various classes, subclasses, and subtypes of this heterogeneous group of proteins. Nonetheless, the detailed mapping of the submolecular location of the various antigenic determinants is, as yet, far from fully developed, with the possible exception of the determinants involved in idiotypic specificities. These are clearly associated intimately with the hypervariable segments of the immunoglobulin variable regions. In addition, a number of specific amino acids of the human and rabbit heavy-chain constant region and some in the variable region of rabbit heavy chains have been correlated with certain allotypic determinants. Further information on the detailed localization of important immunoglobulin determinants must await additional data on tertiary structure from X-ray diffraction analysis of the regions concerned and, very likely, studies involving model peptide analogues of various regions of the native immunoglobulin molecule. It may then be possible to propose a composite antigenic map for an antibody.

IX. References

Appella, E., Rejnek, J., and Reisfeld, R. A., 1969, *J. Mol. Biol.* **41**:473.
Appella, E., Chersi, A., Mage, R. G., and Dubiski, S., 1971, *Proc. Natl. Acad. Sci. USA* **68**:1341.
Appella, E., Roholt, O. A., Chersi, A., Radzimski, G., and Pressman, D., 1973, *Biochem. Biophys. Res. Commun.* **53**:1122.
Atassi, M. Z., 1975, *Immunochemistry* **12**:423.

Atassi, M. Z., 1978, in: *Immunobiology of Proteins and Peptides*, Vol. 1 (M. Z. Atassi and A. B. Stavitsky, eds.), pp. 41–100, Plenum, New York.

Atassi, M. Z., and Lee, C.-L., 1978*a*, *Biochem. J.* **171**:419.

Atassi, M. Z., and Lee, C.-L., 1978*b*, *Biochem. J.* **171**:429.

Atassi, M. Z., Lee, C.-L., and Pai, R.-C., 1976, *Biochim. Biophys. Acta* **427**:745.

Bosma, N. J., DeWitt, C., Hausman, J. V., and Potter, M., 1977, *J. Exp. Med.* **146**:1041.

Brandtzaeg, P., 1971, *Immunology* **29**:323.

Brandtzaeg, P., 1974, *J. Immunol.* **112**:1553.

Brandtzaeg, P., 1976, *Scand. J. Immunol.* **5**:411.

Brandtzaeg, P., 1977, *Immunochemistry* **14**:179.

Brient, B. W., and Nisonoff, A., 1970, *J. Exp. Med.* **132**:951.

Capra, J. D., and Kehoe, J. M., 1974, *Proc. Natl. Acad. Sci. USA* **71**:4032.

Capra, J. D., and Kehoe, J. M., 1975, *Adv. Immunol.* **20**:1.

Capra, J. D., Tung, A. S., and Nisonoff, A., 1977, *J. Immunol.* **119**:993.

Carson, D., and Weigert, M., 1973, *Proc. Natl. Acad. Sci. USA* **70**:235.

Chen, K. C. S., Kindt, T. J., and Krause, R. M., 1974, *Proc. Natl. Acad. Sci. USA* **71**:1995.

Conway, T. P., Dray, S., and Lichter, E. A., 1969*a*, *J. Immunol.* **102**:544.

Conway, T. P., Dray, S., and Lichter, E. A., 1969*b*, *J. Immunol.* **103**:662.

Deisenhofer, J., Colman, P. M., Epp, O., and Huber, R., 1976, *Hoppe-Seyler's Z. Physiol. Chem.* **357**:1421.

Dubiski, S., 1969*a*, *J. Immunol.* **103**:120.

Dubiski, S., 1969*b*, *Protides Biol. Fluids Proc. Colloq.* **17**:117.

Dubiski, S., and Muller, P. J., 1967, *Nature (London)* **214**:896.

Dubiski, S., Rapacz, J., and Dubiska, A., 1962, *Acta Genet. Stat. Med.* **12**:136.

Edelman, G. M., and Gottlieb, P. D., 1970, *Proc. Natl. Acad. Sci. USA* **67**:1192.

Edelman, G. M., Cunningham, B. A., Gall, W. E., Gottlieb, P. D., Rutishauser, U., and Waxdal, M. J., 1969, *Proc. Natl. Acad. Sci. USA* **63**:78.

Farnsworth, V., Goodfleisch, R., Rodkey, S., and Hood, L., 1976, *Proc. Natl. Acad. Sci. USA* **73**:1293.

Feizi, T., Lecomte, J., and Childs, R., 1977, *Clin. Exp. Immunol.* **30**:233.

Fett, J. W., and Deutsch, H. F., 1975, *Immunochemistry* **12**:643.

Fleischman, J. B., 1971, *Biochemistry* **10**:2753.

Fleischman, J. B., 1973, *Immunochemistry* **10**:401.

Forre, Ø., Natvig, J. B., and Kunkel, H. G., 1976, *J. Exp. Med.* **144**:897.

Frangione, B., 1969, *FEBS Lett.* **3**:341.

Gaarder, P. I., and Natvig, J. B., 1970, *J. Immunol.* **105**:928.

Gilman-Sachs, A., and Dray, S., 1972, *Eur. J. Immunol.* **2**:505.

Goding, J. W., Warr, G. W., and Warner, N. L., 1976, *Proc. Natl. Acad. Sci. USA* **73**:1305.

Goodfleisch, R. M., 1975, *J. Immunol.* **114**:910.

Gottlieb, A. B., Seide, R. K., and Kindt, T. J., 1975, *J. Immunol.* **114**:51.

Grey, H., and Kunkel, H. G., 1964, *J. Exp. Med.* **120**:253.

Grey, H., Mannik, M., and Kunkel, H. G., 1965, *J. Exp. Med.* **121**:561.

Grubb, R., 1956, *Acta Pathol. Microbiol. Scand.* **39**:195.

Grubb, R., and Laurell, A. B., 1956, *Acta Pathol. Microbiol. Scand.* **39**:390.

Gutman, G. A., Loh, E., and Hood, L. O., 1975, *Proc. Natl. Acad. Sci. USA* **72**:5046.

Halpern, M. S., and Koshland, M. E., 1970, *Nature (London)* **228**:1276.

Hamers, R., and Hamers-Casterman, C., 1965, *J. Mol. Biol.* **14**:288.

Hanly, W. C., Lichter, E. A., Dray, S., and Knight, K. L., 1973, *Biochemistry* **12**:733.

Horng, W. J., Knight, K. L., and Dray, S., 1976, *J. Immunol.* **116**:117.
Huber, R., Deisenhofer, J., Colman, P. M., and Matsushima, M., 1976, *Nature* **264**:415.
Jaton, J. C., 1974, *Biochem. J.* **141**:15.
Jaton, J. C., 1975, *Biochem. J.* **147**:235.
Jaton, J. C., 1976, *Biochem. J.* **157**:449.
Jaton, J. C., Braun, D. G., Strosberg, A. D., Haber, E., and Morris, J. E., 1973, *J. Immunol.* **111**:1838.
Johnstone, A. P., and Mole, L. E., 1977, *Biochem. J.* **167**:255.
Johnstone, A. P., Thunberg, A. L., and Kindt, T. J., 1978, *Biochemistry* **17**:1337.
Kehoe, J. M., Hurvitz, A. I., and Capra, J. D., 1972, *J. Immunol.* **109**:511.
Kehoe, J. M., Bourgois, A., Capra, J. D., and Fougereau, M., 1974, *Biochemistry* **13**:2499.
Kelus, A. S., and Pernis, B., 1971, *Eur. J. Immunol.* **1**:123.
Kim, B. S., and Dray, S., 1972, *Eur. J. Immunol.* **2**:509.
Kim, B. S., and Dray, S., 1973, *J. Immunol.* **111**:750.
Kindt, T. J., 1975, *Adv. Immunol.* **21**:35.
Kindt, T. J., and Mole, L. E., 1974, in: *Progress in Immunology II*, Vol. 1 (L. Brent and J. Holborow, eds.), p. 13, North-Holland, Amsterdam.
Kindt, T. J., Seide, R. K., Lackland, H., and Thunberg, A. L., 1972, *J. Immunol.* **109**:735.
Kindt, T. J., Seide, R. K., Tack, B., and Todd, C. W., 1973, *J. Exp. Med.* **138**:33.
Klapper, D. G., and Capra, J. D., 1976, *Ann. Immunol. (Inst. Pasteur)* **127**:261.
Knight, K. L., Lichter, E. A., and Hanly, W. C., 1973, *Biochemistry* **12**:3197.
Knight, K. L., Rosenzweig, M., Lichter, E. A., and Hanly, W. C., 1974, *J. Immunol.* **112**:877.
Kunkel, H. G., and Kindt, T. J., 1975, in: *Immunogenetics and Immunodeficiency* (B. Benacerraf, ed.), p. 55, University Park Press, Baltimore.
Kunkel, H. G., Natvig, J. B., and Joslin, F. G., 1969, *Proc. Natl. Acad. Sci. USA* **62**:144.
Laskin, J. A., Gray, A., Nisonoff, A., Klennan, N. R., and Gottlieb, P. D., 1977, *Proc. Natl. Acad. Sci. USA* **74**:4600.
Lee, C.-L., and Atassi, M. Z., 1977a, *Biochem. J.* **167**:571.
Lee, C.-L., and Atassi, M. Z., 1977b, *Biochim. Biophys. Acta* **495**:354.
Litwin, S. D., and Kunkel, H. G., 1967, *J. Immunol.* **99**:603.
Mage, R. G., Young, G. O., and Reisfeld, R. A., 1968, *J. Immunol.* **101**:617.
Mage, R., Lieberman, R., Potter, M., and Terry, W. D., 1973, in: *The Antigens*, Vol. I (Michael Seal, ed.), p. 299, Academic Press, New York.
Malek, T. R., and Knight, K. L., 1977, *Immunochemistry* **14**:493.
Malek, T. R., Peterson, B. E., Hanly, W. C., Knight, K. L., and Friedenson, B., 1978, *J. Immunol.* **120**:950.
Mandy, W. J., and Todd, C. W., 1968, *Vox Sang.* **14**:264.
Mandy, W. J., and Todd, C. W., 1969, *Immunochemistry* **6**:811.
Mandy, W. J. and Todd, C. W., 1970, *Biochem. Genet.* **14**:59.
Margolies, M. N., Strosberg, A. D., Fraser, K. J., Perry, D. J., Brauer, A., and Haber, E., 1974, *Fed. Proc.* **33**:809.
Margolies, M. N., Cannon, L. E., Kindt, T. J., and Fraser, B., 1977, *J. Immunol.* **119**:287.
McBurnette, S. K., and Mandy, W. J., 1974, *Fed. Proc.* **33**: Abstr. No. 2985.
McLaughlin, C. L., and Solomon, A., 1972, *J. Biol. Chem.* **247**:5017.
McLaughlin, C. L., and Solomon, A., 1973, *Science* **179**:580.
Mestecky, J., Schrohenloher, R. F., Kulhavy, R., Wright, G. P., and Tomana, M., 1974, *Proc. Natl. Acad. Sci. USA* **71**:544.
Michaelsen, T. E., Frangione, B., and Franklin, E. C., 1977, *J. Immunol.* **119**:558.

Mihaesco, E., Seligmann, M., and Frangione, B., 1971, *Nature (London) New Biol.* **232**:220.

Milstein, C., 1966, *Nature (London)* **209**:370.

Milstein, C. P., Steinberg, A. G., McLaughlin, C. L., and Solomon, A., 1974, *Nature (London)* **248**:160.

Mole, J. E., Behown, A. S., and Bennett, J. C., 1977, *Biochemistry* **16**:3507.

Mole, L. E., 1975, *Biochem. J.* **151**:351.

Mole, L. E., 1976, *Biochem. Soc. Tr.* **4**:33.

Mole, L. E., Jackson, S. A., Porter, R. R., and Wilkinson, J. M., 1971, *Biochem. J.* **124**:301.

Mole, L. E., Geier, M. D., and Koshland, M. E., 1975, *J. Immunol.* **114**:1442.

Natvig, J. B., 1970, *Immunology* **19**:125.

Natvig, J. B., and Kunkel, H. G., 1968, *Ser. Hematol.* **1**:66.

Natvig, J. B., and Kunkel, H. G., 1973, *Adv. Immunol.* **16**:1.

Natvig, J. B., and Kunkel, H. G., 1974, *J. Immunol.* **112**:1277.

Natvig, J. B., and Turner, M. W., 1971, *Clin. Exp. Immunol.* **8**:685.

Oudin, J., 1956, *C. R. Acad. Sci.* **242**:2606.

Oudin, J., 1960, *J. Exp. Med.* **112**:107.

Oudin, J., 1966, *Proc. R. Soc. London Ser. B* **166**:207.

Pink, J. R. L., Buttery, S. H., de Vries, G. M., and Milstein, C., 1970, *Biochem. J.* **117**:33.

Poljak, R. J., Amzel, L. M., Avey, H. P., Chen, B. L., Phizackerley, R. P., and Saul, F., 1973, *Proc. Natl. Acad. Sci. USA* **70**:3305.

Poljak, R. J., Amzel, L. M., Chen, B. L., Phizackerley, R. P., and Saul, F., 1974, *Proc. Natl. Acad. Sci. USA* **71**:3440.

Poulsen, K., Fraser, K. J., and Haber, E., 1972, *Proc. Natl. Acad. Sci. USA* **69**:2495.

Prahl, J. W., Mandy, W. J., and Todd, C. W., 1969, *Biochemistry* **8**:2712.

Prahl, J. W., Tack, B. F., and Todd, C. W., 1973, *Biochemistry* **12**:5181.

Prendergast, R. A., Grey, H. M., and Kunkel, H. G., 1966, *J. Exp. Med.* **124**:185.

Ropartz, C., Rivat, L., and Rousseau, P. Y., 1964, *Proc. Ninth Congr. Int. Soc. Blood Transf.*, p. 455, Karger, Basel.

Schiffer, M., Girling, R. H., Ely, K. R., and Edmundson, A. B., 1973, *Biochemistry* **12**:4620.

Sela, M., 1969, *Science* **166**:1365.

Silverton, E. W., Navia, M. A., and Davies, D. R., 1977, *Proc. Natl. Acad. Sci. USA* **74**:5140.

Slater, R. J., Ward, S. M., and Kunkel, H. G., 1955, *J. Exp. Med.* **101**:85.

Sogn, J. A., and Kindt, T. J., 1976, *J. Exp. Med.* **143**:1475.

Solomon, A., 1977, *Immunogenetics* **5**:525.

Stemke, G. W., 1964, *Science* **145**:403.

Strosberg, A. D., Fraser, K. J., Margolies, M. N., and Haber, E., 1972, *Biochemistry* **11**:4978.

Thunberg, A. L., Lackland, H., and Hindt, T. J., 1973, *J. Immunol.* **111**:1755.

Tischendorf, F. W., Tischendorf, M. M., and Osserman, E. F., 1970, *J. Immunol.* **105**:1033.

Todd, C. W., 1963, *Biochem. Biophys. Res. Commun.* **11**:170.

Todd, C. W., 1972, *Fed. Proc.* **31**:188.

Tomasi, T. B., Tan, E. M., Solomon, A., and Prendergast, R. A., 1965, *J. Exp. Med.* **121**:101.

Tseng, J., and Knight, K. L., 1975, *J. Immunol.* **115**:454.

Tung, A. S., and Nisonoff, A., 1975, *J. Exp. Med.* **141**:112.

van Haegaerden, M., and Strosberg, A. D., 1976, *FEBS Lett.* **66**:35.

Wang, A.-C., and Fudenberg, H. H., 1972, *Nature (London) New Biol.* **240**:24.

Wang, A.-C., Mathur, S., Pandey, J., Siegal, F. P., Middaugh, C. R., and Litman, G. W., 1978, *Science* **200**:327.

Waterfield, M. D., Morris, J. E., Hood, L. E., and Todd, C. W., 1973, *J. Immunol.* **110**:227.

Weigert, M., Raschke, W. C., Carson, D., and Cohn, M., 1974, *J. Exp. Med.* **139**:137.

Wells, J. V., Fudenberg, H. H., and Givol, D., 1973, *Proc. Natl. Acad. Sci. USA* **70**:1585.

Wilkinson, J. M., 1969a, *Biochem. J.* **112**:173.

Wilkinson, J. M., 1969b, *Nature (London)* **223**:616.

Williams, R. C., and Kunkel, H. G., 1963, *Arthritis Rheum.* **6**:665.

Williams, R. C., and Lawrence, T. G., 1966, *J. Clin. Invest.* **45**:714.

Williams, R. C., Kunkel, H. G., and Capra, J. D., 1968, *Science* **161**:379.

Wolfenstein-Todel, C., Frangione, B., Prelli, F., and Franklin, E. C., 1976, *Biochem. Biophys. Res. Commun.* **71**:907.

World Health Organization Bulletin, 1976, *J. Immunol.* **117**:1050.

3

Combining Regions of Antibodies

Richard B. Weininger and Frank F. Richards

I. Background

A. Introduction

When a mammalian organism is immunized with an antigenic determinant, a highly complex humoral immune response is induced. This consists of a large number of antibodies complementary to the antigenic
determinant. Such antibodies may vary in class and subclass. Furthermore, within a single subclass, there are differences in the energy of
interaction with which each antibody of the population binds the antigenic
determinant. These interactions may be viewed at a single point in time,
although the antibodies expressed at any one time in the immune response
may be only a fraction of the number that the animal is capable of
producing. Certainly, in viewing these antibodies over a period of time,
there are shifts in the populations produced after the initial immunization.

The outstanding feature of the humoral immune response is the high
degree of specificity possessed by this complex population. Indeed, antisera may distinguish between complex chemical structures varying by
a single functional group or between proteins showing a difference of
only a single amino acid residue. The binding activity of antibodies which
provides this specificity is located in two symmetrical combining regions
located at the solvent-exposed ends of the Fab fragments of the immunoglobulin molecule. The combining region itself is in or near a cleft
made up of the NH_2-terminal half of the light chain associated with the

Richard B. Weininger and Frank F. Richards · Department of Internal Medicine, Yale
University School of Medicine, New Haven, Connecticut 06510.

NH$_2$-terminal quarter of the heavy chain. The variations of structure in this region and their relationship to antibody-binding properties will be the theme of this chapter. In particular, we will consider the relationship between the pattern of ligand binding to a single immunoglobulin and the high degree of ligand specificity of the whole immune serum.

B. Antibody Populations

An immune serum is said to be "specific" because it binds most strongly to the immunizing antigen. In addition, this antiserum will commonly show lesser binding energies for ligands with structures resembling that of the inducing antigen. On occasion, the population of antibodies making up an antiserum will contain heteroclitic antibodies which bind a nonimmunizing antigen more strongly (Varga *et al.*, 1973).

The number of immunoglobulins in an immune serum which bind the immunizing antigen, or ligand, may be very large—one may see 50 immunogen-binding bands on isoelectric focusing of such an antiserum. However, the immunoglobulins within such a population do not all react with ligand to the same degree—a wide range of binding constants may be seen in this population (Eisen and Siskind, 1964; Eisen, 1964*a,b*). This suggests a structural heterogeneity which is further complicated by a change of the antibody population with time (Steiner and Eisen, 1966, 1967*a,b*; Macario and Demacario, 1975, Goidl *et al.*, 1975, Lautz and Siskind, 1975). Thus new immunoglobulins appear while others fade, suggesting that at any one time we are seeing only a small proportion of antibodies complementary to the immunizing antigen.

Despite this heterogeneity, however, an immune serum demonstrates a marked specificity and is capable of discriminating between compounds which differ by as little as a single functional group, e.g., stereoisomers or proteins of single amino acid difference (Richards *et al.*, 1975; Reichlin, 1974; Landsteiner, 1938). This combination of wide heterogeneity plus narrow specificity leads one to the conclusion that the number of antibodies (and hence antigens) must be very large.

C. How Many Antibodies and Antigens Exist?

While it is clearly impossible to enumerate the potential antigens to be found in the environment, one may estimate that number based on the following assumption: If we look at the number of chemical compounds which have been catalogued, and the ability of antibodies to discriminate among them, we will have a lower-limit estimate for the number of potential antigens. For example, if we consider only the organic ring compounds, we know there are about 6 million (Wiswesser, 1975). Antisera can readily discriminate among structures of very similar shape or conformation but clearly not among all ring structures. A conservative estimate might be the ability to discriminate among 50% or less of these compounds. Thus a lower-limit estimate of the number of antigens, given these considerations, and for ring compounds only, would be of the order of 10^6.

There have been several experimental approaches to the enumeration of antibody-producing clones which are complementary to a single immunogen. Since this cannot be done directly, various sampling techniques have been tried. Kreth and Williamson (Williamson, 1972) assumed that spleen cells from a mouse, immunized with the determinant nitroiodophenyl (Nip) coupled to a protein carrier, contained all the potential antibody-producing cells. Such cells in very high dilution were injected into irradiated, recipient mice so that one or two anti-Nip cell clones multiplied in each host mouse when the host was challenged with Nip. The host antibodies were subjected to isoelectric focusing (IEF), and the bands representing single anti-Nip antibodies were detected with radioactive Nip. Since the immunoglobulin products of single clones have both characteristic IEF band patterns and characteristic isoelectric points, it is possible to count the number of times a pattern is repeated. Five "repeats" were seen when 337 IEF patterns from four donor mice were examined. The number of repeats expected is inversely proportional to the number of different antibody-producing cell clones. From these results, it is possible to calculate within 90% confidence limits that not less than 3000 and not more than 16,000 different immunoglobulins in one mouse can bind to the Nip determinant.

Quattrochi *et al.* (1969) examined the tryptic peptides from the light chain of 100 different mouse myeloma proteins. They looked for identity of patterns by two-dimensional peptide mapping but were unable to find two that were identical. They concluded that at least 1000 different L chains must exist to account for their results. This is a minimum estimate since it is not known whether the distribution of myeloma light chains is representative of the distribution of light chains in nonneoplastic cells. It is possible that inducing chemical irritant (and also possibly the virus which may be involved in myeloma induction) may have some selective influence on the class and subgroups found, and they may not provide a random sampling of potential antibody producing cells (Potter, 1972; Warner *et al.*, 1974). Other investigators have estimated the number of antibodies induced by trinitrophenyl (Tnp) that also bind dinitrophenyl (Dnp) as being approximately 500 (Pink and Askonas, 1974), suggesting that even when these somewhat more rigid binding criteria are invoked the population of clones able to meet those requirements may be still quite large. Such estimates of 10^3–10^4 distinct antibodies each binding a single small determinant such as Nip or Dnp or Tnp mean that the total antibody repertoire of an animal would have to be extremely large (10^9–10^{10}) since there are upward of several million different antigenic determinants.

Recently, considerable effort has been made to study the arrangement of immunoglobulin genes. Two questions in particular have received attention:

1. How many genes corresponding to the constant and to the variable regions are represented in mouse myeloma cells?
2. Is there evidence of V-C region translocation?

Approaches to counting V-region gene copies have measured hybridization rates of mRNA or cDNA probes to a large excess of genome DNA. It is believed that the rate of hybrid formation in solution under these conditions is dependent on the concentration of complementary DNA sequences. Using probes containing C and V region sequences from myeloma tumor κ and λ chains, most workers interpret their results as compatible with a few (fewer than five) C region genes. Hybridization with probes presumed to represent the V region has also been interpreted as consistent with a small number of V region genes (Williamson, 1973). A number of difficulties cloud these interpretations. A pure mRNA and some knowledge of the base sequence of the messenger as well as more knowledge on the effect of mismatched sequences on hybridization kinetics are needed. It is fair to state that, so far, hybridization experiments have not given unequivocal estimates of the number of V and C region gene copies. This topic has been subject of a lucid review by Williamson. The evidence for somatic V-C region translocation is still indirect. Recent studies by the Basel group indicated that in fetal mouse cells hybridization kinetics were consistent with the presence of separate V and C region-like DNA sequences whereas in myeloma cells there was no evidence of such separation (Tonegawa *et al.*, 1976). Separate C region-like sequences are of course known to occur in β_2-microglobulin (Poulik and Reisfeld, 1975). A more recent finding that there may be an untranslated

DNA sequence of 1250 bases between the V and C regions may also force reinterpretation of previous data (Brack and Tonegawa, 1977).

D. Combining Region Variability

Given the previous estimates of antigen and antibody number, we have a situation whereby an extremely large number of antibodies (10^6–10^9) are apparently generated from a relatively smaller amount of genetic information (coding perhaps for 10^2 germ line genes). Much effort has been devoted to suggest means whereby this number of genes could be amplified and diversified.

Talmage had already pointed out that a high degree of specificity in component immunoglobulins was not a requisite for a highly specific immune serum. In the last 5 years, evidence has accumulated that individual immunoglobulins can bind a number of structurally dissimilar antigens (Rosenstein et al., 1972; Cameron and Erlanger, 1976; Tolleshaug and Hannestad, 1975; Manjula et al., 1976; Rosenstein and Richards, 1976; Secher, 1977; Cameron and Erlanger, 1977) and that such binding is physiologically functional; when two dissimilar antigens bind to one immunoglobulin, either antigen can stimulate the production of that immunoglobulin (Varga et al., 1973). Thus, if each individual antibody molecule were capableof binding n different determinants, the total antibody repertoire of an animal would be reduced by a factor equal to n. The crucial question is: How large is n? This question cannot be answered without considering the energy of interaction between antigen and combining site. Testing of immunoglobulins with banks of antigens has shown that low-energy interactions with intrinsic dissociation constants (K_a) of the order of 1×10^3 liters/mol or less are extremely common, occurring with a frequency of (approximately) 1 per 20–25 compounds tested (4–5%) (Varga et al., 1974; Freedman et al., 1976). Interactions with a K_a of 1×10^5 liters/mol are far less common, occurring only once in approximately 140 compounds tested (0.7%) (Varga et al., 1974a). Since it is difficult to select compounds for testing in a random fashion, these figures to some extent reflect the bias of the experimenter. However, the main point is that the ability to bind more than one antigen with relatively low affinity is probably widely distributed (Parker and Osterland, 1969; Glazer, 1970) while high-affinity binding is relatively infrequent (Varga et al., 1974a; Eisen et al., 1967). Therefore, we may conclude that at least some of the diversity of the antibody response may be accounted for by the presence of polyfunctional antibodies, although at this time we are unable to estimate the magnitude of that contribution.

II. Structural Studies

A. Primary Structure

The amino acid sequences of antibody-combining regions provide us with the means to distinguish one antibody molecule from another; but the sequences themselves offer no information as to which amino acids may be involved in binding to hapten. To learn about hapten contact points directly, we must refer to three-dimensional or affinity-binding studies. However, we may indirectly learn about hapten-binding sequences or residues by looking at similarities or differences in the linear arrangement of amino acids and attempting to correlate them with specific ligand binding.

For instance, when the primary structures of the light- and heavy-chain V regions are compared, certain amino acid sequence patterns become apparent. Analysis of these patterns in both light- and heavy-chain V regions permits the following generalizations to be made: (1) Certain positions are almost always occupied by the same amino acid residue: for instance, positions 5 and 8 in human κ chains are occupied by Thr and Pro, respectively. (2) There are also definite correlations between the occurrence of an amino acid found in one position and of amino acid residues found in certain other positions in the V regions. For instance, in human κ chains, if position 1 is occupied by an Asp residue, position 4 is almost always occupied by Met, position 9 by Ser, etc. However, when Glu is found at position 1, then position 4 will most likely be filled by Leu, position 9 by Gly, and so on. These correlations have recently been aided by the use of computers (Kabat *et al.*, 1976). The same type of correlations holds for V regions in λ light chains and heavy-chain V regions. (3) There are certain positions in each V region which can be occupied by a wide variety of amino acid residues and where the finding of a particular residue (say, at position 35) does not permit one to predict what amino acid would occur, say, at position 54 on the basis of the sequences known at present. These positions have been termed "hypervariable regions" (Wu and Kabat, 1970) and have been implicated as participating in the antigen-binding site. It has been suggested, for instance, that certain hypervariable sequences correlate with binding of the Dnp moiety and others correlate with the ability to bind arsonate (Cebra *et al.*, 1974) or inulin (Vrana *et al.*, 1977). Conversely, in some cases, homogenous immunoglobulins binding the same antigen show differences in their hypervariable region sequences (Margolies *et al.*, 1975). Thus there is not enough information to know how tightly sequence and specificity are coupled or whether all the amino acids in the hypervariable regions actually make contact with the antigen.

The reasons for these apparently contradictory results are not obvious but may be related to the strain of animal from which the antiserum is obtained. For instance, one might expect that antibodies from partially inbred species would have similar hypervariable residues for a given antigen since the gene pool from inbred species is closer to uniformity. On the other hand, a greater diversity in response to the same antigen might be expected from an outbred species and thus provide differences in hypervariable sequences as found by Margolies et al. It is known, however, that these hypervariable regions occur in clusters (Wu and Kabat, 1970). There are three such clusters in light-chain V regions and three such clusters in heavy-chain V regions, although species variations do exist. Data available from affinity and structural studies seem to indicate that these hypervariable clusters are involved in hapten contact, although they are not always the only residues involved, nor is each hypervariable region necessarily involved in hapten contact in every antibody. Finally, it has recently been suggested that the marked variation in length of the third hypervariable region of the heavy chain may point to a special function for this group (Vrana et al., 1977), although that function remains obscure at this time.

Besides correlating residues of the V region with one another, or with binding specificity, one may also attempt to look at the participation of certain amino acid residues in the interaction of ligand with the antibody-combining region. In the next sections, we will examine the techniques used to determine the contact residues of the combining site and to measure the size of that site.

B. Affinity Labeling

Affinity labeling has been applied to immunoglobulins with the hope of being able to identify amino acid residues that make contact with the hapten. This method was first applied to immunoglobulins by Wofsy et al. (1962) and has been used extensively since to study the combining regions of both myeloma proteins and whole antibody populations directed against particular antigenic determinants (Wofsy et al., 1962; Singer and Doolittle, 1966; Knowles, 1972; Givol, 1974; Richards and Konigsberg, 1977).

Affinity reagents consist of reactive moieties which either can be attached to or are an integral part of a haptenic determinant. The effectiveness of such probes depends on maintaining a much higher concentration in or near the combining site than in the environment of reactive amino acid residues which are not in the combining site. Unlike the situation in the serine proteases, there is no evidence for any special reactivity of a single amino acid side chain within the immunoglobulin-combining region. Since concentration differences of the reagent in the solvent and in the environment of the site are crucial for affinity labeling, high affinity of the immunoglobulin for the hapten and a low molar ratio of ligand to immunoglobulin favor specific labeling of the combining region.

In practice, four types of reactive groups have been used as affinity reagents with immunoglobulins. Wofsy et al. (1962) used diazonium fluoroborate, a relatively stable salt which reacts with amino groups and phenolic and imidazole side chains (Wofsy and Parker, 1967). The limited reactivity of these reagents means that the contact residues may not be labeled; instead, the reaction may occur with the most reactive tyrosine, lysine, or histidine residue in or near the combining region. The α-haloketone compounds employed as affinity reagents by Givol, Eisen, and their associates have similar drawbacks (Givol, 1974; Haimovich et al., 1970, 1972; Eisen, 1971); their reactivity with amino acid residues resembles that of the diazonium salts.

Since all affinity reagents are introduced into the aqueous solvent and enter the combining site by diffusion, the rate of hydrolysis of such reagents must be low. This requirement in turn limits both the spectrum of reactivity and the concentrations of the reagent that may be used. Some of these limitations can be overcome, if a nonreactive affinity reagent can be found in the combining site and activated to produce a moiety capable of forming covalent bonds with the antibody. Converse and Richards (1968, 1969) synthesized a Dnp-based diazoketone reagent of the type described earlier by Vaughan and Westheimer (1969) which may be photoactivated to a carbene or a ketene and showed that it reacted with anti-Dnp antibodies. Fleet et al. (1969) introduced another light-activated compound, an aromatic azide, for the same purpose (Fisher and Press, 1974). It is possible to isolate antibody-reagent complexes and activate them, although for this a relatively high binding energy for the hapten-antibody complex is needed. Most reagents highly reactive with proteins will also react readily with water. By generating highly reactive groups in situ, it is possible in theory to modify a large number of different amino acid side chains. Even though no sweeping conclusions are possible from the results of affinity labelig, the following points can be made: (1) In general, modifications occur at or near some of the hypervariable regions, although there are three reports where labeling outside the accepted hypervariable regions has occurred (Richards *et al.*, 1974; Franek, 1973; Klostergaard *et al.*, 1977). Some residues, i.e., the tyrosine at position 33 or 34 in the L chain, are modified in a number of different systems.

To summarize, it is likely that affinity reagents generally modify residues associated with the combining region, but these residues are not necessarily those which are in contact with the antigen.

C. Polymeric Ligand Probes of the Combining Region: How Large Is It?

Kabat devised a method which accurately prediced the size of the combining region of anticarbohydrate antibodies (Kabat, 1960). The principle of the method is as follows: If there is point-to-point contact with antigen in the antibody-combining region, one should be able to raise antibodies to homopolymers of the type $(X-X-X)_n$, where n is a large number. X monomers, dimers, trimers, tetramers, and larger oligomers can be prepared, and their ability to inhibit the reaction between the X polymer and the antibody can be determined. It was reasoned that, on a molar basis, the inhibition of the oligomers should increase until the combining region is completely filled. After that, increasing the size of the competing molecule should have no further effect on inhibition. In his original experiments, Kabat immunized himself with dextran and found that polysaccharide units containing up to five or six glucose units maximally inhibited the dextran-antibody reaction and that, thereafter, increasing the length of the polymer did not increase inhibition. From these data, he suggested that the combining region could be as large as 34 Å × 12 Å × 7 Å (the extended measurement of the isomaltohexose unit). Kabat also noted that there was evidence of heterogeneity in the types of contacts made. With some sera, for instance, the isomaltotriose unit was almost as efficient an inhibitor as the isomaltohexose (Kabat, 1960).

Many laboratories have repeated and extended these studies using other homopolymers such as polyamino acids, random amino acid copolymers, and polynucleotides. The overall conclusions of these studies were that the size of the combining region was compatible with the binding of extended polymers in the size range 25–36 Å × 10–17 Å × 6–7 Å and that in most of the antibodies examined there was some evidence of heterogeneity in the size of the combining regions. Careful quantitative studies by Schechter with antibodies to polyalanine (Schechter *et al.*, 1970) and by Moreno and Kabat (1969) with antibodies to blood group A substance have substantiated the earlier finding that binding energy is incremental with each added monomer unit up to a limiting size and that antibody-antigen complex must have van der Waals contact over a relatively large area of the V region domain. Similar methods have been used to determine if there is a change in the average size of the combining region during changes in antibody population which occur in the maturation of the immune response. In this study, polyasparagine was used as the antigen, and it was concluded that there was some increase in average site dimensions of the antibody-combining region during maturation (Murphy and Sage, 1970).

D. Electron Microscopic Studies of the Antigen-Antibody Complexes

Early biophysical studies had suggested that the viscosity of the IgG molecule was consistent with the interpretation that it is composed of three, independent, mobile units of approximately 50,000 molecular weight each (Noelken *et al.*, 1965). The first convincing demonstration that it was, in fact, Y-shaped and that the two combining regions were located at the ends of the two movalbe arms of the Y came from electron microscopy. The studies of Almeida *et al.*, Lafferty, and Oertilis (Almeida and Waterson, 1969; Lafferty and Oertelis, 1963) showed viruses with threadlike structures forming U-shaped bands on the viral surface, while Feinstein and Rowe (1965) demonstrated ferritin molecules held together by thin, angled molecules. Valentine and Green (1967) used bifunctional DNP haptens which were separated from each other by carbon chains of various lengths. With the bifunctional antigen (Dnp NH[CH$_2$]$_8$NH Dnp) containing eight CH$_2$ groups, cross-linked complexes were obtained in which the combining region of one molecule was joined head to head with the combining region of the next molecule (Fig. 1). The EM field at 400,000 magnification showed predominantly ring-shaped structures of various sizes with knobs protruding outward. These rings were composed of two or more molecules of immunoglobulin joined via their combining regions and held together by the bifunctional antigen. The knobs could be removed with pepsin, an enzyme known to cleave the Fc fragment from the whole immunoglobulin and destroy the fragment. When bifunctional Dnp antigens with five or fewer CH$_2$ groups were tested with protein 315, no ring structures were produced. These electron micrographs showed (1) that antibody molecules were Y-shaped and (2) that the arms were movable about a hingelike region. The failure to form circular structures with short bifunctional haptens suggested strongly that the Dnp-binding site was at least 15 Å below the surface of the protein and that a cleft or cavity was probably present at the free end of the Fab fragment (Green, 1969). The major dimensions of the molecule

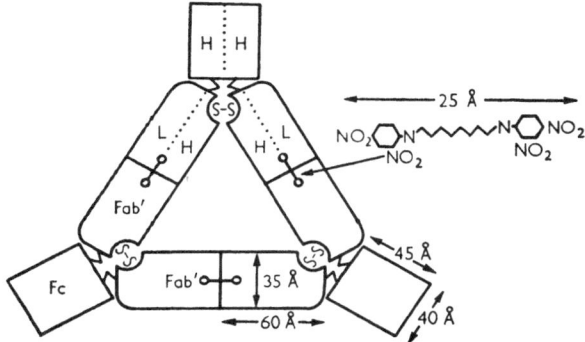

Figure 1. Complexes of anti-Dnp IgG with bivalent Dnp ligands. The electron micrographs on which this diagram is based gave the major dimensions of the IgG molecule and the locations of the combining regions and the Fc fragment. The electron micrographs also demonstrated the flexibility of the Fab region at the hinge region of the molecule. From Valentine and Green (1967); By courtesy of Dr. N. M. Green and the *Journal of Molecular Biology*.

could be measured from the EM photographs; the Fab fragment containing the combining region was estimated as 60 Å long and 35 Å broad (Green, 1969). Careful examination of the IgA protein 315 molecules and of the IgG molecules showed that each Fab region was composed of two compact, round structures, giving visual credence to the domain hypothesis which had been proposed on structural grounds by Edelman, Konigsberg, and their collaborators (Waxdal *et al.*, 1968). Electron microscopic studies of a human IgG1 myeloma protein crystal using an optical averaging method have also confirmed the Y-shaped structure of the whole molecule and the dimensions of the Fab fragment (Labaw and Davies, 1971).

E. X-Ray Crystallography

Northrop had described the first crystalline preparation derived from trypsin-treated antibody in 1942 (Northrop, 1942), and a number of investigators subsequently reported crystalline antibodies or antibody fragments (Nisonoff *et al.*, 1967; Hochman *et al.*, 1973). The first Fab fragment crystals, however, which had potential for high-resolution X-ray analysis became available only in the late 1960s. A human IgG1 myeloma protein, NEW, was analyzed at 2 A resolution by Roberto Poljak and his collaborators at Johns Hopkins Medical School (Poljak *et al.*, 1974), and a mouse IgA myeloma protein, derived from the McPC 603 tumor, was

studied by David Davies's group at the National Institutes of Health at
a resolution of 2 Å (Segal *et al.*, 1974). A third myeloma protein has been
studied extensively at the Argonne National Laboratories by Edmundson, Schiffer, and their collaborators. This is a λ light-chain dimer associated with the McG human myeloma protein (Schiffer *et al.*, 1973;
Edmundson *et al.*, 1974). In addition, a group of researchers from Munich
and the Argonne National Laboratories have compared the structure at
2 Å resolution of two κ L-chain dimers, Au and Rei, which differ in
structure by only 16 amino acid residues (Fehlhammer *et al.*, 1975; Epp
et al., 1975).

At the time of writing, there is available detailed information about
the antigen-combining region complex of one human IgG myeloma
(NEW); one mouse γA combining region–antigen complex (McPC 603)
and three light-chain dimer models of the combining region (from Mcg,
Au, and Re).

Knowledge of the three-dimensional structure of the combining region has answered or can potentially answer a number of questions about
antibody specificity: (1) What is the extent of the region complementary
to antigen? (2) Can several diverse antigen-binding sites be demonstrated
in the combining region? (3) The V region has a common folding pattern
associated with areas of conserved amino acid sequence. In spite of this,
it shows very large variation of antigen-binding specificity. By what
mechanism is structural variation in binding sites created? (4) Why is
antigen binding predominantly to the combining region? What physical
characteristics found in this region, but not elsewhere on the molecule,
facilitate binding? (5) What are the structural consequences of antigen
ligation? Are physiologically important conformational changes found
secondary to antigen binding? If so, are these conformational signals
transmitted to the Fc region or does some other mechanism obtain?

A comparison of the structure of the variable domain shows some
striking similarities between proteins NEW and 603 (Poljak, 1975). First,
the basic immunoglobulin fold of the V region polypeptides is essentially
the same in both proteins, the same fold being found in the light-chain V
region and the heavy-chain V region. The only difference is that the
second L-chain hypervariable region is absent in NEW and the polypeptide backbone brides across the base of the loop. A single S—S bond
links cysteine residues at loci equivalent to positions 26 and 85 on the L
chain. The polypeptide backbone is principally in parallel folds in the
form of β-pleated sheets. There are no substantial α-helical segments.
There are two sets of loops at either end of the V region of each chain
(Figs. 2 and 3). One set of loops makes contact with the first constant
domain; the other set is free in the sense that it is exposed to solvent.

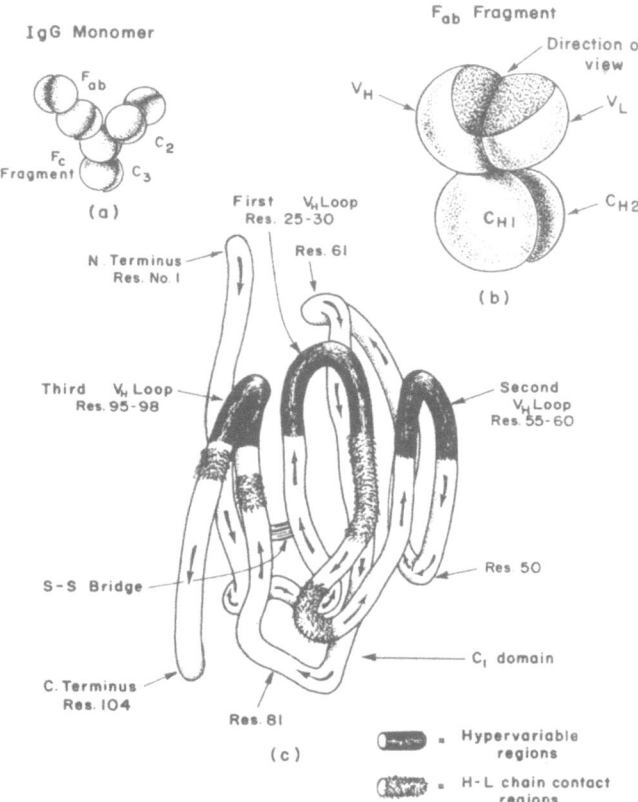

Figure 2. (a) Arrangement of the six domains of the antibody molecule with respect to each other. (b) Detailed diagram of the variable domain showing the V_L-V_H contact surface which is drawn in (c). (c) Polypeptide backbone fold of the heavy chain indicating the areas in contact with the light chain and the approximate location of the hypervariable regions. Redrawn from data on the NEW immunoglobulin molecule from Poljak *et al.* (1973) and Poljak (1975).

These three solvent-exposed loops correspond approximately to the hypervariable regions. Hypervariable regions center on residues 25–30, 50, and 95–100 in the L chain and residues 30, 55–60, and 105–110 in the H chain. It must be remembered that these are not rigidly bounded areas—the extent of hypervariability will depend on whether all light chains, κ or λ, or chains within each κ or λ subgroups are compared; the greater the difference between the groups and subgroups, the more extensive the region of hypervariability. While hypervariable residues in mouse and man occur in the combining region area, there is no evidence to suggest

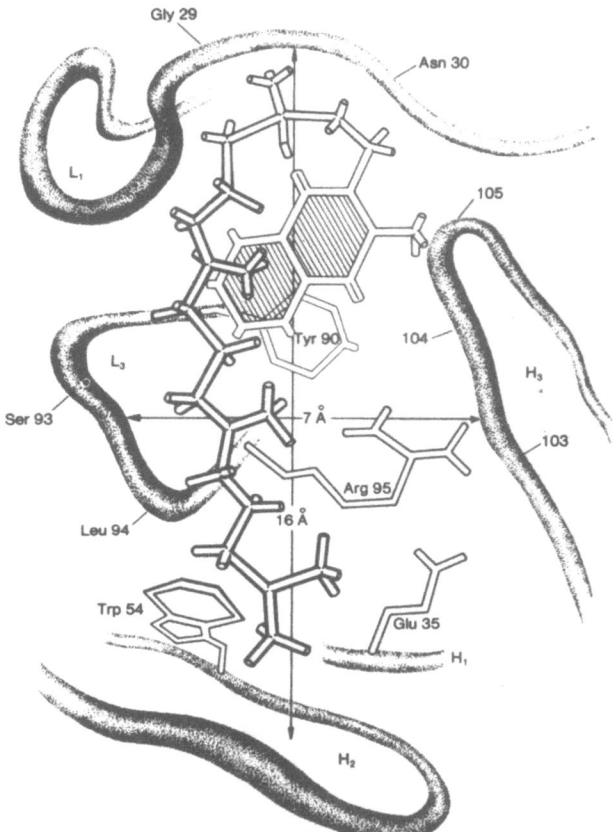

Figure 3. γ-Hydroxyvitamin K_1 bound to the combining region of the human myeloma IgG molecule NEW. L_1 and L_3 are the first and third light-chain hypervariable regions. (L_2 is deleted in this molecule.) H_1, H_2, and H_3 are the three hypervariable regions of the heavy chain. From Amzel et al. (1974).

that these are obligatory contact residues for antigens. The X-ray evidence shows that some hypervariable residues are in contact with antigen; others are close and others do not make contact. Contact is also made by antigen with regions other than the hypervariable ones (Poljak, 1975). In the rabbit the relationship between hypervariability and antigen contact is even less certain (Haber et al., 1975). It is distinctly possible that hypervariability does not reflect only the variation in amino acid sequence needed to bind directly to antigen. Compensatory sequence changes in regions away from the contact residues may also give rise to hypervariability. The predictions made from analysis of variability have proved very valuable in showing the general area in which antigen binding takes place.

In other regions of the backbone polypeptide fold, the side chains of residues are involved in heavy-chain–light-chain interactions. These include residues 35, 37, 42, 43, 86, and 99 in the V_L and C_L, and residues 37, 39, 43, 45, 47, 95, and 108 in the V_H region of protein NEW (Poljak, 1975).

These interacting residues are mainly, although not exclusively, hydrophobic, and their presence does not appear to correlate with H- or L-chain subgroup or L-chain type, suggesting that there is no very rigid restriction on recombination of H and L chains. The V_L and V_H regions are essentially similar in shape. On association they interact in the manner of a Chinese puzzle to form a roughly spherical domain. The solvent-exposed distal end forms an approximately flat plate fringed by the hypervariable loops. Between the areas occupied by the L and H chains on this plate runs a cleft approximately 15–17 A long. In protein NEW, this cleft is shallow (Fig. 4), perhaps 5–6 A deep, while in protein 603 it is 12 Å deep, 15 Å wide, and 20 Å long (Poljak *et al.*, 1974). The light chain of protein 603 is of the κ type and has an insertion of six residues at, or close to, the first hypervariable region. This has the effect of "forcing apart" the V_L and V_H regions and increasing the depth and width of the cleft. In the λ L-chain dimer studied, one L chain takes on a rotational position corresponding to the "H" chain; the other takes the L-chain position (Schiffer *et al.*, 1973; Edmundson *et al.*, 1974). The cleft in these dimers is much deeper, forming a funnel with a cavity at the bottom whose floor is approximately 16–17 Å below the entrance to the

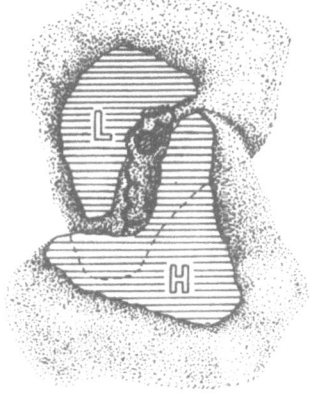

Figure 4.   Scheme of the combining region of protein NEW looking into the long axis of the Fab fragment. The areas labeled L and H are occupied by the light and the heavy chain, respectively. Between lies a depression approximately 5–6 Å deep in which the γ-hydroxyvitamin K_1 molecule is located.

cleft. The κ-chain dimers, Au and Rei, also have a large cavity between the two L-chain regions. An important difference in this region is the presence of tryptophan in Au at position 96 in place of the tyrosine residue found in Rei. The indole ring of tryptophan-96 protrudes into the cavity and looks as if it might impede access of a presumptive hapten to the cavity (Epp et al., 1975; Fehlhammer et al., 1975).

The mouse IgA myeloma protein 603 binds the small molecule phosphorylcholine approximately in the middle of the cleft. The phosphate moiety touches only the heavy chain at tyrosine-33 and arginine-52. The choline moiety lies at the bottom of the cleft, making contact with residues 102–103 of the H chain and residues 91–94 of the L chain; the contact region seems to be predominantly composed of H chain, and it is of interest that phosphorylcholine-binding myeloma proteins which do not share the TEPC 15 idiotype may have L chains which have little resemblance to those found on protein 603 (Poljak, 1975). This suggests that conditions for binding of this small determinant may be relatively nonstringent and are not dependent on a particular L chain, whereas some larger antigens making substantial contact with both L and H chains might show a considerable degree of stringency. It is noteworthy that the hypervariable loops form a very extensive region which frames the sites of hapten attachment. The third hypervariable region of the H chain and the second hypervariable region of the L chain do not make contact with the hapten.

The human IgG myeloma protein NEW binds a γ-hydroxyl derivative of vitamin K_1 (Fig. 3) with K_a of 1.7×10^5 liters/mol. F(ab)' fragment-ligand complexes have been crystallized and analyzed by Fourier difference maps (Amzel et al., 1974; Poljak et al., 1974). Hydroxyvitamin K_1 is a large molecule consisting of a naphthoquinone moiety and a long hydrophobic phytyl side chain. The whole molecule is nestled in the cleft, almost completely filling it. The naphthoquinone residue lies obliquely on the floor of the cleft, making contact with tyrosine residue 90 of the L chain and with the backbone and side chain of H-chain residue 104 and with L-chain residues 29 and 30. When 2-methyl-1:4 naphthoquinone, which is the vitamin K molecule without the phytyl tail, is bound to protein NEW, it occupies an identical site to that occupied when hydroxyvitamin K_1 is bound. Of the total binding energy (approximately 7.2 kcal/mol at 20°C), the naphthoquinone rings provide approximately 4.2 kcal/mol, and it is estimated by the difference that the phytyl tail provides 3.0 kcal/mol. The phytyl tail loops upward and around, making close contact with the L chain at Gly-29 and Asn-30. It then proceeds downward and superficially, making contact with the L chain at residues 93 and 94 and with the H chain at residue 104. At the free end of the chain, contact is made with a constant H-chain tryptophan residue, No. 54. Approximately 10–12 amino acids touch the antigen, and contact is made extensively with both H and L chains over a maximum dimension of perhaps 15 Å (Amzel *et al.*, 1974; Poljak *et al.*, 1974).

The Mcg λ-chain dimer appears to have at least three distinct binding sites. One is located on the rim of the funnel-shaped cleft, a second is at the constriction between funnel and cavity, and a third is at the bottom of the cavity. These sites bind a whole range of compounds including ε-dansyl lysine, colchicine, 1,10-phenanthroline, methadone, morphine, meperidine, 5-acetyluracil, caffeine, theophylline, menadione, triacetin, and other compounds (Schiffer *et al.*, 1973).

Certain general principles are beginning to emerge from the studies so far carried out. These answer, in part, the questions set out at the beginning of this section. It is, however, distinctly possible that further structure elucidation could modify these conclusions: (1) Antigen binding so far observed occurs in the solvent channel between the L- and H-chain areas of the V domain. Since only two antigens have been mapped so far in actual combining regions, we do not yet know whether antigen binding is confined to the channel or can extend outside. Certainly the L-chain dimer model of the combining region suggests that very deep hapten-binding clefts and cavities might exist in some antibodies. More mapping with antibody-antigen complexes will be required before we can define all the region involved in ligation of antigen. (2) Analysis of the protein Fab NEW–hydroxyvitamin K_1 complex suggests strongly that antigen binding is not confined to one small localized contact point but consists of multipoint binding over an extensive region of the immunoglobulin molecule, an observation consistent with the existence of multiple binding sites. If the Mcg model of the immunoglobulin-combining region resembles L-H-chain-combining regions, the clustering of binding sites may also be found in antibodies. (3) It is now clear that both the L and H variable regions as well as the constant regions all have a common polypeptide fold. Each L and each H folded unit has a relatively flat surface which makes contact with the other unit. On assembly each unit makes an angle with the other, i.e., the two units are not completely symmetrical but show one dyad axis. At the free end of the F_V domain, the H and L chains are not in contact, creating a solvent-filled channel. Antigens have been shown to bind to the walls of this channel. The walls of the cleft are composed of six loops (five in protein NEW), the tips of which bear hypervariable residues. The nature of the insertions or deletions of amino acid sequence apparently alters the depth of the cleft, for instance, the "insertion" of six amino acid residues in the first hypervariable loop in κ L chain of the McPC 603 protein "forces apart" the

H- and L-chain regions and gives rise to a deeper cleft. From the three-dimensional models, it has been predicted that variations in the length of the third hypervariable loop (around residue 105) would have the same effect. The pattern of amino acid residue variability found at the tips of the loops resembles the pattern of variable or "permissive" residues found when cytochromes from different species are compared. Here also the loci of greatest variation are found at the tips of outside polypeptide loops. This variability may be permissive in the sense that compensatory changes for differences in cleft structure are visible. It is, however, equally likely that residues at the tips of the loops have some direct functional significance. Haptens appear to bind along the walls of the cleft and not only at the hypervariable residues. The present scanty evidence does not rule out that the binding region could be much more extensive. It appears that the depth of the cleft can be modulated, exposing new binding sites, and that this may be one method of introducing variability in antigen binding. The L-chain dimers show an extremely wide and deep cleft at which a very large number of determinants bind. This effect may be directly related to the large number of combining sites exposed. (4) It is quite unclear why antigen binding occurs primarily at the Fab-combining region, or why most of the ligand binding observed, for example, in an enzyme molecule such as lysozyme, should occur in the cleft in which the substrate binds. Since we know that deep cavities are not required for ligand binding in immunoglobulins, a number of crevices, folds, and channels elsewhere in the molecule might be thought to serve equally well. Frederic Richards (1974) has addressed himself to a similar problem with ribonuclease. He has calculated that the atomic packing densities within the substrate-combining cleft are considerably less than at other solvent-exposed regions of the molecule. This suggests that the vibratory modes of various functional groups in the combining region could occur with greater degrees of freedom and that this might be associated with greater ligating potential. Similar studies carried out with the immunoglobulin molecule would be of great potential interest.

Although X-ray crystallography has so far provided the most extensive insights into the three-dimensional structure of immunoglobulins, it suffers from limitations. One important limitation is the static "average" conformational picture provided of a molecule, which undergoes considerable movement of large regions (Cathou and Dorrington, 1975) and perhaps also exhibits smaller "breathing" movements (Weber, 1975). Other physical methods have added considerably to our knowledge of the dynamics of the molecule.

The properties of all molecules are affected by their environment. With certain molecules, such changes in property between the molecule in solution and the molecule bound to an immunoglobulin-combining region may be observed directly. Such observable physical-chemical alterations on binding may include differences in ionization (Albertson and Phillipson, 1960), solubility properties (Day *et al.*, 1963), increases or decreases of fluorescence either of the protein or of the ligand (Velick *et al.*, 1960) in te rotatory dispersion of light, in the circular dichroism of polarized light, and in the circular dichroism of polarized emitted fluorescent light (Schlessinger *et al.*, 1975). The magnetic properties of the nucleus as well as the electron spin resonance of ligand and ligating molecule may be affected by binding (Dwek *et al.*, 1975a). Sensitive calometric methods can measure changes in enthalpy and indirectly of entropy during antibody-antigen interaction (Johnston *et al.*, 1974). Changes in the rotatory behavior of whole immunoglobulin molecules on binding large antigens can be monitored by depolarization of emitted fluorescence, and even changes in specific molar volume have been observed (Ohta *et al.*, 1970). More recently, the internal patterns of movement of macromolecules—the concerted breaking and re-formation of hydrogen bonds which have been described as the "breathing" of the molecule and which may affect ligand binding—have become accessible to observation. This wealth of physicochemical information cannot be reviewed in detail here: it is covered by specialized reviews (Cathou *et al.*, 1974; Day, 1972). It is perhaps disappointing how little direct information on combining region structure and function this work has yielded in comparison to X-ray diffraction analysis. It seems likely that, as with other proteins, the largest and most important contributions these methods will make is yet to come. It is in the fine analysis of mechanism in macromolecules whose overall anatomy is understood that these methods are most powerful.

Physicochemical probes have given the most information about the combining region, concerning the depth and hydrophobicity of the combining sites, the involvement of light and heavy chains in ligand binding, and the unexpected degree to which small ligands stabilize light- and heavy-chain interaction. Physicochemical methods have also been a mainstay in the assessment of possible conformational changes secondary to antigen binding.

X-ray crystallographic studies quoted elsewhere in this chapter show that in the two antibody V regions so far examined both the small ligand, phosphorylcholine, and a larger one, hydroxyvitamin K_1, appear to make contact with both the L and H chains. Nevertheless, the area of contact of phosphorylcholine with the L chain is small. It is known, however, that L-H chain contacts in the V and C_1 domains of the Fab fragment are extensive, involving many amino acid residues. It is therefore somewhat surprising that small ligands such as the Dnp moiety should stabilize L-H chain interaction to a considerable degree. Light and heavy chains may be isolated from reduced and alkylated IgG in dissociating solvents by gel filtration. Metzger and Singer (1963) found that L- and H-chain yields were considerably reduced when the small Dnp antigen was present in the mixture. Optical rotatory dispersion studies by Cathou and Haber (1967) and Cathou and Werner (1970) showed also that the presence of the Dnp hapten greatly retarded the unfolding of antibody molecules in the dissociating agent, guanidine hydrochloride. Thus antibody without the Dnp ligand unfolds in the presence of 2 N guanidine hydrochloride, while, in the presence of the ligand, binding activity is still intact in the presence of 4 N guanidine hydrochloride. Yet isolated H chains derived from Dnp antibodies still show binding activity albeit with a greatly reduced K_a, which may be due to the presence of new structures resembling combining regions formed from H-chain dimers (Stevenson, 1973).

When tryptophan is excited by UV light at 280 nm, it emits fluorescent light of 345 nm wavelength. Such tryptophan residues are found in close association with the combining region. Introduction of a Dnp group or a folic acid group into the combining region will usually absorb emitted tryptophan fluorescence. The quenching of fluorescence has been used both as a structural tool and as an indication of hapten binding. The wavelength of maximum absorptivity of incident light exhibited by ligands such as Dnp may also be red-shifted by binding to the protein (Eisen, 1964a). The observed spectral changes have suggested to some workers that charge-transfer complexes may be formed between aromatic ligands and residues such as tryptophan. However, convincing evidence for the presence of charge-transfer complexes remains elusive (Rubinstein and Little, 1970). It is now well recognized that a large number of different V regions may bind small ligands such as Dnp, with K_0 ranging from 1 $\times$ 10^{-4} M to 1 $\times$ 10^{-11} M. It is unlikely that such wide range of binding energies can be consistent with one type of Dnp-binding site.

Optical spectrophotometric evidence for conformational changes secondary to antigen binding has been dealt with elsewhere. The introduction of electron spin resonance probes (Stryer and Griffith, 1965; Hsia and Piette, 1969; Piette et al., 1972) has added an additional tool for the study of combining regions. Haptens are used which had been linked to moieties containing the nitroxide spin label. When the hapten is firmly fixed to the nitroxide spin label, it can be shown that it is firmly bound. By producing molecules in which the hapten and the spin label are separated by chemical spacer groups of various lengths, the degree of rotational freedom of the spin label can be estimated as a function of spacer length. Some information on the size or depth of the combining region can be extrapolated from this information. The lanthanide element series bind to both the Fc and the F_V regions of antibody molecules. In rabbit IgG, the Fc-binding constant is around 5×10^{-6} M, while in the combining region K_0 is around 10^{-4} M for gadolinium. It has been shown that in the Dnp-binding IgA myeloma protein the gadolinium (Gd[III]) binding site is close to the Dnp-binding site and that Dnp binding weakens the attachment of lanthanide (Dwek *et al.*, 1975a; Dower *et al.*, 1975). The same workers have also shown by using Piette's technique that the portion of the combining region binding Dnp probably measures $11 \times 9 \times 6$ Å based nitroxide spin labels. Proton nuclear magnetic resonance spectrosopcy at 270 MHz gives a paramagnetic difference spectrum which suggests that about 30 aliphatic and 30 aromatic residues are involved around the Dnp-combining site.

More recently attempts have been made to combine comparative sequence information with magnetic resonance data to build models of the Dnp-binding site in protein 315 (Dwek *et al.*, 1977; Padlan *et al.*, 1974). More definitive methods will be required before it is possible to assess the correctness of the models. A low degree of binding activity for both Dnp-lysine and menadione has been detected in the L—L dimer protein 315, but its relationship to the intact site is not clear (Gavish *et al.*, 1977). Other recent NMR studies have given the interesting information that in phosphorylcholine-binding myeloma proteins the phosphate and methyl moieties at the opposite ends of the hapten have differentiated dissociation rates (Goetze and Richards, 1977a,b).

F. Conformational Changes Secondary to Antigen Binding

There is much evidence to suggest that the combining region of the immunoglobulin itself is the antigen recognition unit of the cell surface receptor on antibody-producing precursor cells (Metzger, 1970). Binding of antigen to this receptor is an obligatory, although not a sufficient step required to turn the precursor cell into a proliferating, antibody-producing set of cells. One possible mechanism by which ligation of antigen to the Fab fragment might be signaled to the cell is if the antigen causes a conformational change in the Fab fragment which, in turn, is transmitted to the Fc fragment. This conformational change in the Fc fragment might be recognized by the Fc receptor on the cell surface. This speculation has given impetus to much work to find conformational changes which follow antigen binding. Several questions have to be answered positively before such changes can be accepted as a valid triggering mechanism.

Among them are: Does antigen induce a conformational change in the Fab fragment? Is it transmitted to the Fc fragment? If so, are any such conformational changes physiologically functional in the sense that they are obligatory for antigen stimulation?

Many studies of direct optical rotatory dispersion, circular dichroism, and the optical properties of emitted fluorescence have indicated that there is a change of symmetry in optically active centers in the Fab region on addition of antigen (Cathou *et al.*, 1974). Moreover, it is known that tryptophan residues, among others, are involved in these changes. It seems reasonable to interpret these studies as showing that some conformational change occurs. It can, of course, be reasoned *a priori* that, unless some exceptional circumstances obtain, any multipoint ligation of a molecule of substantial size will cause at least *some* conformational change in the ligating protein (Weber, 1975). Unfortunately, optical spectroscopic methods do not tell us the extent of these conformational changes.

High-resolution Fourier difference maps constructed from X-ray crystallography data of Fab fragments with and without antigen should demonstrate conclusively the presence or absence of major conformational changes. Protein NEW Fab fragment complexed to hydroxyvitamin K_1, which binds almost over the full length of the cleft, has been analyzed to 3.5 Å resolution (Amzel *et al.*, 1974; Poljak *et al.*, 1974). No conformational changes were detected. Similarly, the IgA immunoglobulin Fab fragment derived from mouse tumor McPC 603 complexed to the smaller antigen phosphorylcholine has also been analyzed (Segal *et al.*, 1974), and no conformational changes could be detected either. It could be that the two proteins studied were atypical or that the conformational changes produced by antigen are less than the limit of resolution of the methods used.

Recently, the transmission of changes from Fab to Fc fragment has been under active investigation. Research workers at the Weizmann Institute have identified and studied the circular dichroic changes derived from the emitted light of UV-stimulated tryptophan residues located in the Fc fragment (Schlessinger *et al.*, 1975). Under the conditions used, the spectral changes in the Fc fragment can be studied separately from those produced in the Fab fragment by interaction with antigen. These studies show that smaller antigens do not produce optical changes arising from the Fc fragment. However, large antigens such as whole proteins or polysaccharides containing 16 or more sugar residues, do produce spectral changes in the Fc region (Jaton *et al.*, 1976).

Recently, workers in the same laboratory (K. J., Willan *et al.*, 1977) have used the binding of gadolinium (Gd[III]) to the Fc fragment as a marker for conformational changes in that part of the antibody molecule. Then, using their homogeneous rabbit anti-(type III pneumococcal polysaccharide) IgG, they confirmed previous work which showed that changes in the solvent proton relaxation rate occurred *only* with greater than 16 saccharide units in the oligosaccharide, although aggregation of the IgG *does* occur at 16 saccharides. For larger saccharides (28 units), both aggregation and proton relaxation rate changes occur—a circumstance the authors attribute to a change in the tumbling time of the IgG rather than a conformational change due to antigen binding.

Thus we are left with a very attractive hypothesis which still remains unproven. The X-ray and spectral studies would seem to indicate that small haptens cause *no* conformational changes. Whether or not the experimental changes caused by the binding of larger molecules reflect Fc alterations is in doubt, although the evidence seems to be pointing against conformational change. The hypothesis is an important one, with implications for several areas of immunology. We look forward to its resolution in the next few years.

III. Structure-Function Relationships

A. Introduction

The relationship between primary amino acid sequence in the V region and antibody specificity is on the one hand very simple: related structures share specificities. On the other hand, it is very complex, since many different unrelated V regions may bind a single antigenic determinant with different degrees of avidity. It is probably naive to expect to find some common structural feature in the V regions of all antibodies to some small determinant X. There may be several anti-X families. The families need bear little resemblance to each other, although within each family the members will have close similarities, sharing idiotypes and perhaps the ability to bind other antigens. The ability to bind X by itself alone is a poor indicator of "consanguinity" since it is the property of many families of antibodies. A large, site-filling antigen which requires interaction at several points and demands stringent binding conditions is more likely to select a smaller set of antibody-producing cell clones, perhaps only one family or even only one clone, which is able to meet these conditions. Again, nonstringent selection conditions which select for binding of a small determinant over a wide range of binding energies will select a relatively large heterogeneous collection of antibody-producing cell clones which are able to meet these nonstringent conditions.

B. Relationships between Primary Structure and Binding Specificity

Antibodies of different ligand-binding specificities may have large regions of the primary sequence in common. It is therefore reasonable to suggest that in these antibodies those regions which show amino acid sequence variability are the regions concerned with binding antigens. However, it does *not* follow from this proposition that those amino acid residues which show the greatest sequence variability are necessarily the contact residues at which antigens bind. Wu and Kabat (1970) analyzed light-chain sequences for variability. They plotted variability at each amino acid position vs. position and obtained a graph showing three regions of greatest sequence variability. They termed these "hypervariable" regions. Capra and Kehoe (1975) performed a similar analysis on heavy-chain variable region sequences and were also able to demonstrate "hypervariable" regions.

Kabat *et al.* (1976, 1977) and his group have recently used computer analysis to show that the frequency distribution of amino acid pairs at or near contact residues is greater than would have been predicted from the random pairing of amino acids. They interpret their findings to show that noncontact residues may hold positions in the primary amino acid sequence which are critical for conformational changes leading to antigen binding. Since, however, the numbers of pairs is small, we must await analyses when a larger number of proteins are available for computer study.

C. Variable Region Groups and Subgroups

Early studies comparing partial amino acid sequences of different myeloma immunoglobulins showed that if one made an attempt to maximize amino acid residue homology, the variable regions of both the κ and λ light-chain groups could be divided into a number of subgroups. Five human λ (V_λ 1–5) and three human κ (V_κ 1–3) subgroups have been described by Smith *et al.* (1971), and Wang *et al.* (1973) have suggested that there may be a fourth subgroup. In the V regions of human heavy chains, three analogous subgroups $V_H 1–3$ have been delineated. Similar analyses on mouse κ chains show tat the number of subgroups and subsubgroups is rather large (Hood *et al.*, 1973). With each group or subgroup, there are amino acid residues which are subgroup specific (found, for instance, only in the $V_\kappa 1$ subgroup), group specific (found only in κ chains), chain specific (found only in L chains), and species specific (found only in dog light chains).

Forre *et al.* (1976) have developed subgroup-specific antisera to human myeloma heavy chains. The antisera were developed from heavy chains whose variable region amino acid sequences were known, thus providing a primary structural basis for the serology. A survey of 167 nonsequenced myeloma proteins showed a ratio of $1:2:3$ for $V_H I : V_H II : V_H III$. This same group (Forre *et al.*, 1977) has detected V_H determinants on the surface of lymphocytes from patients with chronic lymphocytic leukemia. The number of patients studied is too small to allow conclusions to be drawn about distribution of V_H subgroups on the cell surface.

Subgroup-specific antisera to mouse V_H subgroups have recently been reported by Bosma *et al.* (1977), but investigations establishing the presence of these subgroups on the cell surface remain to be done.

Finally, it should be noted that the distribution of V_H subgroups in mn may be influenced to some extent by the ease with which amino acid sequencing can be accomplished. Since the $V_H I$ and $V_H II$ subgroups are blocked (pyrrolidone-5-carboxylic acid at the NH_2-terminus), there are likely to be more sequences available for $V_H III$ heavy chains. Thus we may have to wait for more extensive serology to be done before the exact distribution of subgroups or subsubgroups in man is well established.

D. Hapten Contact and Hypervariable Regions

Several groups of research workers have compared both monoclonal immunoglobulins and antibody populations of known specificity to see if the amino acid sequence in the hypervariable regions can be correlated with antigen-binding specificity. Cebra and his colleagues at Johns Hopkins University have compared the amino acid sequence in the hypervariable regions of guinea pig anti-Dnp and antiarsonate antibodies. These workers use purified antibodies from strain 13 guinea pigs. The hypervariable regions are additionally identified by attachment of radioactive affinity reagents. It is found that distinct sequences occur in the hypervariable regions which correlate with Dnp binding and other sequences occur which correlate with the ability to bind arsonate (Cebra *et al.*, 1974).

Capra *et al.* (1971) examined the light chains from some homogeneous antibodies derived from patients with hypergammaglobulinemic purpura. All these antibodies had IgG-ligating activity. The amino acid residue sequence was identical in some up to residue 40; between others there were only infrequent amino acid differences. The hypervariable regions of most of these proteins closely resembled each other.

In contrast to workers who were able to correlate primary sequence and specificity is the work of Haber and his colleagues. Rabbits are hyperimmunized with type VIII pneumococcal polysaccharide. A percentage of such rabbits show the clonal dominance phenomenon in which the normally heterogeneous antibody response becomes highly restricted or monoclonal. Using this phenomenon, a large number of homogeneous rabbit antibodies with specificity for the type VIII pneumococcal polysaccharide have been isolated. These show the normal variations in binding constants for the antigen. The primary structures of a number of V_L and some V_H regions from these monoclonal immunoglobulins have been determined (Margolies *et al.*, 1975).

Cluster analysis was carried out using both the specific antipneumococcal antibodies and control monoclonal antibodies. The computer searched the sequences for groups or clusters of amino acid residues which were both internally consistent within the experimental (anti-type VIII polysaccharide) group and different from these sequences in the control group. No such clusters could be demonstrated, suggesting that in the rabbit system many different combining regions contribute to the binding of pneumococcal polysaccharide (Haber *et al.*, 1977).

These results are by no means mutually incompatible. If one considers a set of immunoglobulins on neighboring branches of an evolutionary tree, these will have diverged from each other by only a few residues. Among the multiple specificities represented in the combining region, it is quite likely that one function will not have been altered by the few amino acid replacements in the V region. Neighboring branches on such a genetic tree will have a set of proteins with V region structures that closely resemble each other and have a common antigen-binding specificity.

Since, however, other sets of contact amino acids may also bind the same antigen, several dissimilar sets of immunoglobulins will be widely distributed over nonadjacent branches of the tree since they have no necessary close evolutionary kinship. Depending on the method used for selecting the immunoglobulins, sets of immunoglobulins with either similar V regions or dissimilar V regions can be obtained. It is also conceivable that some antigens may be so stringent in their binding requirements that only one set of evolutionarily related clones on adjacent branches may be able to bind the antigen. In brief, it is a logical fallacy to believe that, because antibodies with similar V regions bind a common antigen, this antigen can be bound *only* by that type of V region.

E. Conservation of Variable Regions

When initial comparisons were made between partial L-chain amino acid sequences in mouse and man, it was noted that there was more sequence homology between certain mouse and human L chains than between certain V_L region sequences of two L chains within the species (Smith, 1973). Later work showed great similarity in structure between V regions of inbred and outbred animals of the same species and between the V regions of similar specificity raised in guinea pigs and mice (Capra and Kehoe, 1975). When phosphorylcholine-binding myeloma proteins from humans and mice were compared, extensive similarities of the heavy-chain (but not light-chain) variable regions were found (Riesen *et al.*, 1976). The lack of similarity for L-chain V regions may be related to the particular ligand (phosphorylcholine) where the ligand-binding properties in the mouse myeloma protein McPc 603 is more a function of heavy-chain than of light-chain variable regions (Padlan *et al.*, 1974). Support for this explanation comes from the work of Rivat *et al.*, (1977), who examined variable region markers in several primate species by means of heterologous specific antisera to both light and heavy chains. They were able to show that a greater number of heavy-chain variable regions were preserved from lower primates.

These similarities are not surprising. They may represent, for instance, the *retention* of certain H- and L-chain sequences which ligate some persisting pathogens and thus be subject to selective pressure. Alternatively, they may represent an example of parallel evolution or the development of the same ligating sequence from two originally different sequences under the selective pressure by, perhaps, a common pathogen.

F. Kinetics of Antigen Binding

In the ideal case, the binding of a univalent antigen (hapten) to a single antibody-binding site can be represented by the law of mass action, such that at equilibrium

$$[S] + [L] \rightleftharpoons [S \cdot L]$$

where $[S]$ represents the concentration of antibody-binding sites and $[L]$ represents the concentration of univalent ligand. If 1 mol of sites and 1 mol of ligand are mixed and form x mol of complex, $[S \cdot L]$, then at equilibrium, there will be 1-x mol of sites and 1-x mol of ligand free, with x mol of each in the form $[S \cdot L]$. The binding constant for this equilibrium can be defined as:

$$K_a = \frac{[S \cdot L]}{[S]_{\text{free}} \times [L]_{\text{free}}}$$

From this relationship it can be seen that if 50% of the available antibody-binding sites were associated with ligand then $[S]_{\text{free}} = [S \cdot L]$ and $K_a = 1/[L]_{\text{free}}$.

Thus the binding constant is defined as the reciprocal of the free or unbound ligand concentration resulting in 50% of the available binding sites being associated with ligand. It should be noted that the K_a is *independent* of the antibody concentration. The relationship between bound sites and free sites or between bound ligand and free ligand is not a linear one, but a hyperbolic one. A linear relationship can be derived from this general equation. Let us define the following terms:

1. Let $[L]_{\text{free}} = C$
2. Let $r = \dfrac{\text{mol of ligand bound}}{\text{mol of antibody}}$

   so that $r = \dfrac{[L]_{\text{bound}}}{[Ab]}$

   and $[L]_{\text{bound}} = r \times [Ab]$
   also $[L]_{\text{bound}} = [S \cdot L]$
3. Let the number of binding sites per antibody be n, so that the total site concentration is $n \times [Ab]$
4. It follows from (2) and (3) that the free site concentration $[S]_{\text{free}} = n[Ab] - [L]_{\text{bound}}$

$$K_a = \frac{[S \cdot L]}{[S]_{\text{free}} \times [L]_{\text{free}}} = \frac{[L]_{\text{bound}}}{[S]_{\text{free}} \times [L]_{\text{free}}} = \frac{r[Ab]}{(n[Ab] - [L]_{\text{bound}}) \times C}$$

Dividing top and bottom by [Ab], we obtain

$$K = \frac{r}{(n - [L]_{\text{bound}}/[Ab]) \times C} = \frac{r}{(n - r) \times C}$$

Hence

$$K \times C \times n - K \times C \times r = r$$

and

$$r/C = nK - rK$$

which is a linear relationship between r/C and r whose slope is $-K_a$ and whose y intercept is nK_a.

This useful relationship is known as a Scatchard plot (Scatchard, 1949). From it both the equilibrium binding constant, K_a, and the number of binding sites per antibody, n, can be determined. Since an antibody has a finite number of binding sites, as C increases r/C tends to 0. When C is very large, all of the antibody binding sites are saturated with ligand and $r/C = 0$. Thus the line extrapolates to $r = n$ at $r/C = 0$. Knowing K_a for a particular antibody-ligand interaction enables one to calculate the free energy change associated with binding:

$$\Delta F = -2.303\,RT \log K_a$$

where R is the gas constant and T is temperature in degrees Kelvin. The free energy change associated with binding is composed of two thermodynamic components, enthalpy (heat) and entropy (order):

$$\Delta F = \Delta H - T\Delta S$$

where ΔH is the heat component and ΔS is the order component. Either or both of these can be the driving force the formation of the site-ligand complex. The ΔH contribution can be determined experimentally, either by sensitive calorimetry measurements (Johnston et al., 1974) or by observing the K_a at several different temperatures, since ΔH and K_a are related:

$$\Delta H = \frac{2.303\ R \log\ (K_2/K_1)}{1/T_1 - 1/T_2}$$

If ΔH is 0, then $K_2 = K_1$ and the binding constant is independent of temperature. In this case the driving force for binding is entropy or ΔS.

For the interaction of small haptenic groups such as 2,4-Dnp amino acids and their corresponding antibodies, K_a is temperature dependent.

G. Homogeneous and Heterogeneous Binding

The above treatment is for the ideal case: homogeneous population of binding sites, each with an identical K_a. These results would obtain for a myeloma protein or a pure enzyme. However, naturally raised antibodies are generally not homogeneous species but consist of populations of proteins, each having a distinct K_a for the test ligand. In such a case, a Scatchard binding plot would not be a straight line, but would be a curve, as is shown in Fig. 5.

At low r values, that is, when ligand concentrations are low, only the binding sites with the highest K_a's will start to fill with ligand. Hence the slope of the plot at these values is steep. As ligand concentration

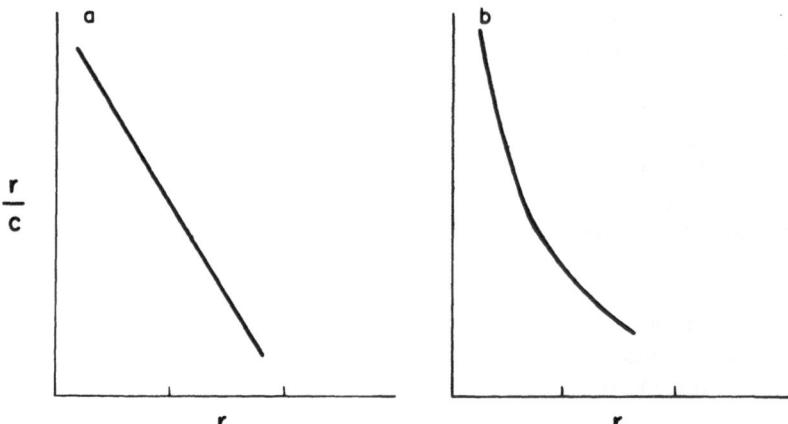

Figure 5.   Scatchard plots of the binding of a small ligand to antibody. (a) Binding of the ligand to homogeneous binding sites. (b) Binding of the ligand to a population of heterogeneous (with respect to binding constant K_a) binding sites.

increases and r starts to approach n, the number of binding sites, the lower and lower affinity sites begin to fill and the slope of the plot decreases. The curve still extrapolates to $r = n$ at $r/C = 0$. An average K_a for the population can be calculated by observing the slope at which r is 50% of saturation.

It is possible to obtain information about the distribution of binding constants, also called the "degree of heterogeneity," by using the Sips distribution function (Nisonoff and Pressman, 1958a,b), relating the fractional saturation of the binding sites to the concentration of ligand.

Since we have already derived the relationship, $r = n\,K_a\,C - C\,K_a\,r$, terms can be arranged to yield

$$r = K_a \cdot C\,(n - r)$$

and

$$\frac{r}{n - r} = K_a C$$

Taking the log of this equation

$$\log \left(\frac{r}{n - r}\right) = \log K_a + \log C$$

a plot of log $[r/n - r)]$ against log C will yield a straight line of slope =

1, and $r/(n - r)$ axis intercept of log K_a. If a population of naturally raised antihapten antibodies is subjected to this analysis, the plot will actually have a slope considerably less than 1. This slope is called the "heterogeneity index" and modifies the equation:

$$\log \left(\frac{4}{n - r} \right) = a \log K_a + a \log C$$

This relationship is truly valid only for a Gaussian type of distribution of binding constants around the mean K_a for the population, and no conclusions can be drawn from the heterogeneity index about the number of antibodies present when the index is less than 1.0. Because of the imprecision of the measurement, even when the index is 1.0 or close to that figure, more than one antibody may be present (Pincus et al., 1968).

The binding equilibrium between antibody binding site and ligand is composed of two rate reactions: a forward reaction, whose velocity, V_1, is

$$V_1 = k_1 [S][L]$$

where k_1 is the forward rate constant (dimensions, sec^{-1} M^{-1}), and a reverse reaction, whose velocity, V_{-5}, is

$$V_{-1} = k_{-1} [S \cdot L]$$

where k_{-1} is the reverse direction rate constant (dimensions, sec^{-1}). At equilibrium $V_1 = V_{-1}$ and $k_1 [S][L] = k_{-5} [SL]$. Therefore,

$$\frac{[SL]}{[S][L]} = \frac{k_1}{k_{-1}} = K_a$$

The ratio of the forward and reverse rate constants equals the equilibrium binding constant. Experimentally, with techniques such as stopped flow, it is easier to determine the forward rate constant. By also determining the equilibrium binding constant, K_a, the reverse rate constant can then be calculated. With relaxation techniques such as temperature jump, both rate constants can be experimentally derived. Using such a method, Pecht (1974) has studied in detail the on and off rates for a series of Dnp ligands binding to protein 315, an IgA$_2$ mouse myeloma protein. The Dnp ligands were synthesized with various modifications in the ring, different alkyl tail lengths, and various degrees of side-chain branching. Pecht found a range of forward and reverse rate constants depending on what changes were made in the various parts of the ligand. All of the forward rates were fast, on the order of $1-5 \times 10^8$ m^{-1} sec^{-1}. The off rates were much slower, varying from 40 sec^{-1} to 1300 sec^{-1}.

The conclusion was that Dnp ligands interacted with the binding site of protein 315 at four subsites:

$$NO_2 \text{—} \langle ring \rangle \text{—} NO_2 \quad NH\text{—}C\text{—}C\text{—}C\text{—}COOH$$

with side groups C (top) and C (bottom) on the first carbon, labeled

$$|\leftarrow\!\!\!\!\!\text{———}S_1\text{———}\!\!\!\!\!\rightarrow|\leftarrow S_2 \rightarrow|\leftarrow S_3 \rightarrow|\leftarrow S_4 \rightarrow$$

S_1 concerned the nature of the ring; S_2 depended on the degree and nature of branching of the side chain; S_3 was a hydrophobic site near the end of the ligand; and S_4 interacted with the charge at the end of the molecule.

Thus even a hapten such as Dnp attached to an aliphatic side chain interacts with the binding site of an antibody over a considerable distance, involving several points of interaction.

IV. Biological Significance of Antigen Binding

A. Polyfunctional Antibody-Combining Regions

In recent years, two lines of evidence have suggested that a single immunoglobulin may be complementary to several structurally dissimilar antigens. Haimovich and DuPasquier (1973) have shown that the tadpole has approximately 1×10^6 lymphocytes yet is able to mount a specific humoral response directed against the Dnp determinant (anti-Dnp). The response to single haptens is usually heterogeneous, involving many different clones of cells which produce anti-Dnp antibody. In order that the antibody reach detectable levels, the number of cells involved in this specific anti-Dnp response must be a very considerable proportion of the total. There is no doubt that the tadpole can respond to many antigens. Thus there seem to be too few cells at any one time to account for the range of immune responses observed. The clonal dilution studies which indicated the presence of many antibodies complementary to one antigenic determinant have been summarized earlier (Williamson, 1972). All these studies may be summarized by stating that if there is only one antihapten specificity per antibody molecule (or per cell), there do not appear to be enough lymphoid cells to account for the number of antigenic specificities. Reciprocally, there appear to be a very large number of clones involved in the production of antibodies against a single haptenic determinant. Over the last decade, homogeneous myeloma proteins which bind antigens have become available. An early finding was that a number of these myeloma proteins bound more than one hepatic determinant. This binding was competitive, and since only one determinant could be bound at a time to a single combining region it was usually assumed that there were common structural features in the competing determinants bound to a single locus on the protein.

Rosenstein and his co-workers examined the combining region of protein 460, a mouse γA myeloma protein which binds competitively the haptens Dnp and menadione. These workers found a —SH group in

relation to the combining region (Rosenstein *et al.*, 1972; Jackson and Richards, 1974). When this —SH group was substituted with a bulky reagent, the ability of protein 460 to bind menadione was impaired, while the ability to bind Dnp remained intact. When the protein was partially denatured with 4.3 M guanidine HCl and then allowed to refold partially, the ability to bind Dnp was ablated while menadione binding remained intact. Other methods for differentially affecting one binding activity were also described. This work suggested, but did not prove, that there were spatially separated sites within the combining region. Later work on the same protein using the technique of fluorescent energy transfer between donor fluorescent probes placed on the —SH groups and the Dnp and menadione molecules bound to their sites showed that there was a minimum separation of 12–14 Å between the Dnp- and menadione-binding sites (Manjula *et al.*, 1976). To support these findings, dextran bead–spacer–Dnp and dextran bead–spacer–menadione columns were constructed with spacer molecules of varying length. The shortest spacer-determinant combination needed to hold protein 460 to the column was determined for both the Dnp and menadione determinants. The difference in length between the two shortest molecules was 1.25 Å, a finding consistent with the separation distance calculated from the energy transfer experiments (Rosenstein and Richards, 1976). There appears to be reasonable evidence that there is substantial spatial separation between two combining sites within the antibody-combining region, making it probable that the combining region is in fact a mosaic of determinant-binding sites.

Even though an individual antibody combining region may bind diverse determinants at different sites, this is not by itself proof that multiple binding is physiologically significant; it is, for instance, possible that binding at only one subsite of the V region cell-surface receptor induces cell proliferation and antibody production. However, experiments have shown that this objection does not appear to be true. In rabbits (Varga *et al.*, 1973) and in mice (Varga *et al.*, 1974*a*), isoelectric focusing can pick out individual immunoglobulin bands which bind two dissimilar haptens. In the same animal, the same double-binding bands can be induced by either of the two antigens (Fig. 6), showing that the binding of both antigens induces cell proliferation and antibody production within the cell clone which binds both antigens (Varga *et al.*, 1973).

Double-binding myeloma proteins appear to have V regions that resemble those of some induced antibodies which bind the same antigens. This is based on the observation that anti-idiotypic sera raised against V region determinants of myeloma proteins will cross-react with their naturally induced counterparts. In fact, this cross-reactivity will occasionally be seen even when the double-binding myeloma protein has arisen in one species and the induced antibodies are from another (Varga *et al.*, 1974*a*). This "species cross-reactivity" stresses the considerable conservation of V region structure, which may be the result of parallel evolution of combining regions.

It is not yet clear how many different antigens are complementary to a single combining region. It has been estimated that when "random" antigens are screened, interactions with a K_0 of approximately 1×10^5 liters/mol occur once in about 140 compounds screened, while weaker interactions in the 1×10^3 liters/mol range occur much more frequently (one in 20 compounds screened). Secher (1977) and Cameron and Erlanger (1977) have recently made similar estimates based on data obtained from various kinds of competitive binding assays. Secher estimates that one antibody may bind ten ligands, whereas Cameron and Erlanger, examining the problem the other way around, find two complementary antigens from a group of 11 tested. The disparities between estimates of the number of binding ligands are likely to be due to selection of antigens, assay procedures, and definitions of significant K levels. Clearly these figures are approximate only since the choice of antigens can never be really random. Nevertheless, the general principle is clear: the higher the interaction energy, the less frequently cross-reactions are found. It is also intuitively clear that if high-energy cross-reactions were very com-

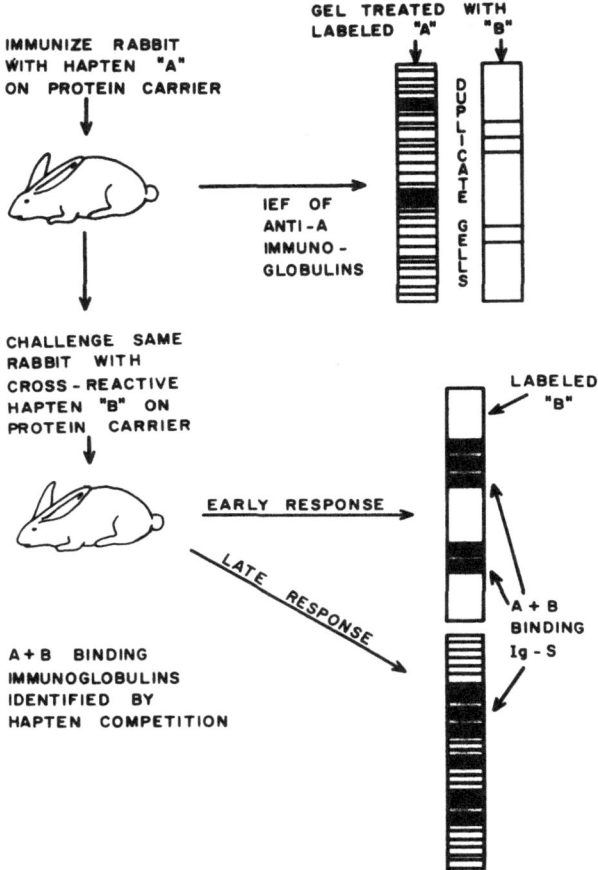

Figure 6. Experimental protocol for determining the presence of immunoglobulins with
polyfunctional combining regions in antihapten antisera.

mon, antibody populations would be like glue, sticking together all biological structures and showing no population specificity.

B. Specificity of Immune Sera

The high degree of specificity of an immune serum has been discussed earlier. It has been a frequent assumption that if a population of
antibodies has apparently exclusive specificity for one antigen, the indi-

vidual antibodies constituting that population must show the same exclusive specificity. In a perceptive article Talmage (1959) showed that this need not be true and that an apparently highly specific population could be derived from members having different specificities. We now know that, in myeloma proteins, individual hapten-combining sites have in fact a high degree of specificity and will, for instance, distinguish Dnp from mononitrophenols and trinitrophenols (Haimovich and DuPasquier, 1973). At the same time, protein 460 will bind a number of unrelated haptens at other sites within the combining region. The consequences of this, however, are exactly as Talmage first suggested. Let us suppose that a single V region may bind 100 different determinants. If the animal is immunized with determinant A, all those cells producing A-binding immunoglobulins of sufficient affinity will respond to the antigenic stimulus by cell proliferation and antibody production. Thus all antibody species produced bind A. Each antibody will also bind 99 other determinants, but these *need not be the same* for each antibody and such ligating activity will be present only at a lower level (i.e., 1%) in the antibody population and will be diluted out. Thus antibody specificity is, in essence, a *population phenomenon*, an average characteristic, rather than the property of each member of the population (see Fig. 7).

C. Epidemiological Considerations

There would be advantages to the animal if a single V region had specificity to more than one antigenic determinant. Thus a single determinant may ensure survival of antibodies complementary to a large number of unrelated antigenic determinants even if those determinants are no longer represented in the environment. "Memory" for a specific antibody to some pathogen may be retained by the presence of a quite different infective agent which need have no common antigenic determinants. This type of "linked" immune response was first recorded many years ago by Weil and Felix, who observed during World War I that many of the German soldiers under their care who had previously been exposed to typhoid fever (*Salmonella typhi*) showed a highly specific increase in antibodies to *S. typhi* when they contracted infection with *Rickettsia prowazekii*, an entirely unrelated organism having no detectible common antigenic determinants (Weil and Felix, 1916). There is a close relationship between this phenomenon and "original antigenic sin" (Fazekas, 1967), the power of a "related" antigen to induce production of antibodies to an antigen introduced long before. This phenomenon may occur both where there are truly "common" determinants and also where

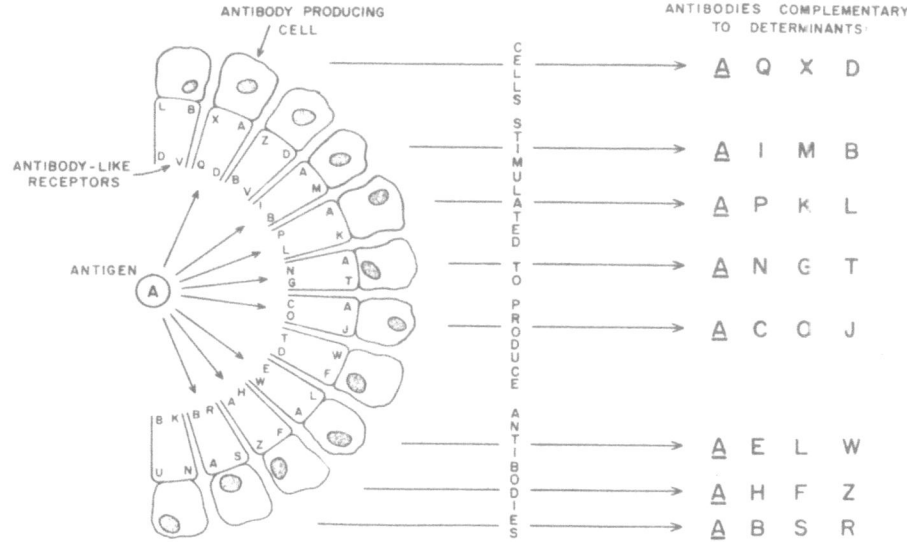

Figure 7. Immune serum specificity as a population phenomenon. Individual B-cell receptors are shown as having properties similar to those of immunoglobulin combining regions. For illustrative purposes, these are drawn as being each complementary to four different antigens; we suppose that this figure is in fact much larger. Stimulation by antigen A causes the cells with A specificity to divide and produce antibodies directed against A. The immune serum produced will therefore react in high titer with antigen A. Each immunoglobulin also has other specificities, but because these need not be the same in every molecule the other specificities B to Z will be diluted out and will react only in low titer.

there are "linked specificities." Since there would appear to be advantage in retaining the capacity for multiple binding, it may well be that the combining region has evolved structurally in such a way as to maximize the determinant-binding potential of the structure.

D. Maturation of Antibody Specificity

Early in the immune response to haptens, the antibody population often shows a lower average intrinsic binding constant for the immunizing antigen than later in the response. One classical pattern of antibody maturation of this type was described by Eisen and Siskind (1964). There is much evidence to suggest that the increase in antibodies of higher average affinity is an active process of recruitment of new antibodies and is not due to selective removal of either high- or low-affinity antibodies (Steiner and Eisen, 1966, 1967a,b). Siskind and Benacerraf (1969) have suggested that early in the immune response when antigen levels are high, effective stimulation of cells producing both low- and high-affinity antibodies will occur. Later in the immune response, when the antigen levels are low, only those cells with high-affinity receptors on their surface, producing high-affinity antibodies, will be stimulated with an increased production of high-affinity antibodies. Segre and Segre (1973) tried to obtain direct confirmation in tissue culture for the role of antigen concentration as the driving force in this process but were unable to do so. It must be emphasized that added antigen per se may also not reflect antigen concentration at the receptor site. Since combination of antigen with the cell surface receptor V region is a reversible reaction, there can be little doubt that the antigen concentration near the receptor must influence the immune response. However, it probably is not the only influence on antibody maturation.

"Polyfunctional" combining regions may play a role in the phenomenon of antibody maturation. When an animal is sensitized to antigen A, a small proportion of the antibodies produced will also bind an unrelated antigen B. Since the antibodies produced were "selected" by antigen A, those immunoglobulins which also bind B will do so on the average with low affinity. When primed with antigen A and then challenged with antigen B, the early anti-B antibodies produced after challenge will be predominantly of the double-binding type which have low average affinity for B. Only later will anti-B antibodies be produced which were "selected" by antigen B and have a higher average binding for this antigen. Hence the antibodies to antigen B will exhibit an increase in the average binding constant with time. The primary challenge with antigen A would have its natural counterpart in the fact that experimental animals are not immunologically virgin and have been subjected to immunological priming by ubiquitous microflora and perhaps also by "self" antigens.

Many examples have now been described of antigens which do not produce classical antibody maturation patterns (Wu and Rockey, 1969; Haber and Stone, 1969; Montgomery et al., 1972; Gopalakrishnan and Karush, 1974; Steward and Petty, 1972; Steward and Voller, 1973). Decreases in the average intrinsic binding constants late in the immune response seem to be a common occurrence, and examples of cyclical changes in antibody affinity have also been described (Macario and Demacario, 1975). Moreover, not only the type and quantity of antigen used but also the mode of administration, the kinetics of cell replication, the antigen carrier, the T-cell controlling mechanism, genetic and infective factors, and the previous immunological history of the host appear to influence the alteration of the antibody population produced. Thus the patterns of antibody maturation are probably the result of many interacting factors, and while they often result in antibody populations of higher affinity late in the immune response, many variations on this theme as well as complete absence of maturation may at times be encountered.

V. Summary

It seems likely that immunoglobulin combining regions have evolved from some archetypal molecule and those forms which are useful to the animal have been retained. It is the entire population of antibody combining regions which forms the antigen recognition repertoire of the humoral immune system, and in such a system not only the properties of individual antibody combining regions but also the properties of the multiprotein system as a whole are important for the defenses of the body against pathogens.

Antibody combining sites may bind a disparate set of structurally related and unrelated ligands. This *multispecificity* can be biologically meaningful: the same clone can be stimulated by different antigens. The most significant impacts of the multispecificity are as follows: (1) It reduces the number of V region genes necessary to code for the total number of combining sites. (2) The cross-stimulation of clones by structurally related and unrelated antigens may be instrumental in the normal maintenance of immune responsiveness and, in addition, may explain the ability to respond to unusual and less ubiquitous antigens. (3) The antigenic history of the animal may contribute to the maturation of the immune response by cross-stimulation of preselected clones of antigenbinding cells.

VI. References

Albertson, P., and Phillipson, L., 1960, *Nature (London)* **185**:38.

Almeida, J. D., and Waterson, A. P., 1969, *Adv. Virus Res.* **15**:307.

Amzel, L. M., Poljak, R. J., Saul, F., Varga, J. M., and Richards, F. F., 1974, *Proc. Natl. Acad. Sci. USA* **71**:1427.

Bell, G. I., 1974, *Nature* **248**:430.

Binz, H., Lindemann, J., and Wigzell, H., 1973, *Nature* **246**:146.

Binz, H., Lindemann, J., and Wigzell, H., 1974, in: *The Immune System, Genes, Receptors, Signals* (E. E. Sercarz, A. R. Williamson, and C. F. Fox, eds.), p. 533, Academic Press, New York.

Bosma, M. J., De Witt, C., Hausman, S. J., Marks, R., and Potter, M., 1977, *J. Exp. Med.* **146**:1041.

Brack, C., and Tonegawa, S., 1977, *Proc. Natl. Acad. Sci. USA* **74**:5652.

Brient, B. W., Haimovich, J., and Nisonoff, A., 1971, *Proc. Natl. Acad. Sci. USA* **68**:3136.

Cameron, D. J., and Erlanger, B. F., 1976, *Immunochemistry* **13**:263.

Cameron, D. J., and Erlanger, B. F., 1977, *Nature (London)* **268**:763.

Capra, J. D., and Kehoe, J. M., 1974, *Proc. Natl. Acad. Sci. USA* **71**:4032.

Capra, J. D., and Kehoe, J. M., 1975, *Adv. Immunol.* **20**:1.

Capra, J. D., Winchester, R. J., and Kunkel, H. G., 1971, *Medicine* **50**:125.

Cathou, R. E., and Haber, E., 1967, *Biochemistry* **6**:513.

Cathou, R. E., and Dorrington, K. J., 1975, in: *Biological Macromolecules,* Series 7, Part C (S. N. Timasheff and G. D. Fasma, eds.), p. 91, Dekker, New York.

Cathou, R. E., and Werner, T. C., 1970, *Biochemistry* **9**:3149.

Cathou, R. E., Holowka, D. A., and Chan, L. M., 1974, in: *Progress in Immunology II,* Vol. 1 (L. Brent and J. Holborow, eds.), p. 63, North-Holland, Amsterdam.

Cebra, J. J., Koo, P. H., and Ray, A., 1974, *Science* **186**:263.

Cesari, I. M., and Weigert, M. G., 1973, *Proc. Natl. Acad. Sci. USA* **70**:2112.

Claflin, J. L., and Davie, J. M., 1975, *J. Immunol.* **114**:70.

Cohen, S., and Porter, R. R., 1964, *Adv. Immunol.* **4**:287.

Converse, C. A., and Richards, F. F., 1968, *Fed. Proc.* **27**:683.

Converse, C. A., and Richards, F. F., 1969, *Biochemistry* **8**:4431.

Cosenza, H., and Kohler, H., 1972, *Proc. Natl. Acad. Sci. USA* **69**:2701.

Cramer, M., and Braun, D. G., 1974, *J. Exp. Med.* **138**:1533.

Crothers, D. M., and Metzger, H., 1974, *Immunochemistry* **9**:341.

Day, E. D., 1972, in: *Advanced Immunochemistry,* 1st ed., Williams and Wilkins, Baltimore.

Day, L. A., Sturtevant, J. M., and Singer, S. J., 1963, *Ann. N.Y. Acad. Sci.* **103**:611.

Dower, S. K., Dwek, R. A., McLaughlin, A. C., Mole, L. M., Press, E. M., and Sunderland, C. A., 1975, *Biochem. J.* **149**:73.

Dwek, R. A., Jones, R., Marsh, D., McLaughlin, A. C., Press, E. M., Price, N. C., and White, A. I., 1975a, *Phil. Trans. R. Soc. Lond.* **B272**:53.

Dwek, R. A., Knott, J. C. A., Marsh, D., McLaughlin, A. C., Press, E. M., Price, N. C., and White, A. I., 1975b, *Eur. J. Biochem.* **53**:25.

Dwek, R. A., Wain-Hobson, S., Dower, S., Gettins, P., Sutton, B., Perkins, S. J., and Givol, D., 1977, *Nature* **266**:31.

Edelman, G. M., and Gall, W. E., 1969, *Annu. Rev. Biochem.* **38**:415.

Edelman, G. M., Cunningham, B. A., Gottlieb, P. D., Rutishauser, U., and Waxdal, M. J., 1969, *Proc. Natl. Acad. Sci. USA* **63**:78.

Edmundson, A. B., Ely, K. R., Girling, R. L., Abola, E. E. Schiffer, M., Westholm, F. A., Fausch, M. D., and Deutsch, H. F., 1974, *Biochemistry* **13**:3816.

Eisen, H. N., 1964a, in: *Immunology,* 2nd ed., Chapter 15, Harper and Row, Hagerstown, Md.

Eisen, H. N., 1964b, in: *Methods in Medical Research,* Vol. 10, p. 115, Year Book Med. Publ., Chicago.

Eisen, H. N., 1971, in: *Progress in Immunology,* p. 243, Academic Press, New York.

Eisen, H. N., and Siskind, G. W., 1964, *Biochemistry* **3**:996.

Eisen, H. N., Little, J. R., Osterland, C. K., and Simms, E. S., 1967, *Cold Spring Harbor Symp. Quant. Biol.* **32**:75.

Epp, O., Lattman, E. E., Schiffer, M., Huber, R., and Palm, W., 1975, *Biochemistry* **14**:4943.

Fazekas De St. Groth, S. 1967, *Cold Spring Harbor Symp. Quant. Biol.* **32**:525.

Fazekas De St. Groth, S., and Webster, R. G., 1966, *J. Exp. Med.* **124**:331.

Fehlhammer, H., Schiffer, M., Epp, O., Colman, P. M., Lattman, E. E. Schwager, P., Steigemann, W., and Schramm, H. J., 1975, *Biophys. Struct. Mechanism* **1**:139.

Feinstein, A., and Rowe, A. J., 1965, *Nature (London)* **205**:147.

Fisher, C. E., and Press, E. M., 1974, *Biochem. J.* **139**:135.

Fleet, G. W., Knowles, J. R., and Porter, R. R., 1969, *Nature (London)* **224**:511.

Forre, ∅., Natvig, J. B., and Kunkel, H. G., 1976, *J. Exp. Med.* **144**:897.

Forre, ∅., Froland, S. S., Natvig, J. B., Michaelsen, T. E., Johnson, P. M., Ly, B., and Laake, K., 1977, *J. Immunol.* **118**:1513.

Francis, T., 1953, *Ann. Intern. Med.* **39**:203.

Franek, F., 1973, *Eur. J. Biochem.* **33**:59.

Freedman, M., Merret, T. R., and Pruzanski, W., 1976, *Immunochemistry* **13**:195.

Gavish, M., Dwek, R. A., and Givol, D., 1977, *Biochemistry* **16**:3154.

Givol, D., 1974, *Essays Biochem.* **10**:73.

Glazer, A. N., 1970, *Proc. Natl. Acad. Sci. USA* **65**:1057.

Goetze, A. M., and Richards, J. H., 1977a, *Proc. Natl. Acad. Sci. USA* **74**:2109.

Goetze, A. M., and Richards, J. H., 1977b, *Biochemistry* **16**:228.

Goetzl, E. J., and Metzger, H., 1970, *Biochemistry* **9**:3826.

Goidl, E. A., Barondess, J. J., and Siskind, G. W., 1975, *Immunology* **29**:629.

Gopalakrishnan, P. V., and Karush, F., 1974, *J. Immunol.* **113**:769.

Green, N. M., 1968, *Adv. Immunol.* **11**:1.

Haber, E., and Richards, F. F., 1967, *Proc. R. Soc. London* **166**:176.

Haber, E., and Stone, M., 1969, *Israel J. Med. Sci.* **5**:332.

Haber, E., Margolies, M. N., Cannon, L. E., and Rosenblatt, M. S., 1975, in: *Molecular Approaches to Immunology*, p. 303, Academic Press, New York.

Haber, E., Richards, F. F., Spragg, J., Austen, K. F., Valloton, M., and Page, L. B., 1967, *Cold Spring Habor Symp. Quant. Biol.* **32**:299.

Haber, E., Margolies, M. N., and Cannon, L. E., 1977, in: *Antibodies in Human Diagnosis and Therapy* (Haber and Krause, eds.), Raven Press, New York.

Haimovich, J., and DuPasquier, L., 1973, *Proc. Natl. Acad. Sci. USA* **70**:1898.

Haimovich, J., Givol, D., and Eisen, H. N., 1970, *Proc. Natl. Acad. Sci. USA* **67**:1656.

Haimovich, J., Eisen, H. N., Hurwitz, E., and Givol, D., 1972, *Biochemistry* **11**:2389.

Haselkorn, D., Friedman, S., Givol, D., and Pecht, I., 1974, *Biochemistry* **13**:2210.

Hew, C.-L., Lifter, J., Yoshioka, M., Richards, F. F., and Konigsberg, W. H., 1973, *Biochemistry* **12**:4685.

Hochman, J., Inbar, D., and Givol, D., 1973, *Biochemistry* **12**:1131.

Heossli, D., Olander, J., and Little, J. R., 1976, *J. Immunol.* **113**:1024.

Hood, L., McKean, D., Farnsworth, V., and Potter, M., 1973, *Biochemistry* **12**:741.

Hsia, J. C., and Piette, L. H., 1969, *Arch. Biochem. Biophys.* **129**:296.

Inbar, D., Hochman, J., and Givol, D., 1972, *Proc. Natl. Acad. Sci. USA* **69**:2659.

Inman, J. K., 1974, in: *The Immune System, Genes, Receptors, Signals* (E. E. Sercarz, A. R. Williamson, and C. F. Fox, eds.), p. 19, Academic Press, New York.

Jackson, P., and Richards, F. F., 1974, *J. Immunol.* **112**:96.

Jaton, J.-C., Huser, H., Riesen, W. F., Schlessinger, J., and Givol, D., 1976, *J. Immunol.* **116**:1363.

Jerne, N. K., 1974, *Ann. Immunol (Paris)* **125c**:373.

Johnston, M. F. M., Barisas, B. G., and Sturtevant, J. M., 1974, *Biochemistry* **13**:390.

Kabat, E. A., 1960, *J. Immunol.* **84**:82.

Kabat, E. A., 1966, *J. Immunol.* **97**:1.

Kabat, E. A., Wu, T. T., and Bilofsky, H., 1976, *Proc. Natl. Acad. Sci. USA* **73**: 617.
Kabat, E. A., Wu, T. T., and Bilofsky, H., 1977, *J. Biol. Chem.* **252:**6609.
Karush, F., 1962, *Adv. Immunol.* **2:**1.
Klostergaard, J., Grossberg, A. L., Krausz, L. M., and Pressman, D., 1977, *Immunochemistry* **14:**37.
Knowles, J. R., 1972, *Acc. Chem. Res.* **5:**155.
Kreth, H. W., and Williamson, A. R., 1973, *Eur. J. Immunol.* **3:**141.
Kuettner, M. C., Wang, A. L., and Nisonoff, A., 1972, *J. Exp. Med.* **135:**575.
Labaw, L. W., and Davies, D. R., 1971, *J. Biol. Chem.* **246:**3760.
Lafferty, K. J., and Oertelis, S., 1963, *Virology* **21:**91.
Landsteiner, K., 1938, in: *The Specificity of Serological Reactions,* p. 1962, Dover, New York.
Lautz, A., and Siskind, G., 1975, *Immunology* **29:**301.
Lieberman, R., Potter, M., Mushinski, E. B., Humphrey, W., Jr., and Rudikoff, S., 1974, *J. Exp. Med.* **139:**983.
Lieberman, R., Potter, M., Humphrey, W., Mushinski, E. B., and Vrana, M., 1975, *J. Exp. Med.* **142:**106.
Lifter, J., Hew, C.-L., Yoshioka, M., Richards, F. F., and Konigsberg, W. H., 1974, *Biochemistry* **13:**3567.
Little, J. R., and Eisen, H. N., 1967, *Biochemistry* **6:**3119.
Macario, A. J. L., and Demacario, E. C., 1975, in: *Current Topics in Microbiology and Immunology,* Vol. 71, p. 125, Springer-Verlag, New York.
Manjula, B. N., Richards, F. F., and Rosenstein, R. W., 1976, *Immunochemistry* **13:**929.
Margolies, M. N., Cannon, L. E., III, Strosberg, A. D., and Haber, E., 1975, *Proc. Natl. Acad. Sci. USA* **72:**2180.
Metzger, H., 1970, *Annu. Rev. Biochem.* **39:**889.
Metzger, H., and Singer, S. J., 1963, *Science* **142:**674.
Michaelides, M. C., and Eisen, H. N., 1971, quoted in H. N. Eisen, *Progress in Immunology,* p. 243, Academic Press, New York.
Montgomery, P. C., Rockey, J. H., and Williamson, A. R., 1972, *Proc. Natl. Acad. Sci. USA* **69:**228.
Moreno, C., and Kabat, E. A., 1969, *J. Exp. Med.* **129:**871.
Murphy, P. D., and Sage, H. J., 1970, *J. Immunol.* **105:**460.
Nisonoff, A., and Pressman, D., 1958*a, J. Immunol.* **80:**417.
Nisonoff, A., and Pressman, D., 1958*b, J. Immunol.* **81:**126.
Nisonoff, A., and Thorbecke, G. J., 1964, *Annu. Rev. Biochem.* **33:**355.
Nisonoff, A., Zappacosta, S., and Jureziz, R., 1967, *Cold Spring Harbor Symp. Quant. Biol.* **32:**89.
Nisonoff, A., Hopper, J. E., and Spring, S. B., 1975, in: *The Antibody Molecule,* Chapter II, p. 448, Academic Press, New York.
Noelken, M. E., Nelson, C. A., Buckley, C. E., III, and Tanford, C., 1965, *J. Biol. Chem.* **240:**218.
Northrop, J. A., 1942, *J. Gen. Physiol.* **25:**465.
Ohta, Y., Gill, T. J., III, and Leung, C. S., 1970, *Biochemistry* **9:**2708.
Padlan, E. A., Segal, D. M., Cohen, G. A., and Davies, D. R., 1974, in: *The Immune System, Genes, Receptors, Signals* (E. E. Sercarz, A. R. Williamson, and C. F. Fox, eds.), p. 7, Academic Press, New York.
Painter, R. H., Sage, H. J., and Tanford, C., 1972, *Biochemistry* **11:**1327.
Parker, C. W., and Osterland, C. K., 1969, *Biochemistry* **9:**1074.

Pecht, I., 1974, in: *The Immune System, Genes, Receptors, Signals* (E. E. Sercarz, A. R. Williamson, and C. F. Fox, eds.), p. 15, Academic Press, New York.

Piette, L. H., Kiefer, E. F., Grossberg, A. L., and Pressman, D., 1972, *Immunochemistry* **9**:17.

Pincus, J. H., Haber, E., and Katz, M., 1968, *Science* **162**:667.

Pink, J. R. L., and Askonas, B. A., 1974, *Eur. J. Immunol.* **4**:426.

Poljak, R. J., 1975, *Nature (London)* **256**:373.

Poljak, R. J., Amzel, L. M., Avey, H. P., Chen, B. L., Phizackerly, R. P., and Saul, F., 1973, *Proc. Natl. Acad. Sci. USA* **70**:3305–3310.

Poljak, R. J., Amzel, L. M., Chen, B. L., Phizackerley, R. P., and Saul, F., 1974, *Proc. Natl. Acad. Sci. USA* **71**:3440.

Porter, R. R., 1958, *Nature (London)* **182**:670.

Porter, R. R., and Press, E. M., 1962, *Annu. Rev. Biochem.* **31**:625.

Potter, M., 1972, *Physiol. Rev.* **52**:631.

Potter, M., and Lieberman, R., 1970, *J. Exp. Med.* **132**:737.

Poulik, M. D., and Reisfeld, R. A., 1976, *Contemp. Top. Mol. Immunol.* **4**:157.

Quattrochi, R., Cioli, D., and Baglioni, C., 1969, *J. Exp. Med.* **130**:401.

Reichlin, M., 1974, *Immunochemistry* **11**:21.

Richards, F., and Konigsberg, W., 1977, in: *Methods in Enzymology,* Vol. XLVI, p. 508, Academic Press, New York.

Richards, F. F., Sloane, R. W., Jr., and Haber, E., 1967, *Biochemistry* **6**:476.

Richards, F. F., Lifter, J., Hew, C.-L., Yoshioka, M., and Konigsberg, W. H., 1974, *Biochemistry* **13**:3572.

Richards, F. F., Konigsberg, W. H., Rosenstein, R. W., and Varga, J. M., 1975, *Science* **187**:130.

Richards, F. M., 1974, *J. Mol Biol.* **82**:1.

Riesen, W. F., Braun, D. G., and Jaton, J.-C., *Proc. Natl. Acad. Sci. USA* **73**:2096.

Rivat, L., Rivat, C., Lebreton, J. P., and Ropartz, C., 1977, *Ann. Immunol. (Paris)* **128**:185.

Rosenstein, R. W., and Richards, F. F., 1976, *Immunochemistry* **13**:939.

Rosenstein, R. W., Musson, R. A., Armstrong, M. Y. K., Konigsberg, W. H., and Richards, F. F., 1972, *Proc. Natl. Acad. Sci. USA* **69**:877.

Rubinstein, W. A., and Little, J. R., 1970, *Biochemistry* **9**:2106.

Ruoho, A. E., Kiefer, H., Roeder, P. E., and Singer, S. J., 1973, *Proc. Natl. Acad. Sci. USA* **70**:2567.

Scatchard, G., 1949, *Ann. N.Y. Acad. Sci.* **51**:660.

Schechter, B., Schechter, I., and Sela, M., 1970, *J. Biol. Chem.* **245**:1438.

Schiffer, M., Girling, R. L., Ely, K. R., and Edmundson, A. B., 1973, *Biochemistry* **12**:4620.

Schlessinger, J., Steinberg, I. Z., Givol, D., Hochman, J., and Pecht, I., 1975, *Proc. Natl. Acad. Sci. USA* **72**:2775.

Schubert, D., Jobe, A., and Cohn, M., 1968, *Nature (London)* **220**:882.

Secher, D., 1977, *Nature (London)* **268**:689.

Segal, D., Padlan, E. A., Cohen, G. H., Rudikoff, S., Potter, M., and Davies, D. R., 1974, *Proc. Natl. Acad. Sci. USA* **71**:4298.

Segre, D., and Segre, M., 1973, *Science* **181**:851.

Singer, S. J., and Doolittle, R. F., 1966, *Science* **153**:13.

Sirisinha, S., and Eisen, H. N., 1971, *Proc. Natl. Acad. Sci. USA* **68**:3130.

Siskind, G. W., and Benacerraf, B., 1969, *Adv. Immunol.* **10**:1.

Smith, G. P., 1973, *The Variation and Adaptive Expression of Antibodies,* Harvard University Press, Cambridge, Mass.

Smith, G. P., Hood, L., and Fitch, W. M., 1971, *Annu. Rev. Biochem.* **40**:969.

Steiner, L. A., and Eisen, H. N., 1966, *Bacteriol. Rev.* **30**:383.

Steiner, L. A., and Eisen, H. N., 1967a, *J. Exp. Med.* **126**:1161.

Steiner, L. A., and Eisen, H. N., 1967b, *J. Exp. Med.* **126**:1185.

Stevenson, G. T., 1973, *Biochem. J.* **133**:827.

Steward, M. W., and Petty, R. E., 1972, *Immunology* **23**:881.

Steward, M. W., and Voller, A., 1973, *Br. J. Exp. Pathol.* **54**:198.

Stryer, L., and Griffith, O. H., 1965, *Proc. Natl. Acad. Sci. USA* **54**:1785.

Talmage, D. W., 1959, *Science* **129**:1643.

Tolleshaug, H., and Hannestad, K., 1975, *Immunochemistry* **12**:173.

Tonegawa, S., Hozumi, N., Matthyssens, G., and Schuller, R., 1976, *Cold Spring Harbor Symp. Quant. Biol.* **41**:877.

Uemara, K.-I., Claflin, J. L., Davie, J. M., and Kinsky, S. C., 1975, *J. Immunol.* **114**:958.

Utsumi, S., and Karush, F., 1964, *Biochemistry* **3**:1329.

Valentine, R. C., and Green, N. M., 1967, *J. Mol. Biol.* **27**:615.

Varga, J. M., Konigsberg, W. H., and Richards, F. F., 1973, *Proc. Natl. Acad. Sci. USA* **70**:3269.

Varga, J. M., Lande, S., and Richards, F. F., 1974a, *J. Immunol.* **112**:1565.

Varga, J. M., Rosenstein, R. W., and Richards, F. F., 1974b, *Fed. Proc.* **33**:810 (abstr.).

Vaughan, R. J., and Westheimer, F. H., 1969, *J. Am. Chem. Soc.* **91**:217.

Velick, S. F., Parker, C. W., and Eisen, H. N., 1960, *Proc. Natl. Acad. Sci. USA* **46**:1470.

Vrana, M., Rudikoff, S., and Potter, M., 1977, *Biochemistry* **16**:1170.

Wang, A. C., Fudenberg, H. H., Wells, J. V., and Roelcke, D., 1973, *Nature (New Biol.)* **243**:126.

Warner, N. L., Potter, M., and Metcalf, D. (eds.), 1974, *International Union Against Cancer,* Workshop No. 1, p. 1, Geneva.

Waxdal, M. J., Konigsberg, W. H., and Edelman, G. M., 1968, *Biochemistry* **7**:1967.

Weber, G., 1975, *Adv. Protein Chem.* **29**:1.

Weil, E., and Felix, A., 1975, quoted in F. F. Richards, W. H. Konigsberg, R. W. Rosenstein, and J. M. Varga, *Science* **187**:130.

Weltman, J. K., and Edelman, G. M., 1967, *Biochemistry* **6**:1437.

Willan, K. J., Wallace, K. H., Jaton, J.-C., and Dwek, R. A., 1977, *Biochem. J.* **161**:205.

Williamson, A. R., 1972, *Biochem. J.* **130**:325.

Williamson, A. R., 1973, *Biochem. J.* **129**:1.

Wiswesser, W. J., 1975, quoted in F. F. Richards, W. H. Konigsberg, R. W. Rosenstein, and J. M. Varga, *Science* **187**:130.

Wofsy, L., and Parker, D. A., 1967, *Cold Spring Harbor Symp. Quant. Biol.* **32**:111.

Wofsy, L., Metzger, H., and Singer, S. J., 1962, *Biochemistry* **1**:1031.

Wu, W. H., and Rockey, J. H., 1969, *Biochemistry* **8**:2719.

Wu, T. T., and Kabat, E. A., 1970, *J. Exp. Med.* **132**:211.

Yguerabide, J., Epstein, H. F., and Stryer, L., 1970, *J. Mol. Biol.* **51**:573.

Yoo, T. J., Roholt, O. A., and Pressman, D., 1967, *Science* **157**:707.

Yoshioka, M., Lifter, J., Hew, C.-L., Converse, C. A., Armstrong, M. Y. K., Konigsberg, W. H., and Richards, F. F., 1973, *Biochemistry* **12**:4679.

4

Biochemistry and Biological Reactions of Complement Proteins

Robert M. Stroud, John E. Volanakis, Shigeharu Nagasawa, and Thomas F. Lint

I. Introduction

Complement research has evolved from the description and discovery of the plasma proteins that make up the system to a new period in which understanding of the relationships of specific fine structural data to functions is being achieved. A few complement protein fragments have been sequenced, as have several key portions of other components. Only as a result of the existence of extensive functional knowledge and specific assays could this new structural knowledge accumulate. Amino acid sequential analyses of more of these important plasma proteins will soon be accomplished by several groups, and detailed knowledge by crystallographic technique is in sight. Furthermore, these biochemical analyses have led to improved insight into the control of certain physiological and biological activities related to this system. The primary goal of most research in this area is pharmacological and/or physiological manipulation of the system to promote beneficial effects while inhibiting the injurious effects presumed to be operative in diseases of man. This goal seems to

Robert M. Stroud and John E. Volanakis · Division of Clinical Immunology and Rheumatology, The University of Alabama in Birmingham, Birmingham, Alabama 35294. **Shigeharu Nagasawa** · Faculty of Pharmaceutical Sciences, Hokkaido University, Sapporo, 060, Japan. **Thomas F. Lint** · Department of Immunology, Presbyterian-St. Luke's Hospital, Chicago, Illinois 60612. This work was supported in part by the Medical Research Service of the Veterans Administration. T. F. L. is supported in part by grants from the Chicago Heart Association and the Schweppe Foundation.

be within reach. The major good effects are those related to host defense against invading organisms. The bad effects are the tissue-destroying aspects of inflammation and cell membrane disruption. These two go hand in hand, and the goal to control one without influencing the other may sound incompatible since inflammation controls the invasion and killing of microbial organisms. However, these events are complex, and with overlapping phenomena there are many potential control points. Also, with supplementary pharmacological agents to eliminate invading organisms, the aim becomes more attractive. Since there is evidence that chronic viral infections may be tolerated by the host unless inflammation occurs, it seems particularly important to manipulate the systems that mediate inflammation in several presumed chronic viral diseases of man, particularly systemic lupus erythematosus and rheumatoid arthritis.

Recently the relationships of complement components to cell membrane receptors, cellular immune responses, and antibody production have been stimulated by the knowledge that some complement component genes are located on the histocompatibility chromosome. It is generally felt that structural analysis may show important unsuspected relationships to other proteins coded for in this area. There is harmony in these immune functions, and the details should soon be known.

This chapter will primarily focus on the biochemistry that is known to date; it will not be exhaustively comprehensive but will attempt to impart knowledge of recent developments in the field.

II. Classical Pathway

A. Complement Nomenclature

Complement nomenclature is still a hurdle for the student, but since there has been an agreement on the classical pathway published by a WHO Committee (WHO, 1970) it is becoming less difficult. There has been wide acceptance of this classical pathway nomenclature, and it is to be hoped that the Committee will soon agree on the alternative pathway. To help guide the reader we have reviewed the multiple terms for the alternative pathway nomenclature which are being used (see Table II), and a brief introduction to the WHO recommended nomenclature will be given here, along with a schematic guide to the various segments of the system (Fig. 1 and Table I). Early classical pathway components are designated by the symbols C1, C4, and C2. C1 consists of subcomponents C1q, C1r, and C1s. The components that are common to both

Table I.

	Classical Pathway
C1q	Recognition component, binds to activators
C1r	Bridges C1q, C1s; enzymatically activates C1s
C1s	Enzymatically activates C4 and C2
C4	Cofactor for C2; necessary for C3 cleavage by C2
C2	Enzymatically cleaves C3; analogous to B
	Alternative Pathway
IF	Proposed recognition component
D	Enzymatically activates B
B	Enzymatically cleaves C3; analogous to C2
C3b	Cofactor for B; necessary for C3 cleavage by B
P	"Properdin"; stabilizes the alternative pathway convertase
	Common to Both Pathways
C3	Major opsonic factor (C3b); necessary for C5 cleavage by B or C2
C5	Initiates membrane attack mechanism; major chemotactic factor (C5a)
C6	
C7	Bind to C5b to produce C5b67; C5b67 attaches to lipid bilayers
C8	
C9	Bind to C5b67 to create a lesion in lipid bilayers

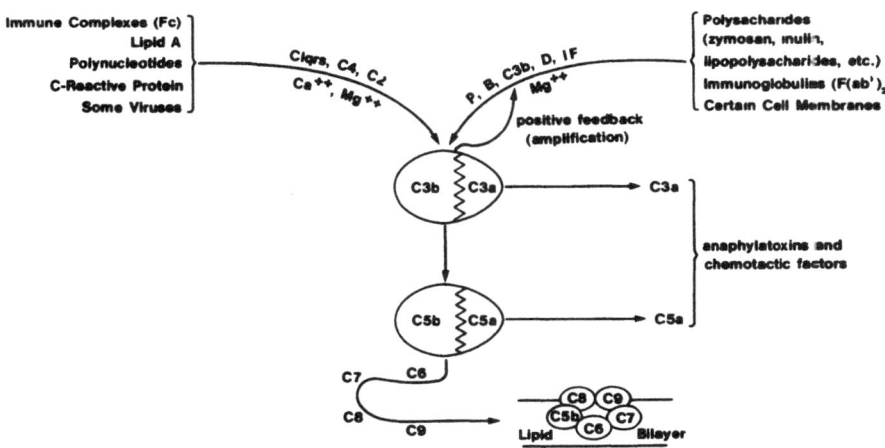

Figure 1. The complement system. Schematic outline of the complement system showing both activating pathways.

systems are C3, C5, C6, C7, C8, and C9. All of these components react in proper numerical order, except for C4 which reacts with C1 prior to C2. Fragments of components are designated by lowercase letters, e.g., C2a, C2b. The activated form of a complement component or assembled group of components is designated with an overbar, e.g., C̄1, C̄4b2a.

When the designation of a symbol is clear, the lowercase letters may be dropped, e.g., C4̲2̲. Peptide chains are designated by Greek letters, and, if altered by a cleavage reduction, a prime is added, e.g., α'. Fragments of peptide chains are designated with numerals, e.g., α'-1, α'-2.

The complement system can be considered in three distinct phases: (1) recognition of an initiating stimulus, (2) assembly of convertases (C3- and C5-cleaving enzymes), and (3) assembly of a membrane attack protein complex (C5b6789 complex). Details of these different areas will be given in subsequent diagrams throughout the chapter.

Since all of the complement molecules are circulating in a noncompetitive or peaceful way in the plasma, there is a requirement for an initial recognition component that receives a disturbing signal. Subsequently a definitive convertase assembly system is turned on so that a C3- and then a C5-cleaving enzyme are produced. These cleaving enzymes have been termed "C3 convertase" and "C5 convertase," and there are distinct although analogous enzymes in both the alternative and classical pathways. After recognition, activation, and assembly, production of the "attack" macromolecule begins with the interaction of C5b with C6 and C7 and subsequently C8 and C9. This molecule is inserted into lipid bilayers and has destructive influences on most cells. However, it has been suggested that it may have some stimulating influence as well (Shearer *et al.*, 1975). The primary assay system for complement components has utilized the cytotoxic effect of C5b6789 on sensitized sheep erythrocytes (EA) or even unsensitized erythrocytes as described in Section IVC. This assay measures the "hemolytic activity" of components, and generally these assays have extraordinary sensitivity. The "one-hit" concept of the cytolytic effect of complement has contributed in a most significant way to the quantitation of these sensitive hemolytic assays and has been a major stimulus to the analysis of the molecular interactions on cell membranes (Mayer, 1973, 1977).

Figure 1 illustrates the two recognition and activation limbs, namely the classical and the alternative pathway. They have homologous functions since both culminate in the assembly of a C3 convertase which results in the cleavage of C3 at exactly the same peptide bond. The enzymes that cleave C3 are factor B in the alternative pathway and C2 in the classical pathway. These two enzymes, in addition to their functional analogy, have shown a remarkable structural similarity and are coded for at approximately the same locus in the histocompatibility chromosome, strongly suggesting that a gene duplication occurred. One should also note that generation of C3b initiates a positive feedback loop which governs the amount of C3 cleaved. The amount of C3 cleaved is important, and the total quantity of C3 that is cleaved is controlled by

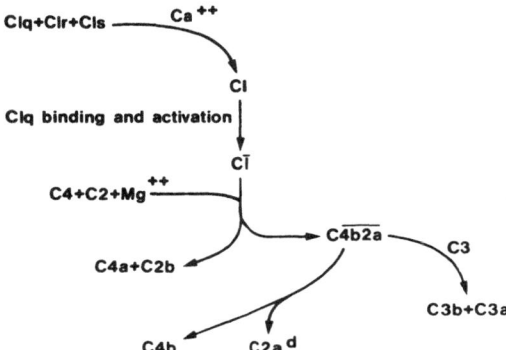

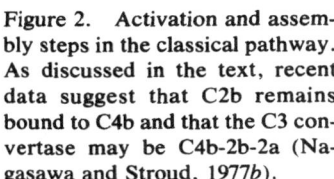

Figure 2. Activation and assembly steps in the classical pathway. As discussed in the text, recent data suggest that C2b remains bound to C4b and that the C3 convertase may be C4b-2b-2a (Nagasawa and Stroud, 1977*b*).

modulating proteins composing the C3b inactivator system. There are other naturally occurring modulators; one is called the "C1 inhibitor" and another is called the "C5, 6, 7 inhibitor." There are probably more to be described. There are also inactivating enzymes for certain biologically active fragments such as the anaphylatoxin inactivator that destroys C3a and C5a activity. These are mentioned in the appropriate sections. Figure 2 illustrates details of the classical pathway.

B. C1 Subcomponent Composition

C1 is a Ca^{2+}-dependent macromolecular complex having a sedimentation rate of 16 S (Ziccardi and Cooper, 1977). It can be dissociated into three subcomponents, C1q, C1s, and C1r, by chelation of Ca^{2+} with EDTA (Lepow et al., 1963). Recently C1t was proposed as the fourth subcomponent of C1 (Assimeh and Painter, 1975), but now there is evidence which directly rules out any effect of C1t on the C1 macromolecule. Apparently C1t copurifies with C1 when affinity chromatography on a Sepharose bed is used (Gigli et al., 1976; Ziccardi and Cooper, 1977; Pepys et al., 1977).

C1q functions as the binding unit to immune complexes of IgG and IgM (Müller-Eberhard and Kunkel, 1961), and, on binding to immune complexes, internal activation of C1r is triggered. Activated C1r, C1r̄, is a DFP-sensitive serine protease and proteolytically activates C1s (Sakai and Stroud, 1974). Activated C1s, C1s̄, is also a DFP-sensitive serine protease. It can react with its natural substrates C4 and C2 to produce the C4b2a convertase whether or not it is bound in the C1q,r,s complex or dissociated from this complex (Haines and Lepow, 1964; Nagaki and Stroud, 1969; Müller-Eberhard and Lepow, 1965).

Because of its lability and spontaneous activation, intact precursor C1 had not been isolated until recently, when, by repeated use of the serine protease inhibitor DFP, it was highly purified from defibrinated human plasma by euglobulin precipitation and gel filtration (Gigli *et al.*, 1976). The molar ratios of C1q, C1r, and C1s in this purified C1 were estimated to be $1:2:2$ by SDS-polyacrylamide gel electrophoresis determined by scanning a gel which had been stained with Coomassie blue (Gigli *et al.*, 1976). However, the optimum hemolytic activity of reconstructed C1 was found to occur at a C1q:C1r:C1s molar ratio of $1:4:4$. A ratio of $1:2:4$ for C1q:C1r:C1s was mentioned (Müller-Eberhard, 1971), and most recently Ziccardi and Cooper (1977) proposed that a single C1q is linked to dimeric forms of C1r and C1s. The possibility that the ratio of C1r or C1s might change during the isolation procedure seems likely since the subcomponents are bound noncovalently. By using quantitative immunochemical techniques, the ratio of the serum concentration of C1q to C1r to C1s is $1:2:2$ in accord with their model.

A partially assembled C1r-C1s complex was purified in its activated form from human plasma (Nagasawa *et al.*, 1974) and was detected immunoelectrophoretically in the serum of patients with urticaria (Laurell, 1976). An active C1 molecule with a sedementation rate of 12 S, "C1-X," which may be missing a portion of C1q, was demonstrated by ultracentrifugation of diluted human serum (Loos *et al.*, 1976a). These data suggest that the C1 macromolecule is not a fixed entity but that the subcomponents are held together in a fragile structure which may be active in several different forms with variable subcomponent composition. C1s is the only necessary subcomponent to possess the hemolytic activity of C1, albeit less efficiently than C$\bar{1}$ (Nagaki and Stroud, 1969).

C1s forms a complex with C1r in the presence of Ca^{2+}, but C1s does not bind to C1q, unless C1r and Ca^{2+} are both present (deBracco and Stroud, 1971; Laurell and Martensson, 1974; Valet and Cooper, 1974b). On the other hand, C1r may bind to C1q in the absence of C1s (Ziccardi and Cooper, 1976a). These data indicate that C1r furnishes a necessary physical link between C1q and C1s in the assembly of the C1 macromolecule; however, an exact understanding of the multiple protein-protein interactions of these five subcomponents, $(C1q)_{,1}$, $(C1r)_2$, $(C2s)_{,2}$, in the C1 macromolecule remains to be elucidated.

1. C1 Activation and Inhibition

The binding of immune complexes to C1 via binding sites on C1q triggers the activation of C1r and subsequently of C1s. This activation is undoubtedly a cascade composed of three internal activation steps; (1)

conformational alteration of C1q on binding to immune complexes, (2) activation of C1r by activated C1q, and (3) proteolytic activation of C1s by C1r. At present, little is known about the proposed conformational change in C1q or C1 when it binds to the Fc portions of IgG and IgM in immune complexes or when physically aggregated. Furthermore, precisely how a conformational change in the C1q molecule could initiate and/or enhance the activation of C1r is not known.

It has intrigued researchers that other nonimmunoglobulin molecules are recognized by C1q. For instance, C reactive protein (CRP) complexed with C polysaccharide or lecithin can interact with C1q and activate C1 (Volanakis and Kaplan, 1974; Claus et al., 1977). Rent et al. (1975) and Fiedel et al. (1976) found that the interaction of heparin with the polyaction protamine markedly stimulates the activation of C1 in whole human serum. These authors suggested the possibility of a nonimmunological activation of C1 by physiological polyanion-polycation complexes which might be formed during an inflammatory reaction. Foreign or host products, e.g., bacteria, viruses, cell surfaces, basement membrane protein, certain proteins from leukocyte granules, and proteins in plasma, might form such complexes. Furthermore, other molecules affect C1 activity. Trasylol, a basic polypeptide trypsin inhibitor found in bovine lung tissue, considerably enhances the ability of C1 to assemble the C3 convertase from C4 and C2 (DeLage et al., 1976). An activity designated "Kf" was separated from human serum. This enhanced one- to threefold the hemolytic activity of activated C1 (Gigli et al., 1971). Kf was proposed to bind to C1, enhancing its reactivity with C4 and C2. Although Kf was supposed to be a fragment generated from plasma kallikrein, the precise molecular nature and mechanism of potentiation by Kf require further study.

Activated C1 can be inhibited by a naturally occurring serum protein, the C1 inhibitor (C1-INH) (Levy and Lepow, 1959), which was characterized as a α-neuraminoglycoprotein (Pensky and Schwick, 1969; Pensky et al., 1961). The inhibition was not reversible and was not associated with enzymatic cleavage of C1 but was accompanied by the formation of a 1:1 stoichiometric complex between the C1-INH and C1s (Nagaki et al., 1974; Harpel and Cooper, 1975). The C1-INH physiologically serves to inactivate any active C1 in circulating blood. It may be more efficient since it also complexes and inhibits C1r (Ziccardi and Cooper, 1976b). It also inhibits a variety of noncomplement plasma proteases. A genetic deficiency of the C1-INH is the hallmark of recurrent hereditary angioneurotic edema (HANE), presumably as a result of the liberation of an active kinin from some point in the chain reaction(s) initiated by activated C1 (Donaldson and Evans, 1963; Donaldson et al., 1970). ϵ-Aminocaproic acid (EACA) was found to inhibit the intrinsic activation of C1 in whole human serum without inhibiting activated C$\bar{1}$ (Soter *et al.*, 1975), and a variety of organic compounds such as substituted benzamidines, pyridinium sulfonylfluorides, synthetic esters, and sulfated polysaccharides inhibit the active site on C1s (Bing *et al.*, 1964; Stroud *et al.*, 1965; Loos *et al.*, 1976*b*).

2. Properties of Subcomponents

a. C1q.   C1q was first isolated by Müller-Eberhard and Kunkel (1961) as a heat-labile 11 S serum protein capable of interacting and precipitating aggregated IgG. Purified C1q (Yonemasu and Stroud, 1971; Calcott and Müller-Eberhard, 1972; Reid *et al.*, 1972; Heusser *et al.*, 1973; Bhattacharyya *et al.*, 1974; Knobel *et al.*, 1975) was found to be an unusual plasma protein with a composition similar to that of collagen. It contains hydroxylysine (2.5 residues per 100 residues) and hydroxyproline (5 residues per 100 residues). These amino acids are found only in the Y position of the repeating collagenlike sequence, $(Gly-X-Y)_n$, in C1q (Reid, 1974). Also, C1q contains glucose and galactose linked to the hydroxyl groups of hydroxylysine as a glucosyl-galactosyl residue (Yonemasu *et al.*, 1971; Calcott and Müller-Eberhard, 1972). There are lesser amounts of fucose, sialic acid, and hexosamines. The $E_{1\,cm}^{1\%}$ at 280 nm is 6.8 (Yonemasu *et al.*, 1971) and the serum concentration is about 75–118 µg/ml (Yonemasu *et al.*, 1971; Ziccardi and Cooper, 1977).

C1q is composed of two nonidentical noncovalently bound subunits composed of three smaller polypeptide chains A, B, and C. The larger noncovalent subunit (molecular weight 55,000–60,000) is a disulfide-linked dimer of A-B chains. The smaller one (molecular weight 42,000–55,000) is a disulfide-linked C-C dimer (Yonemasu and Stroud, 1972; Heusser *et al.*, 1973; Reid and Porter, 1976). On SDS-polyacrylamide gel electrophoresis, the molecular weight of the A, B, and C chains was found to be 29,000, 27,000, and 22,000, respectively (Yonemasu and Stroud, 1972; Bhattacharyya *et al.*, 1974). Based on amino acid compositional data and gel filtration in the presence of guanidine, it was proposed that the A, B, and C chains of C1q are more similar in molecular weight, each being in the range of 23,000–24,000. It was suggested that the apparent discrepancy with results obtained by SDS-polyacrylamide gel electrophoresis was due to a difference in the carbohydrate content of the A, B, and C chains (Reid and Porter, 1976). Thus native C1q is composed of six A-B dimers and three C-C dimers, and the molecular weight of C1q is 410,000 (Müller-Eberhard, 1975). A schematic diagram is shown in Fig. 3.

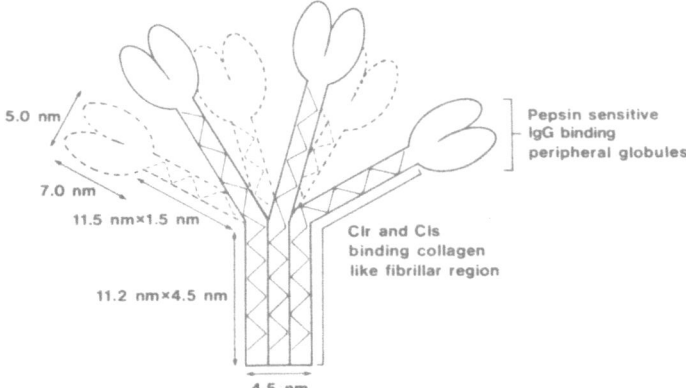

Figure 3. Schematic diagram of C1q. Note the six globular elements which contain immunoglobulin binding sites, the fibrillar portions containing the collagenlike sequences, and the central portion which contains disulfide linkages of A to B chains and C to C chains. Each fibril and globular unit contain an A, a B, and a C chain (Reid and Porter, 1976). The dimensions are taken from Shelton *et al.* (1972).

The three polypeptide chains each have a short NH_2-terminal, non-collagenlike region of three to nine residues followed by a collagenlike internal region of 78 residues and a COOH-terminal noncollagenlike region of about 110 residues (Reid and Porter, 1976). The interchain disulfide linkages in the A-B dimer and the C-C dimer are located in the NH_2-terminal noncollagenlike region of C1q (Reid, 1976).

Electron microscopy of C1q revealed that there are six peripheral globular portions connected by fibrillike strands to a common central portion (Shelton *et al.*, 1972; Knobel *et al.*, 1975). Cleavage of C1q by collagenase and pepsin revealed that the collagenlike region forms the central portion and that the fibrils and noncollagen region make up the peripheral globular portion (Reid, 1976; Reid and Porter, 1976; Brodsky-Doyle *et al.*, 1976). It has been postulated that the collagen portion of each chain (A, B, and C) forms a triple helix (Reid and Porter, 1976). C1r and C1s bind to the collagen region (Reid, 1976) and IgG to the peripheral globular areas (Knobel *et al.*, 1975). The number of monomeric, fluid-phase IgG molecules capable of binding to C1q was shown to be more than ten (Schumaker *et al.*, 1976). Assuming the number of binding sites to be six or an integral multiple of six, the probable number of binding sites was postulated to be 12 or 18. Previously, six had been reported (Calcott and Müller-Eberhard, 1975). The binding site for C1q on IgG is located on the C_H2 domain of the Fc portion (Yasmeen *et al.*,

1976; Colomb and Porter, 1975; Kehoe and Fougereau, 1969). In the case of complement-fixing as well as non-complement-fixing IgM, a 56-residue C_H4 fragment derived from the structurally related $C_\mu4$ domain of IgM was shown to be capable of binding to Cl and presumably to Clq (Hurst *et al.*, 1976). Interesting is the fact that aggregated IgA does not fix Cl, although the Fc of IgA does (Burritt *et al.*, 1977; Iida *et al.*, 1976), suggesting a steric blockade in the intact molecule. This is also a reasonable explanation for the non-complement-fixing IgM molecule (Hurst *et al.*, 1976).

An anionic serum inhibitor of Clq was separated from a partially purified Clq preparation using Con A-Sepharose. The inhibitor exhibited Clq hemolytic activity in a dose-dependent fashion (Conradie *et al.*, 1975) and formed a relatively insoluble inhibitor-Clq complex. The chemical nature of this Clq inhibitor is not known. Certain anionic polymers are known to bind with Clq and inhibit Cl hemolytic activity: liquoid, dextran sulfate, polyvinylsulfate, and heparin (Raepple *et al.*, 1976). Thus molecules that bind to Clq may or may not activate $\overline{Cl}$, indicating that a specific binding activity is necessary for activation.

   b. $\overline{Clr}$. Activated $\overline{Clr}$ was characterized as the proteolytic activator of Cls by Naff and Ratnoff (1968) and highly purified by deBracco and Stroud (1971). The $\overline{Clr}$ is a β-globulin with a molecular weight of 168,000 (gel filtration). This value suggests the possibility of a dimer formation, since the molecular weight of $\overline{Clr}$ was estimated to be approximately 100,000 on SDS-polyacrylamide gel electrophoresis (Takahashi *et al.*, 1975*b*; Ziccardi and Cooper, 1976*b*). Dimer formation was subsequently shown by Zicccardi and Cooper (1977). Activated $\overline{Clr}$ is composed of two polypeptide chains (molecular weights 60,000–68,000 and 35,000–47,000) connected by disulfide linkages (Takahashi *et al.*, 1975*b*; Ziccardi and Cooper, 1976*b*; Sim *et al.*, 1977). The serum content of $\overline{Clr}$ was found to be 90–110 μg/ml by deBracco *et al.* (1974) and 34 μg/ml by Ziccardi and Cooper (1977).

Until recently, it was questioned whether Clr exists in a precursor zymogen form or is in a naturally activated state in the native Cl macromolecule. The two-chain structure of active $\overline{Clr}$ suggested the presence of a zymogen form of Clr consisting of a single polypeptide chain as in the case of other serine proteases (Takahashi *et al.*, 1975*b*). This was confirmed by the isolation of precursor Clr as a noncovalent dimeric form of a single polypeptide chain with a molecular weight of 95,000 (Ziccardi and Cooper, 1976*a*; Gigli *et al.*, 1976). Precursor dimeric Clr had a molecular weight of 190,000 on gel filtration and a sedimentation rate of 7.0 S (Valet and Cooper, 1974*b*; Ziccardi and Cooper, 1976*b*). Precursor dimeric Clr does not activate Cls. The Cls-activating function is associated with the conversion of each of the single chains into two disulfide-linked polypeptide chains (Ziccardi and Cooper, 1976b). Although trypsin was thought to bring about this cleavage, this interpretation has been retracted (Ziccardi and Cooper, 1976a). Ca^{2+}, liquoid, DFP, and the C1-INH inhibited the spontaneous activation of C1r (Ziccardi and Cooper, 1976a). Spontaneous activation of C1r was found to conform to the second-order autocatalytic rate law. This indicated that autocatalytic activation of C1r was possible (Takahashi et $al.$, 1976a), although a similar kinetic phenomenon to C1s (Morgan and Nair, 1975) was subsequently found not to hold true on direct experiment (Gigli et $al.$, 1976).

Since the autocatalytic activation of trypsinogen was explained by the formation of "active trypsinogen" by a bimolecular self-self interaction (Kay and Kassell, 1971), a similar biomolecular interaction of the zymogen form of C1r seems possible and would be compatible with the autocatalytic activation of C1r. This is attractive since there are two C1r molecules in the C1 macromolecule (Ziccardi and Cooper, 1976b, 1977). Two moles of C1r binds with 1 mol of C1q (Gigli et $al.$, 1976; Ziccardi and Cooper, 1977); therefore, a possible mechanism of C1 activation by immune complexes may be as follows: First, the binding of immune complexes to C1q causes a conformational change in C1q, allowing or promoting the close association of two C1r molecules. Next, an active site is formed in one member of the dimer which in turn activates by proteolytic cleavage its partner. On the other hand, Taylor et $al.$ (1977) have recently proposed that activation is dependent on the presence of traces of $\overline{C1r}$.

The proteolytic activation of C1r occurred on addition of aggregated IgG to C1 reconstituted from C1q, C1r, and C1s in the presence of Ca^{2+}. Neither C1q,C1s, nor aggregated IgG alone activated C1r (Ziccardi and Cooper, 1976b; Gigli et $al.$, 1976).

The C1s activator activity of $\overline{C1r}$ decreased when $\overline{C1r}$ combined with C1q and C1s in the presence of Ca^{2+} (Ratnoff and Naff, 1969; Ziccardi and Cooper, 1976a). The reason for the failure of $\overline{C1r}$ in the reconstituted C1 to activate C1s is not known. Also, $\overline{C1r}$ is inhibited in the presence of Ca^{2+} even without C1q (Ratnoff and Naff, 1969; Gigli et $al.$, 1976; Volanakis and Stroud, unpublished).

The molecular weight and amino acid composition of $\overline{C1r}$ were the same as those of precursor C1r, thus excluding the possibility that liberation of a large activation peptide occurs during the autocatalytic activation of C1r (Sim and Porter, 1976; Ziccardi and Cooper, 1976b).

Although the natural substrate of $\overline{C1r}$ is C1s, $\overline{C1r}$ was found to hydrolyze N-substituted esters of arginine and to a lesser extent lysine Naff and Ratnoff, 1968). Sim et $al.$ (1977), using highly purified $\overline{C1r}$, could not show that $\overline{C1r}$ hydrolyzed many of several *N*-benzyloxycarbonyl-L-amino-acid-*p*-nitrophenyl esters tested.

The substrate specificity of $\overline{C1r}$ suggests that $\overline{C1r}$ activates C1s by cleaving a Lys-X or an Arg-X peptide bond on the C1s molecule. The X amino acid in the cleaved peptide bond of C1s was shown to be isoleucine (Takahashi *et al.*, 1975*a*).

The C1s-activator activity as well as the esterolytic activity of $\overline{C1r}$ could be inhibited by DFP, and the DFP-sensitive active site of $\overline{C1r}$ was located on the light-chain portion having isoleucine as its amino terminus (Takahashi *et al.*, 1975*b*). The $\overline{C1r}$ activity was also inhibited by the C1-INH (Ratnoff *et al.*, 1969), which forms a covalently linked 1 : 1 molar ratio complex with $\overline{C1r}$ via the light chain of $\overline{C1r}$ (Nagaki *et al.*, 1974; Ziccardi and Cooper, 1976*a*).

The serum of two patients with a C1r deficiency showed a very low C1 activity, although the C1q and C1s concentrations were normal (Pickering *et al.*, 1970; Day *et al.*, 1972). It was further shown that there was an inadequate association of these C1 subcomponents, confirming the necessity of C1r for the physical linkage between C1q and C1s (deBracco and Stroud, 1971). Ziccardi and Cooper (1977) made similar observations with purified components.

   c. C1s. The identification of precursor C1s and its activation by $\overline{C1r}$ were shown by Naff *et al.* (1964) and Naff and Ratnoff (1968). Precursor C1s was isolated in relatively large yields by Sakai and Stroud (1973), who showed that the single chain of C1s was cleaved by $\overline{C1r}$ into two polypeptide chains connected by disulfide bonds. This limited proteolytic activation of C1s has been confirmed by many investigators (Valet and Cooper, 1974*a*; Takahashi *et al.*, 1975*a*; Ziccardi and Cooper, 1976*a*; Gigli *et al.*, 1976). The polypeptide chain structure of $\overline{C1s}$ is the same as that of $\overline{C1r}$; and the molecular weight of the light chain of $\overline{C1s}$ is less than that of $\overline{C1r}$ by 7000–10,000 (Takahashi *et al.*, 1975*a,b*; Ziccardi and Cooper, 1976*a,b*). Sim *et al.* (1977) reported that the molecular weights of the two chains of $\overline{C1s}$, as measured by gel filtration in guanidinium chloride, were identical to those of $\overline{C1r}$. The apparent difference on gels presumably is due to carbohydrate variation. C1s has a serum concentration of 27–36 μg/ml, and the $E_{1\,cm}^{1\%}$ at 280 nm is 16.9 (Nagaki and Stroud, 1970).

The single polypeptide chain of precursor C1s is cleaved by $\overline{C1r}$ at an X-Ile peptide bond, and the NH$_2$-terminal and COOH-terminal portions of C1s become the heavy and light chains of activated $\overline{C1s}$, respectively (Takahashi *et al.*, 1975*a*). The first 20 amino acid sequences of the light chain of $\overline{C1s}$ are homologous to those of other serine proteases, and there is striking homology with C1r, trypsin, and chymotrypsin (Sim *et al.*, 1977). Considering that the terminal light-chain isoleucine in these serine proteases is essential for expression of their proteolytic function, it is likely that the cleavage of an X-Ile peptide bond in C1s by C̄1̄r̄ is an essential step for the generation of the functional activity of C1s. Equimolar concentrations of C1s and C̄1̄r̄ were required for full activation of C1s. This lack of a significant turnover of C1s by C̄1̄r̄ was explained by the fact that these two molecules bind to each other (Valet and Cooper, 1974*a*). However, it was recently shown that complete activation of C1s occurred at any ratio of C̄1̄r̄/C1s if the time of incubation of C1s with C1r is prolonged (Gigli *et al.*, 1976). This confirms an observation of Sakai and Stroud (1974) that virtually undetectable quantities of C1r could lead to C1s activation. Although the natural substrates of C̄1̄s̄ are C4 and C2, C̄1̄s̄ also hydrolyzes a series of *N*-substituted esters of arginine, lysine, and tyrosine (Naff and Ratnoff, 1968), suggesting that C̄1̄s̄ possesses specificities similar to those of trypsin and chymotrypsin. This mixed specificity is very unusual in serine proteases.

An arginine ester, *p*-tosyl-L-arginine methyl ester (TAMe), inhibited the function of C̄1̄s̄ to cleave C2 (Stroud *et al.*, 1965), but a tyrosine ester, *N*-acetyltyrosine ethyl ester (ATEe), only slightly inhibited the cleavage of C4 by C̄1̄ (Shimada and Tamura, 1972). These results suggested that the chymotrypsinlike specificity of C1s for synthetic esters bears no relation to the proteolytic function of C̄1̄s̄.

The esteroproteolytic activity of C̄1̄s̄ was inhibited by DFP (Haines and Lepow, 1964) and the C1-INH (Levy and Lepow, 1959). The DFP-sensitive active site of C̄1̄s̄ was shown to reside on the light chain (Sakai and Stroud, 1974), and the C1-INH formed a covalently bound equimolar complex with C̄1̄s̄ via the light chain of C̄1̄s̄ (Nagaki *et al.*, 1974; Harpel and Cooper, 1975). The active enzyme center of C̄1̄s̄ is composed of a highly hydrophobic area that is capable of binding simple hydrocarbons which contain no functional group (Canady *et al.*, 1976; Bing *et al.*, 1964) and an anionic binding site through which positively charged amino acid esters interact with C̄1̄s̄ (Bing, 1969).

Leupeptin, a trypsin inhibitor of actinomycetes, inhibited the esterase activity of C̄1̄s̄ for arginine as well as tryosine esters, but chymostatin, a chymotrypsin-specific inhibitor of actinomycetes, was not inhibitory (Takahashi *et al.*, 1976b).

The autocatalytic activation of C1s was studied by Morgan and Nair (1975). Their C1s preparation spontaneously activated and followed the autocatalytic rate law during this spontaneous activation. The lag phase portion of the sigmoidal activation curve was shortened by increase of the C1s content and by addition of activated C̄1̄s̄. However, Gigli *et al.* (1976) did not find any activation of C1s by C̄1̄s̄.

The amino acid composition of C1s was similar to that of activated C̄1̄s̄ (Sim *et al.*, 1976), indicating that at least a major activation peptide was not released on activation by C$\overline{1}$r. It was also demonstrated that the amino acid composition of C1s is essentially the same as that of C1r.

It has been a subject of specific interest to determine whether C$\overline{1}$s has two distinctive active sites, one which cleaves C4 and the other C2. Based on data showing that there is no competitive inhibition between C4 and C2, Strunk and Colten (1974) proposed that C1 may possess two distinctive active sites. Also, Kondo *et al.* (1972) reported that the C1-INH and heat treatment abolished the C2-cleaving activity of C$\overline{1}$ while leaving its C4-cleaving activity intact. Considering that the C1-INH inhibits C$\overline{1}$ by forming a stoichiometric complex with C$\overline{1}$s via its active site, these data suggested the presence of two active sites in C$\overline{1}$s or two types of C$\overline{1}$s, which have different specificity for C4 and C2. On the other hand, the preliminary data by Barkas et al. (1973) showed that C$\overline{1}$s has only one active serine site.

While C$\overline{1}$s readily cleaves C2 and C4 in free solution, macromolecular C$\overline{1}$ does not cleave C2 unless C4 or C4b is also present (Gigli and Austen, 1969*a*). It was shown that C$\overline{1}$r inhibits the C2-cleaving activity of C$\overline{1}$s, and the inhibition by C1r was overcome by the addition of C4 (Gigli and Austen, 1969*b*). Based on this evidence, it was suggested that the reactive site for C2 on C$\overline{1}$s may be sterically hindered in the C$\overline{1}$ macromolecule by the presence of C$\overline{1}$r in close proximity to the C2-reactive site of C$\overline{1}$s. On binding of C4 to C$\overline{1}$, an allosteric change presumably occurs, allowing the access of C2 to the C$\overline{1}$s subcomponent in the C$\overline{1}$ macromolecule (Gigli and Austen, 1969*b*). An alternative explanation is that C4 or C4b forms a complex with C2 and modifies C2 allosterically to allow it to be accessible to C$\overline{1}$s in the C$\overline{1}$ macromolecule. Strunk and Colten (1974) also proposed that the potentiation of C2 cleavage by C$\overline{1}$s in the presence of C4 was due to the availability of a site for product deposition, augmenting removal of the product from the enzymatic site. Binding of C4 to C$\overline{1}$s was reported by Taubman (1975), who showed that C$\overline{1}$s has a C4-binding site in addition to its enzyme site, since C4 bound to DFP-inactivated C$\overline{1}$s. Loos *et al.* (1976*b*) were able to show that sulfated polysaccharides inhibited the cleavage of C4 and C2 but did not affect synthetic ester cleavage, suggesting an important secondary binding site for the natural substrates.

C. Other Proteins of the Classical Pathway

1. C4

The isolation of C4 was described by Müller-Eberhard and Biro (1963), Schreiber and Müller-Eberhard (1974), Nagasawa *et al.* (1976), and Bolotin *et al.* (1977). The protein is a β-globulin and has a sedimentation rate of 10 S. The serum content is 400 μg/ml (Kohler and Müller-Eberhard, 1967), and the $E_{1\,cm}^{f\%}$ at 280 nm is 8.3 (Nagasawa and Stroud, 1977b).

C4 is composed of three polypeptide chains (α, 95,000; β, 78,000; γ, 33,000) connected by disulfide bonds, and the molecular weight of intact C4 is 210,000 (Schreiber and Müller-Eberhard, 1974). The three-chain structure is very unusual for plasma proteins, and Hall and Colten (1977) have suggested that it is synthesized as a single polypeptide chain. The NH_2 terminals of the α, β, and γ chains are Asp, Lys, and Glu, respectively, and the NH_2-terminal sequences have been partially determined (Bolotin *et al.*, 1977).

A genetically determined structural polymorphism was detected in C4, and at least seven different patterns were reported (Rosenfeld *et al.*, 1969). The polymorphism of C4 was formed by varying combinations of three subtypes, C, A, and A_1 (Rosenfeld *et al.*, 1969). A C4 structural gene was shown to be linked to the HLA gene complex on chromosome 6, as in the case of C2, C8, and factor B of the alternative pathway (Teisberg *et al.*, 1976; Bitter-Suermann *et al.*, 1977).

$C\overline{1s}$ activates C4 by cleaving an X-Ala peptide bond (Nagasawa *et al.*, 1976) on the α chain of C4, producing a small NH_2-terminal fragment, C4a (molecular weight 8600) and a larger C4b portion (molecular weight 190,000) (Patrick *et al.*, 1970; Budzko and Müller-Eberhard, 1970).

C4b is further cleaved by a plasma protease, the C4b inactivator (Cooper, 1975a), in the presence of a macromolecular weight cofactor (Shiraishi and Stroud, 1975; Nagasawa *et al.*, 1976) into a large fragment, C4c, and a small fragment, C4d. The C4b inactivator is the same protein as the C3b inactivator (Nagasawa and Stroud, 1977c; Cooper, 1975a). By the action of this C4b inactivator system the α' chain of C4b is cleaved into a large α'-1 fragment (molecular weight 58,000) and a small α'-2 fragment, (molecular weight 28,000). The large α'-1 fragment has been called "C4d," and the small α'-2 fragment remains bound to the β and γ chains by disulfide linkages to form C4c (molecular weight 140,000) (Nagasawa *et al.*, 1976) (Fig. 4). The known functions of C4 are twofold: (1) assembly of a new protease (C3 convertase), with C2 in the presence of $C\overline{1s}$, and (2) immune adherence.

On cleavage of C4 by $C\overline{1s}$, C4b acquires two binding sites, a labile site which allows the C4b to attach itself to cell membranes and a stable site which enables cell-bound C4 to react with a C4b receptor on human erythrocytic and lymphocytic cells, producing immune adherence (Cooper, 1969; Bokisch and Sobel, 1974). The labile binding site is thermodynamically unstable and quickly loses its binding ability. Conse-

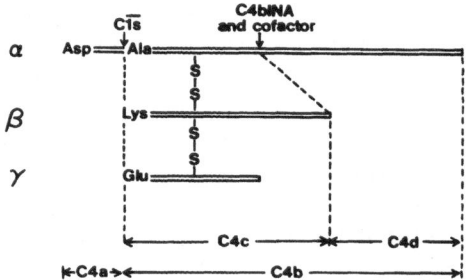

Figure 4.   Cleavage patterns of C4 and C3. Schematic diagram of the stepwise-limited proteolysis of C4 and C3 by plasma enzymes. The fragments are shown and the sites of cleavages are designated by arrows. The C3b-INA and C4b-INA are the same protein and utilize the same cofactor (Nagasawa and Stroud, 1977*b*). The number and absolute position of the disulfide bond(s) are not known.

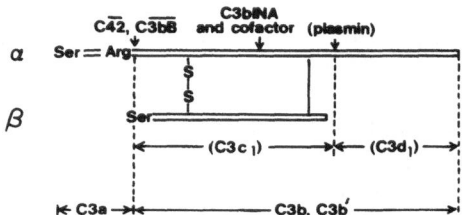

quently, only a small portion of the C4b becomes bound and tʌe residual C4b remains unbound in the fluid phase as an inactive fragment. The receptor for C4b on human erythrocytes and B lymphocytes reacts with either cell-bound or fluid-phase C4b via the stable binding site on C4b (Bokisch and Sobel, 1974). Similar receptors were shown to be present on polymorphonuclear leukocytes (Ross and Polley, 1974). Since the attachment of immune complexes to phagocytic cells is usually followed by phagocytosis of these complexes, the C4b receptor should play a role in the immune clearance of such complexes. The observed reduced clearance of immune complexes in C4-deficient guinea pig sera may be explained by the lack of C4b-dependent immune clearance in addition to an inability to reach the C3b stage of C activation (Ellman *et al.*, 1971). The immune adherence and cytotoxic activities of C4b are inactivated after the cleavage of the α' chain by the C4b inactivator (Cooper, 1975*a*) and its cofactor (Shiraishi and Stroud, 1975). The labile binding site probably is located on the C4d portion, since the C4d fragment remains bound to cells even after the dissociation of the C4c portion from cells by the action of the C4b inactivator (Cooper, 1975*a*).

   In addition to its stable binding site to cells, C4b has a stable binding site by which C4b binds C2 or C̄1s-activated C2 in order to assemble the C3 convertase, C̄4b2a (Müller-Eberhard *et al.*, 1967). The cofactor role of C4b in the generation of C3-cleaving activity in the assembled C3 convertase is to provide a receptor site for C3 and/or to induce the proper conformational exposure of the active site in C2a, allowing it to cleave C3. The binding site for C2 seems to locate on the α chain of C4b, since the presence of C2 on C4b protected the α' chain from cleavage by the C4b inactivator (Cooper, 1975a).

It is not yet known whether C4a has biological activity analogous to that observed for C3a and C5a, although some C4a preparations were found to have a smooth muscle contracting activity (Budzko and Müller-Eberhard, 1970).

2. C2

Of all the early classical pathway complement components, C2 has the lowest serum concentration, approximately 25-30 μg/ml. Human C2 was purified by Polley and Müller-Eberhard (1968) and was found to be a β-globulin with a molecular weight of 115,000 and a sedimentation rate of 5.5 S. Recently, C2 was purified by affinity chromatography using a C4b-Sepharose column (Nagasawa and Stroud, 1977a). This method is a modification of the particulate affinity adsorption method, using EAC14 cells for isolation of guinea pig C2 (Mayer et al., 1970). Human C2 was found to be a single polypeptide chain with a molecular weight by sedimentation equilibrium of 100,000. Alanine is the NH$_2$-terminal amino acid (Nagasawa and Stroud, 1977a). The $E_{1\,cm}^{1\%}$ at 280 nm of C2 is 8.9. C$\bar{1}$s cleaves C2 into two antigenically distinct fragments, a large fragment, C2a (molecular weight 73,000), and a small fragment, C2b (molecular weight 34,000) (Nagasawa and Stroud, 1977b). Using the affinity method, C2 was purified from a single donor and resolved into three components on isoelectric focusing between Ph 6.0 and 6.3 (Nagasawa and Stroud, 1977a), confirming Alper's observations on whole serum (Alper, 1976).

The functions of C2 are (1) to furnish the active enzyme site for C3 convertase and C5 convertase and (2) possibly to participate in the generation of a vasoactive mediator, the so-called C-kinin, which participates in the edema formation of hereditary angioneurotic edema (HANE) (Klemperer et al., 1969).

3. Assembly of C3 Convertase

Neither C2 nor the large fragment, C2a, has any proteolytic activity on C3 until C2a binds to C4b in the fluid phase or on cell surfaces (Stroud et al., 1965; Müller-Eberhard et al., 1967). In order to assemble C3 convertase, it is necessary to cleave C2 with C$\bar{1}$ or C$\bar{1}$s in the presence of C4 or C4b, because the binding site for C4 has a very short half-life and undergoes a rapid conformational change into inactive C2i. The molecular form of the C3 convertase has been generally accepted to be a 1:1 complex of C4b and C2a (Müller-Eberhard *et al.*, 1967). This was based on the fact that the assembled C3 convertase had a molecular weight of approximately 300,000. This was less than the combined molecular weight of C4b and C2 by about 40,000. A C2 fragment, released from the C3 convertase in a time-dependent fashion (a process called "decay"), was found to be smaller (by 30,000–40,000 molecular weight) than native C2. This fragment was called "C2a," and since only the C2a fragment could be recovered from C4b the C3 convertase was considered to be C4b-C2a (Müller-Eberhard *et al.*, 1967; Polley and Müller-Eberhard, 1968; Stroud *et al.*, 1966). C2b could not be found in these earlier studies, and no information was available as to its role, if any, in the assembly of the C3 convertase. C2b was considered to accumulate in the surrounding fluid. Recently, contrary to this concept, it was shown that when the C4b-C2 complex was activated with C$\overline{1}$s, only the C2a portion was found in the surrounding fluid as a result of the decay-dissociation of C3 convertase, while the C2b fragment was found to remain noncovalently bound to C4b (Nagasawa and Stroud, 1977*b*). This suggests that C2b contains a stable finding site for C4b. Since native C2 can bind to C4 or C4b (Sitomer *et al.*, 1966), it seems possible that under physiological conditions, C2 binds to C4b, then the C4b-C2 complex is activated by C$\overline{1}$ to generate a C3 convertase, C4b-C2b-C2a. The assembly of C3 convertase is enhanced by the presence of Mg^{2+}, but chelation of Mg^{2+} with EDTA does not dissociate the assembled C3 convertase (Müller-Eberhard *et al.*, 1967).

Native C2, as well as the C2a fragment, hydrolyzed N-substituted esters of lysine. The esterase activity of native C2 was only slightly increased after conversion to C2a by C$\overline{1}$s (Cooper, 1975*b*). The most susceptible ester was acetylglycyl-L-lysine methyl ester (AGLMe) with a K_m of 1.8×10^{-2} M. The ability of C3 convertase to cleave C3 (K_m of 1.8×10^{-6} M) was competitively inhibited with AGLMe, exhibiting a K_i of 1×10^{-2} M. This suggested that the esteratic active site on C2 is related to the proteolytic activity of C3 convertase (Cooper, 1975*b*). The trypsinlike specificity of C2 or C2a is consistent with the data that the COOH-terminal amino acid of C3a released from C3 by C3 convertase is arginine (Budzko *et al.*, 1971). C2 is also the enzyme in the macromolecular convertase C$\overline{423}$ that cleaves C5.

Several protease inhibitors from plasma, tissue, and plant sources did not inhibit the esterase and C3 convertase activity (Cooper, 1975*b*). Recently, Medicus *et al.* (1976*a*) proposed that C2a is a serine esterase, since the C5 convertase activity, $\overline{C423}$, was partially inhibited by a high concentration of DFP. Also, pretreatment of native C2 with a high concentration of DFP slightly decreased the C2 hemolytic activity. It was not clear whether C3 convertase activity was also inhibited by DFP. Compared with other serine proteases, the rate of inactivation by DFP was much slower and required a high concentration of DFP. Further study is necessary to conclude that C2a has a DFP-sensitive serine residue at its active center, since nonserine proteases such as papain and bromelain can be inhibited with high concentrations of DFP.

A possible involvement of —SH groups in the hemolytic function of C2 was proposed by Leon (1965), who showed that treatment of C2 with p-chloromercuribenzoate results in the loss of C2 hemolytic activity.

The hemolytic activity of C3 convertase is abrogated by the time- and temperature-dependent decay-dissociation of the assembled $\overline{C4b2a}$ complex (Borsos et al., 1961). The stability of this C3 convertase is greatly enhanced when C2 has been treated with iodine. Specifically, the half-life of the C3 convertase is lengthened from 10 min for $\overline{C42}$ to 200 min for $\overline{C4,2}^{oxy}$ (the conventional symbol for the convertase made with iodine-treated C2, Polley and Müller-Eberhard, 1967). In addition, treatment of C2 with iodine enhanced ten- to twentyfold the hemolytic activity of C2. It was proposed that C2 contains two —SH groups which are positioned in close proximity to each other and form an intramolecular disulfide bond on oxidation with iodine (Müller-Eberhard, 1975). Thus it appears that iodine-oxidized C2 acquires an extraordinary increase in binding strength to C4b and consequently in C3-cleaving activity.

Another possible function of C2 is in relation to the liberation of a kinin mediator (C-kinin) in the serum of patients with HANE (Donaldson et al., 1969, 1970). It was found that HANE results from a severe deficiency of the C1-INH protein or from structurally abnormal and functionally inactive C1-INH (Donaldson et al., 1963; Harpel et al., 1975). Thus activated $\overline{C1}$ is increased in the serum of these patients, and on incubation a dialyzable and heat-stable mediator is released which increases vascular permeability and contracts smooth muscle without causing tachyphylaxis. The activity was inactivated by carboxypeptidase B and, unlike bradykinin, by trypsin, suggesting that the active principle is a polypeptide distinct from bradykinin, C3a and C5a anaphylatoxins (Donaldson et al., 1969). The liberation of this activity required $\overline{C1}$, C4, and C2 and was inhibited by added C1-INH or antiserum to C4 or C2 but not by anti-C3 (Donaldson et al., 1969, 1970). In addition, the active principle was detected in the incubation mixture of refined $\overline{C1s}$, C4, and C2 (Klemperer et al., 1969). Intradermal injection of active $\overline{C1s}$ increased vascular permeability in normal but not in C2-deficient patients (Klemperer *et al.*, 1967, 1968). Based on this evidence it was proposed that a kininlike polypeptide is probably released from C2 at least in HANE (Donaldson *et al.*, 1970).

On considering that liberation of the C-kinin in the serum of HANE patients was blocked by soybean trypsin inhibitor and EACA, compounds which do not inhibit C1s, another plasma protease, such as plasma kallikrein or plasmin, appeared to be involved in the liberation of the C-kinin (Nilsson *et al.*, 1966; Lundh *et al.*, 1968; Sheffer *et al.*, 1972). Furthermore, the disease responds to treatment with the plasmin inhibitors trasylol and EACA (Sheffer *et al.*, 1972; Frank *et al.*, 1972).

Since the C-kinin has never been completely purified, its chemical nature is not conclusively known. The conclusion that the C-kinin is a fragment from C2 must await further study with highly purified C4 and C2.

4. C3

C3 is the most abundant protein of all the complement components (80–130 mg/100 ml). It has been purified and studied by many investigators (Nilsson and Müller-Eberhard, 1965; Molenar *et al.*, 1973; Tack and Prahl, 1976). The molecular weight of C3 is 190,000, and it is composed of two polypeptide chains bridged with disulfide linkages; the α chain, with a molecular weight of 120,000, and the β chain, with a molecular weight of 75,000 (Nilsson *et al.*, 1975; Bokisch *et al.*, 1975). The NH_2 terminals of the α and β chains are serine, and the COOH terminal of at least one of the two chains is alanine (Tack and Prahl, 1976). The partial specific volume is 0.736 ± 0.003 ml g^{-1} and the $E_{1\,cm}^{1\%}$ at 280 nm is 9.7 (Tack and Prahl, 1976).

Both the classical and alternative pathway C3 convertases, $\overline{C42}$ (Müller-Eberhard *et al.*, 1967) and $\overline{C3bBb}$ (Müller-Eberhard and Götze, 1972), cleave the α chain of C3 to produce the large fragment, C3b (molecular weight 180,000), and the small fragment, C3a (molecular weight 9000) (Budzko *et al.*, 1971; Bokisch *et al.*, 1975; Hugli *et al.*, 1975*a*). Liberation of a C3a-like fragment was also observed with trypsin and plasmin (Bokisch *et al.*, 1969).

The NH_2- and COOH-terminal amino acids of C3a are serine and arginine, respectively, indicating the location of C3a on the NH_2-terminal portion of the α chain and liberation after the cleavage of an arginyl-X peptide bond by the C3 convertases (Budzko *et al.*, 1971).

C3a is a highly cationic single polypeptide chain containing 77 amino acids and has a 40% helical structure (Hugli *et al.*, 1975*a,b*; Hugli, 1975). Its primary structure was determined by Hugli (1975). Other characteristics of C3a include a high half-cystine content (six residues of the total of 77 residues), four of which were present as a cysteinylcysteinyl sequence (positions 22, 23 and 56, 57), and the unusual concentration of six basic amino acid residues among the 14 residues at the COOH-terminal end of C3a (Hugli, 1975).

C3b is further cleaved by a serum protease, the C3b inactivator (Tamura and Nelson, 1967), also called "KAF" (Lachmann and Müller-Eberhard, 1968). The two fragments, C3c and C3d, were described as the products of this C3b cleavage (Ruddy and Austen, 1971), but their polypeptide structures were not elucidated. Originally, C3c and C3d were identified as the C3 fragments which accumulated on prolonged incubation of whole human serum (West et al., 1966). The structures of C3c and C3d isolated from whole human serum were characterized by Bokisch et al. (1975) as follows: C3c (molecular weight 140,000) is composed of the intact β chain linked by disulfide bonds to at least three polypeptide fragments derived from the α' chain, and C3d (molecular weight 25,000) is a single polypeptide chain derived from the amino-terminal portion of the α' chain of C3b.

However, recent experiments using purified C3b and C3b-INA showed that C3b-INA alone failed to cleave C3b in the fluid phase and required a macromolecular weight cofactor for the cleavage of C3b in the fluid phase (Nagasawa and Stroud, 1977c). Since the cofactor was identical to the macromolecular cofactor for C4b-INA (Shiraishi and Stroud, 1975), it was called the "C4b-C3b-INA" cofactor (Nagasawa and Stroud, 1977c). The C3b-INA and cofactor cleaved a single peptide bond on the α' chain of C3b to produce a new C3b derivative, C3b', which is composed of three polypeptide chains connected by disulfide linkages. Two of these are fragments of the α' chain, designated "α'-1" (molecular weight 70,000) and "α'-2" (molecular weight 45,000), and the third is the intact β chain. After this cleavage, the ability of C3b to interact with $\bar{D}$ to cleave B is lost (Nagasawa and Stroud, 1977c), but the molecular weight and mobility are unchanged. Plasmin cleaves C3b', but not C3b, to form $C3c_1$ (molecular weight 140,000) and $C3d_1$ (molecular weight 45,000), which are subsequently cleaved during longer incubation into the lower molecular weight fragments $C3c_2$ (molecular weight 130,000) and $C3d_2$ (molecular weight 32,000), respectively (Nagasawa and Stroud, 1977c). These cleavages are shown schematically in Fig. 4.

Gitlin et al. (1975) reported that the reaction of C3b-INA with C3b is twofold in nature: the first rapid cleavage produces a C3b derivative "C3bi," which is composed of an α' chain (molecular weight 85,000) and a β chain (molecular weight 70,000) connected by an unknown number of disulfide linkages. The second slow cleavage produces a C3c-like fragment composed of two 70,000 polypeptide chains connected by di-sulfide linkages. Whether the second slow reaction is mediated by C3b-INA or a trace contamination such as plasmin remains to be resolved, but the final fragment is similar to the plasmin-produced $C3c_1$ or $C3c_2$.

At least four functions have been ascribed to C3 fragments: (1) anaphylatoxin, C3a, (2) a molecular unit of the C5 convertase, C3b, (3) interaction and binding to lymphocytes and phagocytes, C3b, and (4) amplification of C3 cleavage by initiating the feedback or amplification loop of the alternative pathway, C3b (see Fig. 5).

5. C3a Anaphylatoxin

Many biological functions have been attributed to C3a anaphyla-toxin. It has the ability to release histamine from mast cells and thereby to increase vascular permeability, cause an intradermal wheal and ery-thema, and contract smooth muscle with tachyphylaxis (Dias Da Silva and Lepow, 1967; Bodammer and Vogt, 1970; Lepow *et al.*, 1970; Wuep-per *et al.*, 1972; Bokisch *et al.*, 1969). Whether it has a direct effect on smooth muscle is somewhat uncertain. Recent studies have shown that the smooth muscle activity resides in a smaller fragment (Erickson *et al.*, 1977).

The biological activity of C3a can be abolished irreversibly on the release of a COOH-terminal arginine residue by carboxypeptidase B or reversibly by denaturation with guanidine and β-mercaptoethanol (Hugli *et al.*, 1975a,b).

6. C5 Convertase

The cleavage of C3 by either classical or alternative C3 convertase is accompanied by the generation of a labile and stable functional site on the C3b molecule. This labile binding site of C3b has a very short half-life, and only a small amount of C3b combines with the membrane receptor before this activity is spontaneously lost. Presumably this is a rapid conformational change. Most of the C3b which fails to collide with the receptor becomes inactive and accumulates in the surrounding fluid (Müller-Eberhard *et al.*, 1966b). On binding of C3b via the labile binding site to cells bearing C42, a new protease—C5 convertase, C423b—is generated (Cooper and Müller-Eberhard, 1970; Shin *et al.*, 1971a; Ham-mer *et al.*, 1976). This C5 convertase was also reported to be assembled in the fluid phase by C4,2 and C3b. The active site of this C5 convertase resides in the C2 portion (Cooper and Müller-Eberhard, 1970; Goldlust *et al.*, 1974; Shin *et al.*, 1971a). The C5 convertase cleaves an arginyl-X peptide bond to release a small fragment, C5a (molecular weight 11,000), from the NH_2-terminal portion of the α chain of C5 (Nilsson *et al.*, 1975; Fernandez and Hugli, 1976). The C5-cleaving activity can be inhibited by a high concentration of DFP (Medicus *et al.*, 1976*a*).

7. Immune Adherence

C3b is reactive with cells having C3b receptors (leukocytes, lymphocytes, renal epithelial cells, etc.). Immune adherence of antigen-antibody complexes and the production of lymphokines can be mediated by this binding through a stable C3b site (Nelson, 1953). Furthermore, there is a possible relationship to antibody synthesis (Pepys *et al.*, 1976). The C3b receptors have been found on monocytes (Huber et al., 1968), B lymphocytes (Ross *et al.*, 1973) and macrophages (Lay and Nussenzweig, 1968; (Bianco *et al.*, 1970). C3b bound to Sepharose can be used as an affinity preparative column for separation of T and B cells (Casali and Perussia, 1977).

The C3 receptor solubilized from lymphoid cells was shown to rely on both protein and lipid moities for the expression of C3-binding activity (Dierich and Reisfeld, 1975).

The fixation of a cleavage product of C3 to the surface of activating substances or immune complexes is a critical step for the rapid ingestion by phagocytes. The molecular nature of the opsonically active C3 fragment has not yet been clarified. It has been reported that the opsonically active C3 fragment is composed of two polypeptide chains of the same molecular weight connected by disulfide linkages; one is the intact β chain and the other is a fragment of the α chain having a molecular weight of 70,000. Consequently it has a similarity to the plasmin-produced C3c (Nagasawa and Stroud, 1977*c*). The opsonically active fragment also has a free —SH group related to its function (Stossel *et al.*, 1975).

Immune phagocytosis is usually caused by a synergistic role of C3b and IgG. The role of C3b as an opsonin is primarily to establish contact between C3b-bearing particles and phagocytes (Ehlenberger and Nussenzweig, 1977).

Of four guinea pig C3 fragments, C3a, C3b, C3c, and C3d, made with trypsin, only C3b is capable of stimulating spleen cells to elaborate a macrophage chemotactic factor which is similar in molecular size to the chemotactic factor generated after stimulation by lipopolysaccharides (Koopman *et al.*, 1976).

The major significance of C3 in host defense against pathogenic bacteria has been documented by the observation of recurrent severe infections in patients with a genetic C3 deficiency (Alper *et al.*, 1976) and in a single patient with a C3 deficiency due to hypercatabolism of C3 caused by the lack of C3b-INA (Alper *et al.*, 1970). In the latter patient the amplification loop is continuously operative because of inadequate control of the C3b concentration; thus C3 is consumed in this irrelevant turnover.

III. Alternative Pathway

A. Introduction

As presently conceived, the alternative complement pathway (Fig. 5) carries out two interrelated functions. On the one hand, it constitutes a positive feedback amplification loop whereby the major fragment of C3 cleavage, C3b, initiates the formation of additional C3-cleaving enzymes. On the other hand, as originally described by Pillemer (1955) and Pillemer *et al.* (1954, 1955), the alternative pathway provides a mechanism for recruiting the biological activities of the late-acting complement components independently of the classical pathway activation sequence. The former function of the alternative pathway is the best understood of the two and can be discussed in molecular terms: C3b derived from C3 cleavage through one of several possible ways interacts with serum enzymes B and D to form a new C3-convertase designated C3bBb. The second function of the alternative pathway, i.e., the formation of a C3- and C5-cleaving enzyme without the participation of C1, C4, and C2, has not been completely elucidated. It has been firmly established that interaction of fresh serum with certain polysaccharides or other activators of

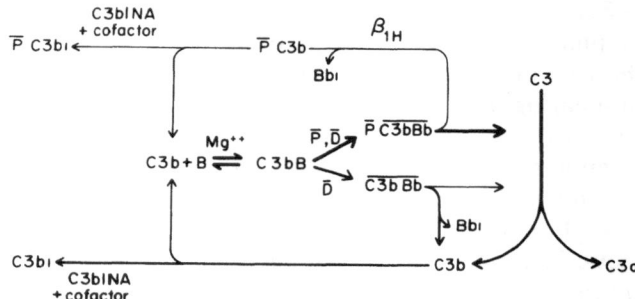

Figure 5. Alternative pathway of complement activation: amplification loop. Schematic outline of the alternative pathway and the positive feedback loop initiated by C3b. Because of the uncertainty over whether all activating substances utilize the same initial steps, these steps have not been included.

the alternative pathway results in the formation of multiunit C3 and C5 convertases in the absence of C4 and/or C2. The evidence for this comes from many experiments using a variety of methods and activators. For example, the pattern of complement activation by bacterial lipopolysaccharides (LPS) was examined in detail, and it was found that incubation of serum with LPS resulted in profound consumption of each one of the C3–C9 components with little or no consumption of C1, C4, and C2 (Bladen et al., 1967; Gewurz et al., 1968). It was subsequently shown that on incubation of LPS with guinea pig serum an intermediate termed "LPS-X" was formed with C3 convertase activity. This C3 convertase showed features in common with the classical pathway EAC42 convertase. However, C2 was not present in LPS-X, since it was not affected by treatment with antiserum to C2, at concentrations that completely blocked C3 cleavage by EAC42 (Marcus et al., 1971). These experiments and the finding that LPS can activate C3–9 in C4-deficient serum (Frank et al., 1971) provided more definitive evidence that C4 and C2 are not essential components of the C3 convertase assembled on LPS. Similar data were obtained with guinea pig γ_1-immunoglobulins, which in complex with specific antigens can activate the alternative pathway (Osler et al., 1969; Sandberg et al., 1970); consumption of C3–9 by γ_1-immunoglobulin complexes was shown to proceed in C4-deficient guinea pig serum (Sandberg et al., 1972). Finally, activation of complement by zymosan was also shown to be independent of C4 and C2 (Brade et al., 1973, 1974; Nicholson et al., 1974). The molecular interactions initiating the assembly of these enzymes remain to be resolved. A distinct serum protein termed "initiating factor" (IF) (Schreiber et al., 1976a) has been recently proposed as the recognition protein of the alternative pathway. IF on interaction with activating substances forms a C3-cleaving enzyme depending on the presence of C3, B, D, and Mg^{2+} (Medicus et al., 1976c). The physicochemical and functional characterization of this factor is still incomplete. Another possible mechanism for the assembly of the initial alternative pathway C3 convertase has emerged from experiments demonstrating the formation of such an enzyme on interaction of native C3 with B and Active D̄ (Fearon and Austen, 1975d). The efficiency of C3 cleavage by this enzyme is considerably enhanced by properdin, which prevents its spontaneous decay-dissociation (Fearon and Austen, 1975a; Schreiber et al., 1975). This C3-dependent convertase generates the initial C3b necessary for the assembly of the C3b-dependent enzyme. The alternative pathway-activating substances such as zymosan play a stabilizing role protecting the C3b-dependent convertase from the action of the natural serum inactivators C3-INA and β1H (Fearon and Austen, 1977).

Irrespective of its exact mechanism, activation of the alternative pathway results in the generation of all the biological activities that are elicited from C3–C9 by classical pathway activation. This indicates that the alternative pathway plays a central role in host defense against pathogens, especially early after infection when adequate levels of specific antibody are not available. Opsonization of bacteria by C3b is believed to be of great importance in that respect. The fact that activators of the alternative pathway are widely distributed among both gram-negative (Pillemer *et al.*, 1955; Bladen *et al.*, 1967) and gram-positive (Tauber *et al.*, 1976) bacteria supports the view that this pathway might indeed represent a broad, nonspecific defense system. In fact, it has been suggested that the alternative pathway might have evolved as a primitive defense system before adaptive immunity. This hypothesis is supported by the finding that certain lower vertebrates and invertebrates lacking immunoglobulins, as well as C1, C4, and C2, show evidence for the presence of a complement-like lytic system. Lysis of mammalian erythrocytes by the hemolymph of these animals can be induced by a pathway initiated by cobra venom factor (CoVF), a known activator of the human alternative pathway (Day *et al.*, 1970).

B. Nomenclature

A provisional nomenclature for the alternative pathway was agreed on by the Complement Nomenclature Committee at the Second International Congress of Immunology (Brighton, United Kingdom, 1974). New factors and activities have since been reported. The pathway has been previously referred to as the "properdin pathway," "alternate pathway," "C3-activator system," "C3 bypass," or "C3 shunt." The components or factors of this pathway are designated by capital letters. Descriptive names used previously are given in Table II. In conformity with the nomenclature of the classical pathway, active factors are indicated by an overbar, e.g., $\bar{D}$ for enzymatically active D. Fragments produced during activation by peptide bond cleavage are designated by the symbol of the factor followed by lowercase letters, e.g., Ba, Bb.

C. Proteins of the Alternative Pathway

1. B

B was originally characterized as one of the serum factors required for C3 destruction by the zymosan-activated properdin system. It was

Table II.   Factors Involved in the Alternative Pathway: Symbols and
Synonyms

Symbol	Synonyms
B	Properdin factor B, β_2-glycoprotein II, heat-labile factor (HLF), C3 proactivator (C3PA), glycine-rich β-glycoprotein (GBG), unknown factor (UF)
D	Factor D, C3-proactivator convertase (C3PAse), GBGase
P	Properdin
C3	Factor A, hydrazine-sensitive factor (HSF)
IF	Initiating factor
C3-Nef	C3 nephritic factor, nephritic factor (NF)
C3b-INA	C3b inactivator, factor C (?), conglutinin-activating factor (KAF)
β_{1H}	C3b inactivator accelerator

shown to be distinct from the known classical pathway complement components and completely destroyed by heating at 50°C for 30 min (Blum *et al.*, 1959). B has been purified and characterized structurally and functionally under various descriptive names, including "β_2-glycoprotein II" (Haupte and Heide, 1965)," glycine-rich β-glycoprotein" (GBG) (Boenisch and Alper, 1970*b*), and "C3 proactivator" (C3PA) (Götze and Müller-Eberhard, 1971). The functional and structural identity of these different preparations with B was subsequently established (Goodkofsky and Lepow, 1971; Alper *et al.*, 1973). B is a glycoprotein containing 10.6% carbohydrate consisting of 5.4% hexose, 4.2% acetyl-hexosamine, 0.9% acetylneuraminic acid, and 0.1% fucose. The galactose:mannose molar ratio was found to be 1:1. The amino acid composition is characterized by a high (8.35%) glycine content (Boenisch and Alper 1970*b*). A sedimentation coefficient $s_{20,w}$ of 6.2 was reported by Boenisch and Alper, 1970b) and of 5.4 by Lynen *et al.* (1973). A molecular weight of 93,000 was calculated from ultracentrifugal data (Lynen *et al.*, 1973). Following reduction with 1% 2-mercaptoethanol in the presence of 8 M urea and 1% SDS or oxidation with performic acid, B migrates on SDS-polyacrylamide gels as a single polypeptide chain (Ziegler *et al.*, 1975; Götze, 1975). The electrophoretic mobility of B on either agar gel or cellulose acetate at pH 8.6 is that of a β-globulin. Its normal serum concentration is 27.4 ± 9.2 mg/dl (mean ± SD) and its $E_{1\,cm}^{1\%}$ at 280 nm is 6.2 (Boenisch and Alper 1970*b*). By isoelectric focusing, the isoelectric point of B was calculated to be 5.7 by Lynen *et al.* (1973) and 6.6 by Fearon and Austen (1975*d*). Heating B at 50°C for 30 min results in loss of not only its functional activity but also its antigenicity (Lynen *et al.*, 1973). Electrophoretic studies using agarose gels indicate that B is polymorphic in humans, with two common alleles designated GB^F and Gb^S (Alper *et al.*, 1972). A close linkage between B and the major histocompatibility complex in man was shown by Allen (1974). Genetically determined polymorphism of B under the control of at least six codominant alleles occupying a single autosomal locus has been demonstrated in the rhesus macaque (Ziegler *et al.*, 1975).

B on reaction with C3b, the major fragment of C3 activation, forms a Mg^{2+}-dependent, reversible complex (Nicholson *et al.*, 1975). The C3bB complex has been recently shown to be stoichiometric at a molar ratio of 1:1. Its molecular weight was calculated by microdisk electrophoresis on polyacrylamide gradient gels at 307,000 (Vogt *et al.*, 1977). Similar Mg^{2+}-dependent, reversible complexes had been previously described between B and a protein in cobra venom termed "cobra venom factor" (CoVF) (Cooper, 1973; Vogt *et al.*, 1974). CoVF is a 6.5 S β-glycoprotein with a molecular weight of 144,000 (Nelson, 1966; Müller-Eberhard *et al.*, 1966a; Müller-Eberhard and Fjellström, 1971) which on interaction with normal serum activates the late-acting complement components C3–9 without affecting C1, C4, and C2 (Flexner and Noguchi, 1903; Ritz, 1912; Klein and Wellensiek, 1965). Recently Alper and Balavitch (1976) demonstrated that CoVF is antigenically related to human C3 and suggested that it might represent cobra C3b. During alternative pathway activation, a single arginyl-lysine peptide bond on B is cleaved by the catalytic action of $\bar{D}$ (Nagasawa *et al.*, 1977). Cleavage of B by $\bar{D}$ requires its prior complexing with C3b or CoVF (Müller-Eberhard and Götze, 1972; Hunsicker *et al.*, 1973). As a result, two unequal-size fragments are generated termed "Bb" and "Ba" (Götze and Müller-Eberhard, 1971). The two fragments have different electrophoretic mobilities and have been demonstrated by immunoelectrophoresis, molecular sieve and ion-exchange chromatography, sucrose density ultracentrifugation, and SDS-polyacrylamide gel electrophoresis. The largest fragment, Bb, has a γ mobility on agar gels at pH 8.6 and contains 1.3–1.5% sialic acid (Boenisch and Alper, 1970a; Haupt and Heide, 1965). Bb has an extinction coefficient $E_{1\,cm}^{1\%}$ of 10.0–11.0 at 280 nm and a sedimentation coefficient $s_{20,2}$ of 3.7–4.3. Its molecular weight was calculated by low-speed sedimentation equilibrium at 59,600 (Nagasawa *et al.*, 1977). Values of 55,000 (Ziegler *et al.*, 1975) and of 63,000 (Götze, 1975) were obtained by SDS-polyacrylamide gel electrophoresis. Its amino acid composition is characterized by a high (7.65%) glycine content. The smaller fragment of B, Ba, has an α mobility on agarose gels at pH 8.6 (Boenisch and Alper, 1970b; Götze and Müller-Eberhard, 1971). Its molecular weight was calculated to be 27,600 by low-speed sedimentation equilibrium (Nagasawa *et al.*, 1977) and 30,000 by SDS-polyacrylamide gel electrophoresis (Götze, 1975).

Functionally, B is the alternative pathway equivalent of C2. The two proteins have many functional and structural properties in common, suggesting a common ancestral gene (Fig. 6). Both proteins form Mg^{2+}-dependent reversible protein-protein complexes, C2 with C4b, B with C3b. They are both cleaved into two unequal molecular weight fragments by the action of a serine esterase, C2 by $\overline{C1s}$, B by $\overline{D}$. Following cleavage, the largest fragment, C2a or Bb, forms Mg^{2+}-independent complexes endowed with esterolytic and endopeptidase activity. Both enzymes C4b2a and C3bBb have identical substrate and bond specificity cleaving an arginyl-X peptide bond on the α chain of C3 (Hugli, 1975). C2a and Bb contain the catalytic center of the respective enzyme. Both C4b2a and C3bBb bind additional C3b, which modifies their substrate specificity from C3 to C5. Finally, both C2 and B have in their native state esterolytic activity against N-substituted lysine esters. B cleaves the synthetic esters acetylglycyl-L-lysine methyl ester (AGLMe), N-α-acetyl-L-lysine methyl ester (ALMe), and N-ϵ-carbobenzoxyl-L-lysine methyl ester (CBZLMe) but not the arginine ester N-α-acetyl-L-arginine methyl ester (AAMe) (Cooper, 1971; Vogt *et al.*, 1977). The trypsin inhibitors from bovine lung (Trasylol), soybean and lima bean, as well as ovomucoid and *p*-nitro-

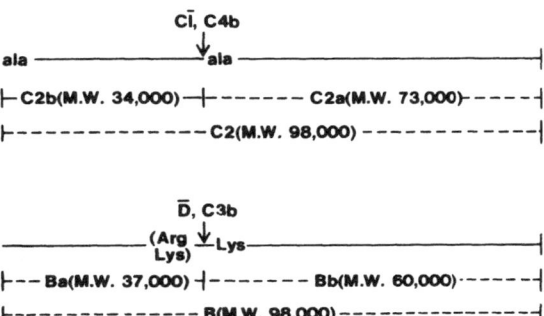

Figure 6.   C2 and factor B. Schematic diagram illustrating the similarity of the analogous convertase enzymes in the classical pathway (C2) and the alternative pathway (B). Factor B and C2 have similar esterase activity. When combined with their respective cofactors, both cleave C3 to produce C3a and C3b. Gene maps show remarkably close loci, and their physical and chemical features are similar. These facts suggest a gene duplication. The molecular weights were determined by SDS gels (Nagasawa and Stroud, unpublished data). The requirement for C3b in B cleavage by $\overline{D}$ is absolute, whereas the requirement for C4b in the cleavage of C2 by $\overline{C1}$, although enhancing, does not appear to be absolute

phenyl-*p'*-guanidine benzoate do not inhibit the action of B on C3 (Götze and Müller-Eberhard, 1976). The sensitivity of B to diisopropylfluorophosphate (DFP) remains controversial. Fearon *et al.* (1974*a*) reported that treatment of B with 10^{-3} M DFP followed by dialysis did not affect its hemolytic activity. Similarly, treatment of EAC43bBb cells with 10^{-3} M DFP followed by washing did not affect their ability to lyse upon subsequent addition of C5–9. Götze (1975) also reported that treatment of the CoVFBb enzyme with 10^{-2} M DFP did not influence its biological activity, i.e., its ability to cleave C3. Finally, Vogt *et al.* (1977) found that 10^{-3} M DFP had no effect on the esterolytic activity of native B using AGLME as substrate. In contrast to these data, Medicus *et al.* (1976*a*) reported that the CoVFBb C3 convertase was sensitive to DFP. However, inactivation of the enzyme required much higher concentrations of DFP and longer incubation times that other serine esterases. Perhaps more importantly, incorporation of [^{3}H]-DFP into native B was also shown at a 0.7 mol/mol ratio after 60 min incubation at 37°C.

2. D

D is a trace serum protease with serine esterase activity. Although usual purification procedures yield enzymatically active D̄ (Müller-Eberhard and Götze, 1972; Fearon *et al.*, 1974*a,b*; Dieminger *et al.*, 1976; Volanakis *et al.*, 1977) the zymogen form of the enzyme has also been isolated from human plasma (Fearon *et al.*, 1974*a*). Active D̄ has a molecular weight of 22,900 by sedimentation equilibrium (Volanakis *et al.*, 1977). Values of 25,000 (Fearon *et al.*, 1974*a*) and 21,500 ± 700 (Dieminger *et al.*, 1976) were obtained by gel-filtration and of 24,000 by SDS-polyacrylamide gel electrophoresis (Götze, 1975). D̄ has an apparent sedimentation coefficient of 3.0S by sucrose density gradient ultracentrifugation (Müller-Eberhard and Götze, 1972). Its electrophoretic mobility from serum has been variably reported as that of an α-globulin using pevikon block electrophoresis at pH 8.6 or β- to γ-globulin using agarose immunoelectrophoresis at pH 8.6. By isoelectric focusing, its isoelectric point was found at pH 7.4 (Fearon and Austen, 1975*d*) or 7.8 (Dieminger *et al.*, 1976). D̄ consists of a single polypeptide chain, since reduced and alkylated preparations exhibit a single protein band on SDS-polyacrylamide gel electrophoresis (Götze, 1975; Volanakis *et al.*, 1977). By the dansyl chloride method, isoleucine was determined as the NH$_2$ terminus (Volanakis *et al.*, 1977). D̄ is a protease catalyzing limited proteolytic cleavage of B, resulting in the generation of the C3 convertase C3bBb. Its action on B depends on the presence of C3b, the major fragment of C3 cleavage, or CoVF (Müller-Eberhard and Götze, 1972; Hunsicker *et* *al.*, 1973). It has been suggested that a susceptible peptide bond on B is exposed by the formation of a Mg^{2+}-requiring protein-protein complex of B and C3b or CoVF (Müller-Eberhard and Götze, 1972; Cooper, 1973; Vogt *et al.*, 1974). Formation of the C3 convertase on the surface of a red cell results from interaction of C3b-bearing cells with purified B and D in the presence of Mg^{2+} (Fearon *et al.*, 1973). On subsequent interaction of these EAC3bBb cells with the late-acting complement components (C3–9, the cells are lysed. This hemolytic reaction can be used as a sensitive assay of the proteolytic activity of D̄ preparations. D̄ also has esterolytic activity against certain synthetic amino acid esters of arginine and lysine (Dieminger *et al.*, 1976; Volanakis *et al.*, 1977). Benzoyl-L-arginine methyl ester (BAMe) was the most sensitive substrate among those tested. The substrate profile of D̄ was distinct when compared to that of C1̄s, C1̄r, plasmin, urokinase, and trypsin. Both the hemolytic (Fearon *et al.*, 1974a) and esterolytic (Volanakis *et al.*, 1977) activity of D̄ were irreversibly inhibited by 10 mM DFP, suggesting that both activities reside in the same active center. This hypothesis is also supported by the finding that *p*-tosyl-L-arginine methyl ester HC1 (TAMe) competitively inhibited B cleavage by D̄ (Fearon and Austen, 1975b). Inhibition of B cleavage was also observed with ALMe and AGLMe (Dieminger *et al.*, 1976). Reduction and alkylation of D̄ inhibited its activity irreversibly, indicating that intrachain disulfide bond(s) are essential for the expression of enzymatic activity (Volanakis *et al.*, 1977). The trypsin inhibitors from bovine lung (Traysylol®), soybean and lima bean, and ovomucoid (Götze and Müller-Eberhard, 1976) and also 10^{-2} M tosyl-L-lysine chloromethyl ketone (TLCK) (Fearon *et al.*, 1974a) have no effect on D̄. Finally, D̄ failed to cleave casein, hemoglobin, fibrin, and elastin (Götze and Müller-Eberhard, 1976). The DFP-resistant zymogen of the enzyme (D) has been isolated from human plasma (Fearon *et al.*, 1974a). Precursor D can be activated to D̄ by trypsin. The natural activator of D has not been identified to date. The molecular weight of D was estimated by Sephadex filtration at 25,000, indicating that no large fragment is released during the activation process.

3. Properdin

Properdin (from the Latin verb *perdere*—to destroy) was first recognized as a distinct serum protein related to complement by Pillemer and associates in the early 1950s (Pillemer *et al.*, 1954). It was shown to play an essential role in the then described properdin pathway, which was conceived as an alternative mechanism for the activation of the late-acting complement components not requiring antibody, C1, C4, and C2.

Thus properdin was thought to be an important component of host defense and to "participate in such diverse activities as the destruction of bacteria, the neutralization of viruses, and the lysis of certain red cells" (Pillemer *et al.*, 1954). An important initial observation was that properdin under appropriate conditions and in the presence of Mg^{2+} ions and other serum proteins could bind to zymosan, an insoluble polysaccharide derived from yeast cell walls. Binding of properdin to zymosan from serum and subsequent elution with high ionic strength buffer was used as a first step in its purification (Pensky *et al.*, 1968). Properdin is among the most basic serum proteins, migrating cathodally to all serum proteins on electrophoresis on cellulose acetate strips at pH 8.6 (Pensky *et al.*, 1968). Although its exact isoelectric point has not been determined, it appears to be greater than 9.5 (Götze and Müller-Eberhard, 1974) Properdin is a glycoprotein-containing 9.8% carbohydrate composed of hexose (3.8%), fucose (0.7%), hexosamine (1.5%), and sialic acid (3.8%) (Minta and Lepow, 1974). By sedimentation equilibrium its molecular weight was calculated to be 216,000 (Pensky *et al.*, 1968), using an assumed partial specific volume of 0.75. Minta and Lepow (1974), using a partial specific volume of 0.7 calculated from the amino acid and carbohydrate composition, reported a molecular weight of 184,000 for purified properdin. For the same partial specific volume these two values are very similar. A sedimentation coefficient $s_{20,2} = 5.2$ and a diffusion constant $D_{20,2} = 2.15 \times 10^{-7}$ cm²/sec were calculated for properdin from ultracentrifugal data (Pensky *et al.*, 1968). These values in conjunction with the molecular weight indicate a highly asymmetrical molecule. No NH_2-terminal amino acid could be detected in properdin by the dansyl chloride method (Minta and Lepow, 1974). On electrophoresis on SDS-containing gels and on gel filtration on Sepharose 4B in the presence of 6 M guanidine hydrochloride, properdin migrates as a homogeneous protein with an approximate molecular weight of 45,000–53,000 (Götze and Müller-Eberhard, 1974; Minta and Lepow, 1974). These data indicate that the native molecule is composed of four identical noncovalently bound subunits. The normal serum concentration of properdin is 1.48 ± 0.39 mg/dl (Minta *et al.*, 1973).

Properdin purified either by absorption to and elution from zymosan (Pensky *et al.*, 1968; Minta and Lepow, 1974) or by euglobulin precipitation followed by conventional chromatographic techniques (Götze and Müller-Eberhard, 1974; Fearon *et al.*, 1974*b*) is apparently in an activated state ($\bar{P}$). Added to normal human serum, $\bar{P}$ can initiate the assembly of a C3-cleaving enzyme requiring the participation of native C3, factors B and D, and Mg^{2+} (Götze and Müller-Eberhard, 1974). Precursor properdin (P), defined by its inability to initiate by itself C3 cleavage on reaction with normal human serum, was recently purified by Minta (1976) and also by Götze et al. (1977). The former method used a neutral euglobulin precipitation of serum followed by reversed affinity chromatography. The purified precursor P differed from $\bar{P}$ in several respects. P was shown to be a 6.1 S β_2-globulin composed of four subunits with a 57,900 molecular weight. In contrast, $\bar{P}$ was a 5.1 S γ_2-globulin with a subunit molecular weight of 53,000. In addition, on double diffusion analysis, antigenic differences between P and $\bar{P}$ were observed, suggesting that certain antigenic determinants on P were absent from $\bar{P}$ (Minta, 1976). Conversion of P to $\bar{P}$ was achieved by mild treatment with plasmin or trypsin. These data indicated that properdin is present in serum in a precursor-inactive form and that its activation is effected by a limited proteolytic cleavage. A normal human serum protein termed "properdin convertase" was described by Stitzel and Spitzer (1974) as a natural activator of P. Following its activation by zymosan, properdin convertase can directly activate properdin either in serum or in the purified state. Such activation by properdin convertase is associated with a cathodal shift in the electrophoretic mobility of properdin (Spitzer et al., 1976). Properdin activated by this mechanism was reported to activate C3 and C5 in the fluid phase without a requirement of B and D (Stitzel and Spitzer, 1974; Spitzer et al., 1976). At present it does not appear that properdin activated by properdin convertase is similar physicochemically and functionally to plasmin- or trypsin-activated properdin. It should also be noted that purified properdin used for these studies should be in an "activated" state according to the criteria of other workers, since it was purified by the use of zymosan. In contrast to these data, Götze et al. (1977) reported recently that P and $\bar{P}$ were identical by several physicochemical parameters: the two forms of properdin had the same electrophoretic mobility, identical sedimentation characteristics on sucorse density gradients, and subunits of identical molecular weight (50,000). Precursor P was purified from serum via QAE-Sephadex chromatography followed by Sepharose 6B filtration and reversed affinity chromatography. Activation of P to $\bar{P}$ was achieved by interaction with cell-bound C3 convertase, C3bBb (Medicus et al., 1976b). These data suggested that activation of properdin is due to a partially reversible conformational change of the molecule rather than to limited proteolytic cleavage. Further characterization of P and $\bar{P}$ is apparently necessary in order to fully understand the activation process. However, it seems possible that both proteolytic cleavage and conformational changes might be necessary for the full expression of properdin activity.

Activated properdin has an apparent affinity for C3 and its activation fragments. Under appropriate conditions of pH and ionic strength, and in the presence of factor B and Mg^{2+}, $\bar{P}$ formed precipitation lines in reaction with C3 in agar (Ziegler *et al.*, 1976). These precipitates were dissimilar to antigen-antibody lattices in that they involved not only C3 and $\bar{P}$ but also agar. Direct interaction between $\bar{P}$ and C3 in the fluid phase has been demonstrated by Chapitis and Lepow (1976) using sucrose density gradient ultracentrifugation. Purified $\bar{P}$ on reaction with C3 or its fragments C3b or C3c formed heavier sedimenting complexes. The formation of these complexes did not require the presence of metal ions. $\bar{P}$ was also shown to bind to red cell-bound C3b (Fearon and Austen, 1975c), causing agglutination of the red cells (Schreiber *et al.*, 1975). This last finding indicated the presence of more than one binding site on $\bar{P}$ for C3b. These interactions of $\bar{P}$ with C3 and its fragments are apparently related to its physiological role, which is to stabilize the alternative pathway C3- and C3b-dependent C3-cleaving enzyme.

4. C3 Nephritic Factor (C3Nef) and Initiating Factor (IF)

C3Nef and IF are discussed together because they are immunochemically related (Vallota *et al.*, 1974) and perhaps the latter represents the precursor form of the former (Schreiber *et al.*, 1976a). C3Nef is an incompletely characterized protein present only in some pathological sera, specifically in sera from certain patients with renal diseases (Spitzer *et al.*, 1969; Vallota *et al.*, 1970) or with partial lipodystrophy (Sissons *et al.*, 1976). Its presence was first suggested by Pickering *et al.* (1968), who demonstrated that sera from patients with acute and chronic forms of glomerulonephritis were "anticomplementary." The anticomplementary activity was shown to be thermolabile and to cause consumption of the six terminal complement components (C3–9) on incubation with normal guinea pig serum. It was subsequently shown that sera from children with a form of glomerulonephritis termed "hypocomplementemic membranoproliferative" (West *et al.*, 1965) contained a factor designated C3Nef which under appropriate conditions effected cleavage of C3 (Spitzer et al., 1969). C3 cleavage could be quantitated by measuring immunochemically the reduction of the B antigenic determinant of C3, which is present only in the native molecule (West *et al.*, 1961). C3Nef was shown to be a thermolabile pseudoglobulin which in the presence of Mg^{2+} formed C3-cleaving complexes with a thermolabile normal serum pseudoglobulin, later identified with B (Vallota *et al.*, 1970; Ruley *et al.*, 1973). C3Nef migrates on cellulose acetate and pevikon block elctrophoresis at pH 8.6 as a γ-globulin. Its sedimentation rate was estimated by sucrose density gradient centrifugation to be approximately 7 S (Vallota *et al.*, 1974). A molecular weight of 170,000 was calculated for C3Nef from SDS-polyacrylamide gel electrophoresis data. Following reduction the main protein band had an apparent molecular weight of 85,000. These data suggest that C3Nef is composed of two disulfide-linked and probably identical polypeptide chains (Shcreiber *et al.*, 1976*b*). An isoelectric point of 8.75–8.95 was calculated by isoelectric focusing (Daha *et al.*, 1976). Data showing that C3Nef-like activity in the serum of a patient with hypocomplementemic proliferative glomerulonephritis was associated with an IgG_3-rich, IgG fraction suggested that C3Nef might indeed be an "altered" form of IgG_3 (Thompson, 1972*a*). This hypothesis was further supported by the finding that patients with membranoproliferative glomerulonephritis had a relative increase of serum IgG_3 (Thompson, 1972*b*). More recently, though, Vallota *et al.* (1974) distinguished C3Nef from IgG immunochemically, using antisera specific for various immunoglobulin determinants, including antisera to IgG_3. It should be noted, however, that most of the literature data on the function of C3Nef have been obtained using preparations contaminated with IgG.* Functionally, C3Nef is similar although not identical to activated properdin ($\bar{P}$). Like $\bar{P}$, C3Nef binds to the C3bBb enzyme both in the fluid phase and on the surface of red cells (Schreiber *et al.*, 1975; Daha *et al.*, 1977). In the latter case, C3Nef binding causes agglutination of the red cells similarly to $\bar{P}$. However, whereas $\bar{P}$ has been shown to bind to C3b, the exact binding site on the C3bBb complex for C3Nef is not known. Similarly to $\bar{P}$, C3Nef binding to C3bBb results in stabilization of the enzyme, extending its half-life at 30°C ten- to fifteenfold (Daha *et al.*, 1976). C3Nef-stabilized C3 convertase in contrast to $\bar{P}$-stabilized C3 convertase is relatively resistant to β1H-induced decay. β1H, as will be discussed below, is one of the control proteins of the alternative pathway causing acceleration of the decay of $\bar{P}$-stabilized C3bBb (Weiler *et al.*, 1976).

Although C3Nef is present only in pathological sera, adsorption of a normal serum with insolubilized antiserum to C3Nef resulted in impairment of the alternative pathway function (Vallota *et al.*, 1974). This experiment suggested the presence of a normal serum analogue of C3Nef, which was named "initiating factor" (IF). It was subsequently shown that IF is essential for the activation of the alternative pathway by zymosan and inulin, and it was proposed as the recognition protein of the pathway (Schreiber *et al.*, 1976*a*). Partially purified IF was shown to have a β mobility on agarose electrophoresis at pH 8.6 and a 7 S sedimentation rate on sucrose density gradient ultracentrifugation. Its apparent molecular weight is 70,000–120,000 by Sephadex G-150 filtration and 170,000 by SDS-polyacrylamide gel electrophoresis. Following reduction

* See addendum at end of this chapter.

with dithiothreitol in the presence of 8 M urea and 1% SDS, a molecular weight of 85,000 was obtained by SDS-polyacrylamide gel electrophoresis. These data suggest a two-polypeptide-chain structure for IF (Schreiber *et al.*, 1976a). Thus C3Nef and IF in addition to immunochemical cross-reactivity exhibit similar molecular weights and polypeptide chain structure. However, the two proteins have different electrophoretic mobilities and functional characteristics. As mentioned, C3Nef added to normal serum causes cleavage of C3, a property not shared by IF. This led to the suggestion that C3Nef might represent the activated form of IF. In fact, it was shown that incubation of IF for 5 hr at 4°C in pH 2.2 glycine-HCl buffer resulted in change of its electrophoretic mobility from β to γ. In addition, acid-treated IF exhibited C3Nef-like activity, being able to cause cleavage of C3 on addition to normal human serum (Schreiber *et al.*, 1976a).

5. C3b Inactivator (C3b-INA)

C3b-INA is the main control protein of the alternative pathway, effectively blocking the amplification loop by inactivating C3b (Fig. 4). It has a β electrophoretic mobility on pevikon block electrophoresis at ` pH 8.6 (Lachmann and Müller-Eberhard, 1968) and a molecular weight of 91,000 calculated by SDS-polyacrylamide gel electrophoresis (Fearon, 1977). An approximate sedimentation coefficient of 5.5–6.0 S was estimated by sucrose density gradient ultracentrifugation and a diffusion coefficient of 5×10^{-7} cm²/sec by Sephadex G-200 gel filtration (Lachmann and Müller-Eberhard, 1968). It is composed of two disulfide-linked polypeptide chains with molecular weights of 55,000 and 41,000 as calculated by SDS-polyacrylamide gel electrophoresis (Fearon, 1977). Electrophoretic studies indicate that C3b-INA is polymorphic, with at least four protein bands present on alkaline polyacrylamide gels. C3b-INA appears to be an endopeptidase which in the presence of a macromolecular cofactor cleaves a peptide bond on the α chain of C3b (Tamura and Nelson, 1967; Lachmann and Müller-Eberhard, 1968; Ruddy and Austen, 1969, 1971; Nagasawa and Stroud, 1977c). Its mechanism of action has been described in detail in a previous section of this chapter. C3b-INA is thermostable, resisting heating at 56°C for 4 hr (Tamura and Nelson, 1967). It is also resistant to treatment with 15 mM hydrazine, 0.1 mM iodine, 10 mM iodoacetamide, 10 mM dithionite, 5 mM diisopropyl fluorophosphate (DFP), and soybean trypsin inhibitor (Lachmann and Müller-Eberhard, 1968) as well as N-ethylmaleimide (Ruddy and Austen, 1969). Its activity is irreversibly inhibited by reduction-alkylation and also by potassium metaperiodate (Lachmann and Müller-Eberhard, 1968). Sodium cyanate at concentrations of 0.5–5.0 mM also causes irreversible inactivation of C3b-INA probably due to carbamylation (Schultz and Arnold, 1975). Finally, its function is inhibited in 1 M EACA (Vogt *et al.*, 1975). Treatment of cell-bound C3b with the antitrypanosomal drug antrypol (Suramin®) renders it resistant to the action of C3b-INA (Tamura and Nelson, 1967) even after the cells have been washed to remove the drug (Lachmann *et al.*, 1973*b*). The biological significance of this inactivator is best illustrated by a patient genetically deficient in this protein (Alper *et al.*, 1970; Abramson *et al.*, 1971). This patient suffered from a marked susceptibility to pyogenic infections and exhibited low C3 and factor B levels due to continuous uncontrolled activation of the amplification loop. This defect was reproduced *in vitro* by immunochemical depletion of C3b-INA from serum (Nicol and Lachmann, 1973). The result was spontaneous activation of the alternative pathway with consumption of factor B and C3.

6. β_{1H}

β_{1H} is another control protein of the alternative pathway modulating the activity of the C3-cleaving enzyme(s). It was first recognized as a distinct serum protein when crude C3 β_{1C} preparations were analyzed immunochemically (Nillson and Müller-Eberhard, 1965). Its name designates its electrophoretic mobility on agarose gels at pH 8.6. β_{1H} is a glycoprotein containing 15–20% carbohydrate (Ruddy *et al.*, 1977). Reduction and alkylation followed by SDS-PAGE indicate that β_{1H} is composed of a single polypeptide chain (Whaley and Ruddy, 1976*a*). Its isoelectric point was calculated at 6.9 by isoelectric focusing (Ruddy *et al.*, 1977). The normal serum concentration of β_{1H} has been reported to be 516 ± 89 μg/ml (Weiler *et al.*, 1976), representing approximately 1% of the total serum protein. The molecular weight of β_{1H} was calculated at 150,000 by sedimentation equilibrium, using an assumed partial specific volume of 0.733. Considering the high carbohydrate content of β_{1H}, its actual molecular weight might be lower than 150,000. A similar value was also obtained by SDS-polyacrylamide gels, whereas a 300,000 molecular weight was calculated by Sephadex gel filtration. By analytical untracentrifugation a sedimentation coefficient of $s_{20,2} = 5.6$ and a diffusion coefficient $D_{20,2} = 2.8 \times 10^{-7}$ cm²/sec were calculated (Whaley and Ruddy, 1976*a*; Ruddy *et al.*, 1977). An apparent density of greater than 1.2 g/ml was indicated by NaBr density gradient centrifugation. These combined data suggest an asymmetrical molecular structure. The extinction coefficient of β_{1H} $E_{1\,cm}^{1\%} = 13.1$ at 280 nm.

The function of β_{1H} appears to be twofold: (1) it accelerates the cleavage of C3b by C3b-INA, thus preventing the assembly of the C3b-dependent C3 and C5 convertases, and (2) it shortens the half-life of the properdin stabilized C3-cleaving enzyme C3bBb by apparently enhancing the release of the Bb subunit of the enzyme (Weiler *et al.*, 1976; Whaley and Ruddy, 1976*a,b*; Ruddy and Whaley, 1977). These activities of β_{1H} are destroyed by trypsin and also by heating at 56°C for 20 min. However, β_{1H} is resistant to treatment with DFP, soybean trypsin inhibitor, N-ethylmaleimide, phospholipases B and C, or 0.1 mM iodine (Whaley and Ruddy, 1976*a*; Ruddy *et al.*, 1977). No recognizable enzymatic activity has been detected in β_{1H}. It appears that its activity depends on its ability to bind to C3b (Ruddy and Whaley, 1977).

IV. The Complement Attack Mechanism

The last five components (C5–C9) of the complement system compose what has been called the "membrane attack mechanism" (Müller-Eberhard, 1972), for it is the action of these proteins, functioning as a unit, which causes a lesion in the target membrane capable of producing lysis. This is shown schematically in Fig. 7. The attack mechanism was also recently reviewed in detail by M. Mayer in a Harvey Lecture (1977).

A. Proteins of the C Attack Mechanism

The individual proteins of the C attack mechanism have been purified and characterized, and some of their physical properties are shown in Table III.

1. C5

C5 is 200,000 molecular weight glycoprotein composed of two dissimilar polypeptide chains linked by one or more disulfide bonds. Its molecular weight has been variously estimated at between 180,000 and 220,000 (Nilsson and Müller-Eberhard, 1965; Nilsson *et al.*, 1972, 1975). The cleavage of C5 by various proteolytic enzymes is the only known enzymatic step of the C attack sequence.

C5a, an 11,000 molecular weight fragment generated on cleavage from the amino-terminal end of the heavy (α) chain of C5 (Nilsson *et al.*, 1975), is a potent chemotactic factor (Snyderman *et al.*, 1969) and anaphylatoxin (Cochrane and Müller-Eberhard, 1968; Wissler, 1972; Fernan-

**Table III.   Components of the C Attack proteins
from Human Serum: Summary of Properties**

Component or chain		Molecular weight	Relative electrophoretic mobility
C5		220,000	β_1
	α chain	140,000	
	β chain	80,000	
C6		128,000	β_2
C7		121,000	β_2
C8		164,000	γ_1
	α chain	77,000	
	β chain	63,000	
	λ chain	13,700	
C9		79,000	α
S		88,000	α_1
C5b–9		1,000,000	α

dez and Hugli, 1976). It contains three intrachain disulfide bonds, is composed of about 25% carbohydrate (Fernandez and Hugli, 1976), and has substantial α-helical content (Morgan *et al.*, 1974). The carboxyl-terminal arginine residue is essential for biological activity (Vallota *et al.*, 1973; Fernandez and Hugli, 1976). C5b, the larger fragment, has an affinity for cell membranes (Cooper and Müller-Eberhard, 1970) as well as for C6, and its production initiates the assembly of the attack unit (Lachmann and Thompson, 1970; Götze and Müller-Eberhard, 1970; Arroyave and Müller-Eberhard, 1973).

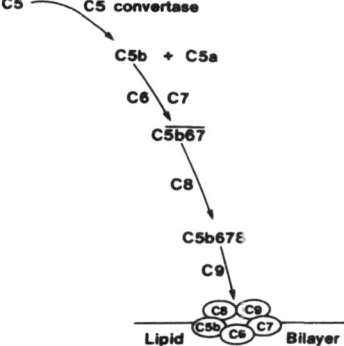

Figure 7.   Assembly of the membrane attack macromolecule. Schematic diagram illustrating how the cleavage of C5 is the key event in initiating assembly. Cleavage of C5b must be near or on a membrane for efficient assembly in a lipid bilayer. Bound C3b potentiates the membrane binding significantly (see text).

2. C6

C6 is composed of a single polypeptide chain with a molecular weight estimated to be between 111,000 and 128,000, and a sedimentation coefficient of 5.7 S (Podack *et al.,* 1976*a*). It has the ability to bind to and stabilize C5b and does not appear to be cleaved during this or any subsequent reaction.

3. C7

C7 is a single polypeptide chain with a molecular weight between 102,000 and 121,000 and a sedimentation coefficient of 5.6 S; like C6, it has β_2 electrophoretic mobility (Podack *et al.,* 1976*a*). It has the capacity to bind to the C56 complex, forming C567 with a labile membrane-binding site. An unconfirmed report (DeLage *et al.,* 1973) suggested that native C7 has esterolytic activity toward tributyrin.

4. C8

C8, the key molecule of the C attack mechanism, has γ_1 electrophoretic mobility, a molecular weight of 163,000, and a sedimentation coefficient of 8 S (Kolb and Müller-Eberhard, 1976). The binding of C8 to a cell-bound C567 complex results in membrane damage, and C9 serves to accelerate this action (Stolfi, 1968; Tamura *et al.,* 1972). C8 is composed of three polypeptide chains, with the 77,000 molecular weights γ chain bound to the 13,700 α chain by one or more disulfide bonds, while the 63,000 β chain is bonded to the α-γ complex by noncovalent forces (Kolb and Müller-Eberhard, 1976).

The C8 α chain was found to be highly resistant to iodination in the native molecule, although it was readily iodinated after dissociation. This suggested that the α chain was "buried" within the β and γ chains, possibly because of a high content of hydrophobic residues, which might favor the interaction of the α chain with lipid membranes (Kolb and Müller-Eberhard, 1976). Circular dichroism studies indicate that the molecule has some α helical secondary structure (Kolb *et al.,* 1976).

5. C9

The last component of the complement attack sequence, C9, is a 79,000 molecular weight α-globulin with a sedimentation coefficient of 4.5 S (Hadding and Müller-Eberhard, 1969). It is composed of a single polypeptide chain (Kolb and Müller-Eberhard, 1975*b*) and appears to act by adsorbing to bound C8 (Kolb and Müller-Eberhard, 1974).

B. Activation of the C Attack Mechanism

Since the C attack mechanism seems to assemble spontaneously on cleavage of native C5, any enzyme which can produce C5b may activate the sequence. However, the most thoroughly studied activators are the complex enzymes of the complement system for which C5 can be considered the "natural" substrate.

The classical pathway C5 convertase is C4b2a3b (Cooper and Müller-Eberhard, 1970; Götze and Müller-Eberhard, 1970; Shin *et al.*, 1971a; Goldlust *et al.*, 1974). The proteolytic site for C5 resides in the C2a fragment, just as the proteolytic site for C3 is found in the C2a portion of the C3 convertase, C4b2a. The presence of C3b in the enzyme changes the substrate specificity of C2a from C3 to C5; C3b provides the binding site for C5 on the enzyme (Shin *et al.*, 1971a,b; Goldlust *et al.*, 1974). Activation of the alternative pathway also generates a C5 convertase, which is analogous in many respects to the classical C4b2a3b enzyme. It consists of activated factor B and at least two molecules of C3b (Medicus *et al.*, 1976b) and may be written as $(C3b)_nBb$. Bb provides the catalytic site for the cleavage of both C3 and C5, and as in the classical pathway enzymes the addition of more molecules of C3b changes the substrate specificity from C3 to C5. The decay rate of the enzyme may be slowed considerably by the addition of properdin (P) or nephritic factor (C3Nef), which retard the decay-loss of Bb from the enzyme (Medicus *et al.*, 1976b).

The requirement for two associated C3b molecules in the alternative pathway C5 convertase seems to restrict formation of this enzyme to the surface of particulate C activators where association of C3b may occur more readily. Even in the presence of stabilizing factors such as P, fluid-phase C5 convertase activity is very low. However, cobra venom factor, a C3b analogue (Alper and Balavitch, 1976), forms an efficient fluid-phase C5 convertase in association with factor B, perhaps because of the association or aggregation of the CoVF-Bb enzyme (Medicus, 1977).

Other enzymes may also possess C5 convertase activity. For example, it has been reported that a fragment of properdin generated by the action of an enzyme, properdin convertase, can directly cleave C5 in the absence of other serum cofactors (Spitzer *et al.*, 1976). Plasmin and trypsin have been shown to generate C567 when incubated with the purified components (Arroyave and Müller-Eberhard, 1973), and leukocyte lysosomal enzymes have been shown to generate chemotactic activity from C5, presumably C5a (Goldstein and Weissmann, 1974); it is likely that they also generate C5b (Arroyave and Müller-Eberhard, 1973) and initiate the assembly of the C attack mechanism.

C. Interactions of the C Attack Proteins

The purified, native components of the C attack mechanism were shown to interact *in solution*, and this information enhanced the understanding of the probable structure of the activated assembly. C5 was found to have an affinity for C6, C7, and C8, while C9 interacted only with C8 (Nilsson and Müller-Eberhard, 1965; Arroyave and Müller-Eberhard, 1973; Kolb *et al.*, 1973). It was therefore postulated that the binding of C6 to C5b allows the firm attachment of C7 to C5b with little direct interaction between C6 and C7. C8 could then attach to the C567 complex through C5b, and C9 would then complete the sequence by absorbing to C8.

Many of these concepts were confirmed by studying the interactions of the activated C attack components, either on the cell surface (Kolb *et al.*, 1972) or in free solution (Kolb *et al.*, 1973). Using radiolabeled proteins, it was found that C5b, C6, and C7 reacted in a 1:1:1 ratio (Götze and Müller-Eberhard, 1970; Arroyave and Müller-Eberhard, 1973) and that this trimolecular complex then bound one molecule of C8; the use of specific antisera suggested that the bound C8 is closely associated with each component of the C567 complex (Kolb and Müller-Eberhard, 1973). A maximum of six C9 molecules could then bind to the C8. These ratios were confirmed by the isolation and characterization of the C5b–9 complex formed in solution by the activation of complement in whole serum (Kolb and Müller-Eberhard, 1975*b*). The complex was usually unsaturated with respect to C9 and could even be assayed by its ability to bind additional C9 (Kolb and Müller-Eberhard, 1973). Analysis of the functional activity of C9 on cell-bound C8 indicated that at least two (Kitamura *et al.*, 1976) or three (Kolb and Müller-Eberhard, 1974) molecules of C9 were required to produce hemolysis with human components, though only one C9 molecule was required when guinea pig components were used (Rommel and Mayer, 1973; Kitamura and Inai, 1974). The sigmoidal dose-response curves of C9 uptake and C9-induced lysis indicated that a positive cooperative interaction of C9 molecules occurred during the binding process (Kolb and Müller-Eberhard, 1974).

The isolated C5b–9 complex has an estimated molecular weight of 1,040,000, a sedimentation coefficient of 23 S, and α electrophoretic mobility (Kolb and Müller-Eberhard, 1975*b*). The complex could be isolated following activation of either the classical or alternative C pathways (Podack *et al.*, 1976*b*) and, surprisingly, contained an extra "unknown" protein (Kolb and Müller-Eberhard, 1975*b*; Podack *et al.*, 1976*b*). This molecule was thought to be either a complement inhibitor or a "serum equivalent" of the C5b–9 membrane binding site, and has been called the

"S protein" (Podack *et al.*, 1977). It is incorporated into the C5b–9 complex at the C7-binding level, and three S molecules are present in each complex (Kolb and Müller-Eberhard, 1975*b*; Podack *et al.*, 1976*b*). The S protein has a high carbohydrate content, a molecular weight of 88,000, and α_1 electrophoretic mobility (Podack *et al.*, 1977). The S protein and C9 probably contribute most of the net surface charge to the C5b–9 complex, since they, like C5b–9, have α electrophoretic mobility, even though C5b, C6, C7, and C8 behave as β- or γ-globulins.

The C5b–9 complex is stable enough to undergo the rigors of purification, but the components are all bound by noncovalent forces, since they are readily dissociated by sodium dodecylsulfate (Kolb and Müller-Eberhard, 1975*b*). Analysis of the C5b–9 complex showed that it was antigenically deficient with respect to native C5, C6, and C8, indicating that these components were partly "buried" in the complex, while C7 and C9 antigenic determinants were fully expressed. In addition, neoantigens, not present on the isolated native components, were expressed (Kolb and Müller-Eberhard, 1975*a*). These new antigenic determinants could also be found on the C567 complex (Podack *et al.*, 1976*c*) and their presence could be used as an indication of assembly of the C attack mechanism.

When C5b binds to C6 in solution, a stable bimolecular complex C56 is formed, and it can be used to initiate the assembly of the C attack complex. C56 can be generated in some sera on addition of alternative pathway activators (Thompson and Rowe, 1968; Thompson and Lachmann, 1970; Lachmann and Thompson, 1970; Goldman *et al.*, 1972; Baker *et al.*, 1975*b*). It seems that a relative excess of C5 and C6 over C7 is required to consume all of the C7, with the remaining C5 and C6 then being available to form C56 (Lachmann and Thompson, 1970). C56 can also be made by reacting the classical pathway C5 convertase with purified C5 and C6 (Götze and Müller-Eberhard, 1970; Goldman, 1974). The subsequent interaction of C56 with C7 results in the formation of C567 complexes, which display a short-lived membrane binding site, estimated to remain active for less than 0.1 sec at 37°C (Götze and Müller-Eberhard, 1970). On interaction with an erythrocyte membrane the stable EC567 intermediate is formed, which is then susceptible to lysis on the addition of C8 and C9. Thompson and Rowe (1968) called this sequence of events "reactive lysis," and the study of this phenomenon has added much to our knowledge of the C attack mechanism. Hemolytically inactive C567 complexes still retain chemotactic activity (Ward *et al.*, 1966; Lachmann *et al.*, 1970*a*). Reactive lysis allows functional analysis of the terminal C sequence without the presence or prior participation of earlier-acting components. In addition to erythrocytes, bacteria (Goldman and

Austen, 1974), liposomes (Lachmann *et al.*, 1970*b*), and nucleated cells (Baker *et al.*, 1977) have been shown to be susceptible to reactive lysis. Studies on reactive lysis of liposomes have provided one demonstration that a lipid bilayer alone can serve as the "receptor" for C5b–9, with no protein other than the five terminal C components being necessary for lysis to occur (Lachmann *et al.*, 1970*b*, 1973*a*).

D. Interaction between the C Attack Proteins and Membranes

While cleavage of C5 produces a fragment (C5b) with binding affinity for a membrane, the sequential buildup of the C5b–9 complex seems to be an unlikely mechanism for the expression of complement-mediated membrane damage. Instead, it seems as though C567 (or C5b–9) acts as a functional unit to produce lysis. Evidence for this view comes from multiple experiments. C5b is much more efficient at initiating lysis when C6–9 are present (Nilsson and Müller-Eberhard, 1967; Cooper and Müller-Eberhard, 1970), and EC5b or EC56 intermediate cells are virtually impossible to produce. However, EC567 intermediates are readily formed when C56 and C7 are present together with the target cells (Thompson and Rowe, 1968; Lachmann and Thompson, 1970; Götze and Müller-Eberhard, 1970). Only a small amount (1–10%) of the C5b produced by a cell-bound enzyme EAC423b becomes attached to the cell, and even this C5b has very limited hemolytic activity, decaying with a half-life of 2.3 min at 37°C (Cooper and Müller-Eberhard, 1970; Shin *et al.*, 1971*a*).

The interaction of C567 or C5b–9 with the membrane seems to occur through hydrophobic binding. It has been postulated (Mayer, 1972) that C5b–9 produces lysis by insertion of the entire complex into the lipid bilayer, perhaps thereby producing the characteristic annular lesion visualized on electron microscopic examination of complement-treated membranes (Borsos *et al.*, 1964; Humphrey and Dourmashkin, 1969). Evidence for an insertional mechanism of C567 attachment was provided by trypsin-stripping experiments. Radiolabeled C5 was readily removed from EAC1-6 cells by trypsin, suggesting that the C56 was exposed on the cell surface. When C7 was added, however, this stripping was greatly reduced (Hammer *et al.*, 1975). The isolated C567 complex has been reported to aggregate through hydrophobic interaction (Podack *et al.*, 1976*c*). These experiments provided evidence that the attachment of C7 to C56 produced an alteration in the C567 complex that allowed it to insert into the hydrophobic regions of the lipid bilayer. More recently, similar data have been obtained for C8 and C9 insertion (Hammer *et al.*, 1977).

Additional evidence was obtained with the use of antisera specific to the terminal C components or to the C5b–9 neoantigens. Since EC$\overline{567}$ were agglutinated by these antisera, it suggested that at least some of the antigenic determinants of the C$\overline{567}$ complex were exposed on the surface of the cell (Kolb and Müller-Eberhard, 1975a; Podack *et al.*, 1976c). These data do not exclude an insertional mechanism, however, but may suggest that C$\overline{567}$ is only partially buried in the membrane.

E. Control of the Complement Attack Mechanism

The C attack proteins are subject to control by three mechanisms that also limit the activity of the early-acting components: decay of labile binding sites, breakdown of active components to inactive products by enzymes, and inhibition by control proteins which do not act enzymatically.

As mentioned earlier, C5b has only transient hemolytic activity, and unless it is stabilized by C6 it rapidly decays, both in the fluid phase and on the target cell surface (Cooper and Müller-Eberhard, 1970; Shin *et al.*, 1971a,b). The evanescence of the membrane-binding site on the C$\overline{567}$ complex has been commented on by several investigators (Lachmann and Thompson, 1970; Götze and Müller-Eberhard, 1970; Goldman *et al.*, 1972).

C5b (and perhaps complexes containing C5b) are probably also susceptible to enzymatic cleavage and inactivation. It has been shown (Kolb and Müller-Eberhard, 1975b; Podack *et al.*, 1976b) that the isolated C5b–9 complex contains a fragment termed "C5c," which is probably a breakdown product of C5b. It was proposed that the structural similarity of C3b, C4b, and C5b might indicate that they could be inactivated by the same enzyme, the C3b inactivator (Müller-Eberhard, 1975). The C3b inactivator has already been shown to cleave C4b as well as C3b in the presence of a cofactor (Cooper, 1975a; Stroud and Nagasawa, 1977c).

Several inhibitors of the individual attack components have been described, but none is well characterized. A C6 inactivator which blocks cell-bound but not fluid-phase C6 has been reported but only partially characterized (Tamura and Nelson, 1967; Nelson and Biro, 1968; Goldlust *et al.*, 1974). A C7 inhibitor has been found in two patients with C7 deficiency (Wellek and Opferkuch, 1975; Lint *et al.*, 1976b), but a definitive characterization is still lacking. A C$\overline{56}$ inhibitor has also been described, but its characterization remains to be completed (Lint *et al.*, 1975). A molecule derived from inactive C8 has been reported to act as a specific C8 inhibitor (Stolfi, 1968), but its occurrence *in vivo* is questionable. Also, hemolytically inactive complexes of C$\overline{567}$, C$\overline{5678}$, and

C5b–9 have been shown to inhibit the classical C pathway, probably by competing with their active counterparts for native C8 and C9 (Koethe *et al.*, 1973; Kolb and Müller-Eberhard, 1973).

Despite the short half-life of the C567 complex formed in solution, this complex is quite capable of initiating extensive membrane damage to bystander erythrocytes (Götze and Müller-Eberhard, 1970; Lachmann and Thompson, 1970; Goldman *et al.*, 1972; McLeod *et al.*, 1974; Baker *et al.*, 1975b) and nucleated cells (Baker *et al.*, 1977). There are several control mechanisms which hold this "contagious" lytic capacity of C567 in check. The most thoroughly studied are a group of serum C567 inhibitors (C567-INH) which prevent the attachment of fluid-phase C567 complexes to target cells (McLeod *et al.*, 1974, 1975a,b). This inhibitory activity is shared by several serum proteins (McLeod *et al.*, 1975a), including all classes of lipoproteins (Lint *et al.*, 1977). C567-INH activity is also a property of many polyanions (Baker *et al.*, 1977) and is neutralized by both synthetic (McLeod *et al.*, 1975b; Baker *et al.*, 1975a) and naturally occurring (Baker *et al.*, 1976) polycations. Counteraction of C567-INH activity in whole serum has been shown to allow enhanced lysis of bystander cells (McLeod *et al.*, 1975c; Lint *et al.*, 1976a). C567-INH is unique in that it can be manipulated by external agents such as polyanions and polycations, making the C attack mechanism amenable to pharmacological manipulation by these agents. Recently the S protein has been reported to act as a C567 inhibitor, although its mechanism of action has not been elucidated (Podack *et al.*, 1977).

Cell-bound C3b has been shown to enhance the hemolytic activity of C567 (Hammer *et al.*, 1976; Tamura and Baba, 1976), probably by providing a binding site for C56 or C567. This binding near the cell surface would greatly increase the likelihood that C567 could attach to its lipid membrane-binding site before decay and might also allow the C567 complex to "escape" from C567 inhibitors. This mechanism probably explains the observation that reactive lysis of cells with guinea pig C56 and C7 could not be obtained unless C3b was first bound to the target cells (Goldlust *et al.*, 1974).

V. Conclusion

This review was completed prior to the Seventh International Complement Workshop. We have made a few additions after the Workshop and updated the text. Notably the agreement by several groups that C3Nef is an immunoglobulin capable of reacting with the C3bBb convertase was added. We would also call notice to the increased interest in cell-bound and macrophage-synthesized components. It was particularly of interest that Reid reported C1 synthesis by fibroblasts and suggested that there is a pro-C1q molecule. Loos found C1 synthesis by macrophages. Factor D and thrombin derivatives were noted to have functional and immunochemical similarities by Davis, and more fine structural detail about all components is accumulating. Interest in the C56789 "doughnut" theory of Mayer is increasing with several new methods of study. Future biological applications of new knowledge to control immune and bone marrow cell functions seem particularly exciting.

VI. Addendum

At the Seventh International Complement Workshop (St. Petersburg, Florida, November 1977), five different groups of investigators presented data indicating that C3Nef is an IgG autoantibody with specificity for conformational antigenic determinants on the C3 convertase C3bBb. D. M. Scott, N. Amos, J. G. P. Sissons, and D. K. Peters reported that C3Nef binds to immobilized staphylococcal protein A and that C3Nef activity is not restricted only to the intact molecule but is also present in its $F(ab')_2$ and Fab fragments prepared by digestion with pepsin and papain, respectively. M. R. Daha, K. F. Austen, and D. T. Fearon demonstrated that specifically purified C3Nef reacted with anti-γ, anti-IgG1, anti-IgG2, anti-κ, and anti-λ sera but not with anti-μ, anti-α, and anti-δ sera. In addition, reduction and alkylation of C3Nef followed by SDS-PAGE revealed that it consisted of two polypeptide chains migrating with the heavy and light chains of purified IgG. Similarly, D. G. Williams reported that purified C3Nef reacted with antisera against more than one IgG subclass and with both anti-κ and anti-λ sera. In contrast, R. D. Schreiber and H. J. Müller-Eberhard presented data on a purified C3Nef which exhibited characteristics of a monoclonal IgG antibody with unique antigenic determinants; it contained only a type of λ chain and had no κ chains, its Fc portion was antigenically deficient, and it had a larger (60,000 molecular weight) heavy chain than ordinary IgG. Finally, A. E. Davis, III, E. W. Gelfand, P. H. Schur, F. S. Rosen, and C. A. Alper reported that C3Nef from certain patients contained only λ antigenic determinants, that from others had only κ, and that from still others had both λ and κ. They concluded that C3Nef is an IgG antibody with restricted light-chain type and subclass. They also reported that C3Nef from a pregnant patient crossed the placenta to her fetus.

In conclusion, there appears to be general agreement as to the IgG nature of C3Nef and its antibody specificity for unique antigenic determinants on the C3bBb complex. Since initiating factor (IF) was originally defined on the basis of its reactivity with anti-C3Nef serum, there new reports on the antibody nature of C3Nef raise a number of important questions concerning the nature, occurrence, and function of IF.

ACKNOWLEDGMENTS

Thanks are due Ms. Rhoda P. Cummings and Dr. Patricia J. Baker for their assistance in the preparation of the manuscript.

VII. References

Abramson, N., Alper, C. A., Lachmann, P. J., Rosen, F. S., and Jandle, J.H., 1971, *J. Immunol.* **107:**19.

Allen, F. H., Jr., 1974, *Vox Sang.* **27:**382.

Alper, C. A., 1976, *J. Exp. Med.* **144:**1111.

Alper, C. A., and Balavitch, D., 1976, *Science* **191:**1275.

Alper, C. A., Abramson, N., Johnston, R. B., Jr., Jandle, J. H., and Rosen, F. S., 1970, *New Engl. J. Med.* **282:**349.

Alper, C. A., Boenisch, T., and Watson, L., 1972, *J. Exp. Med.* **135:**68.

Alper, C. A., Goodkofsky, I., and Lepow, I. H., 1973, *J. Exp. Med.* **137:**424.

Alper, C. A., Colten, H. R., Gear, J. S. S., Rabson, A. R., and Rosen, F. S., 1976, *J. Clin. Invest.* **57:**222.

Arroyave, C. M., and Müller-Eberhard, H. J., 1973, *J. Immunol.* **111:**536.

Assimeh, S. N., and Painter, R. H., 1975, *J. Immunol.* **115:**482.

Baker, P., Lint, T. F., McLeod, B., Behrends, C., and Gewurz, H., 1975*a*, *J. Immunol.* **114:**554.

Baker, P. Rubin, L., Lint, T. F., McLeod, B. and Gewurz, H., 1975*b*, *Clin. Exp. Immunol.* **20:**113.

Baker, P., Lint, T. F., Siegel, J., Kies, M. W., and Gewurz, H., 1976, *Immunology* **30:**467.

Baker, P. J., Lint, T. F., Mortensen, R. F., and Gewurz, H., 1977, *J. Immunol.* **118:**198.

Barkas, T., Scott, G. K., and Fothergill, J. E., 1973, *Biochem. Soc. Tr.* **1:**1219.

Bhattacharyya, S. N., Passero, M. S., and Lynn, W. S., 1974, *Biochim. Biophys. Acta* **342:**343.

Bianco, C., Patrick, R., and Nussenzweig, V., 1970, *J. Exp. Med.* **132:**702.

Bing, D. H., 1969, *Biochemistry* **8:**4503.

Bing, D. H., Cory, M., and Doll, M., 1964, *J. Immunol.* **113:**584.

Bitter-Suermann, D., Krönke, M., Brade, V., and Hadding, U., 1977, *J. Immunol.* **118:**1822.

Bladen, H. A., Gewurz, H., and Mergenhagen, S. E., 1967, *J. Exp. Med.* **125:**767.

Blum, L., Pillemer, L , and Lepow, I. H., 1959, *Z. Immunitätsforsch Exp. Ther.* **118:**349.

Bodammer, G., and Vogt, W., 1970, *Int. Arch. Allergy Appl. Immunol.* **39:**648.

Boenisch, T., and Alper, C. A., 1970*a*, *Biochim. Biophys. Acta* **214:**135.

Boenisch, T., and Alper, C. A., 1970*b*, *Biochim. Biophys. Acta* **221:**529.

Bokisch, V. A., and Sobel, A. T., 1974, *J. Exp. Med.* **140**:1336.
Bokisch, V. A., Müller-Eberhard, H. J., and Cochrane, C. G., 1969, *J. Exp. Med.* **129**:1109.
Bokisch, V. A., Dierich, M. P., and Müller-Eberhard, H. J., 1975, *Proc. Natl. Acad. Sci. USA* **72**:1989.
Bolotin, C., Morris, S., Tack, B., and Prahl, J., 1977, *Biochemistry* **16**:2008.
Borsos, T., Rapp, H. J., and Mayer, M. M., 1961, *J. Immunol.* **87**:310.
Borsos, T., Dourmashkin, R. R., and Humphrey, J. H., 1964, *Nature (London)* **202**:251.
Brade, V., Lee, G. D., Nicholson, A., Shin, H. S., and Mayer, M. M., 1973, *J. Immunol.* **111**:1389.
Brade, V., Nicholson, A. Bitter-Suermann, D., and Hadding, U., 1974, *J. Immunol.* **113**:1735.
Brodsky-Doyle, B., Leonard, K. R., and Reid, K. B., 1976, *Biochem. J.* **159**:279.
Budzko, D. B., and Müller-Eberhard, H. J., 1970, *Immunochemistry* **7**:227.
Budzko, D. B., Bokisch, |V.|A., and Müller-Eberhard, H. J., 1971, *Biochemistry* **10**:1166.
Burritt, M. F., Nickolas, J., Satish, S., and Tomasi, T. B., Jr., 1977, *J. Immunol.* **118**:723.
Calcott, M. A., and Müller-Eberhard, H. J., 1972, *Biochemistry* **11**:3443.
Canady, W. J., Westfall, S., Wirtz, G. H., and Robinson, D. A., 1976, *Immunochemistry* **13**:229.
Casali, P., and Perussia, B. M., 1977, *Clin. Exp. Immunol.* **27**:38.
Chapitis, J., and Lepow, I. H., 1976, *J. Exp. Med.* **143**:241.
Claus, D. R., Siegel, J., Petras, K., Osmand, A. P., and Gewurz, H., 1977, *J. Immunol.* **119**:187.
Cochrane, C. G., and Müller-Eberhard, H. J., 1968, *J. Exp. Med.* **127**:371.
Colomb, M., and Porter, R. R., 1975, *Biochem. J.* **145**:177.
Conradie, J. D., Volanakis, J. E., and Stroud, R. M., 1975, *Immunochemistry* **12**:967.
Cooper, N. R., 1969, *Science* **165**:396.
Cooper, N. R., 1971, in: *Progress in Immunology* (B. Amos, ed.), pp. 567–577, Academic Press, New York.
Cooper, N. R., 1973, *J. Exp. Med.* **137**:451.
Cooper, N. R., 1975*a*, *J. Exp. Med.* **141**:890.
Cooper, N. R., 1975*b*, *Biochemistry* **14**:4245.
Cooper, N. R., and Müller-Eberhard, H. J., 1970, *J. Exp. Med.* **132**:775.
Daha, M. R., Fearon, D. T., and Austen, K. F., 1976, *J. Immunol.* **16**:1.
Daha, M. R., Austen, K. F., and Fearon, D. T., 1977, *Fed. Proc.* **36**:1244 (abstr).
Day, N. K. B., Gewurz, H. Johannsen, R., Finstad. J., and Good, R. A., 1970, *J. Exp. Med.* **132**:941.
Day, N. K., Geiger, H., Stroud, R. M., deBracco, M., Mancado, B., Windhorst, D., and Good, R. A., 1972, *J. Clin. Invest.* **51**:1102.
deBracco, M. M. E., and Stroud, R. M., 1971, *J. Clin. Invest.* **50**:838.
deBracco, M. M. E., Christian, C. L., and Stroud, R. M., 1974, *Clin. Exp. Immunol.* **16**:453.
DeLage, J.-M., Lehner-Netsch, G., and Simard, J., 1973, *Immunology* **24**:671.
DeLage, J.-M., Simard, J., and Lehner-Netsch, G., 1976, *Immunology* **31**:601.
Dias Da Silva, W., and Lepow, I. H., 1967, *J. Exp. Med.* **125**:921.
Dieminger, L., Vogt, W., and Lynen, R., 1976, *Z. Immunitätsforsch.* **152**:231.
Dierich, M. P., and Reisfeld, R. A., 1975, *J. Immunol.* **114**:1676.
Donaldson, V. H., and Evans, R. R., 1963, *Am. J. Med.* **35**:37.
Donaldson, V. H., Ratnoff, O. D., Dias Da Silva, W., and Rosen, F. S., 1969, *J. Clin. Invest.* **48**:642.
Donaldson, V. H., Merler, E., Rosen, F. S., Kretschmer, K. W., and Lepow, I. H , 1970, *J. Lab. Clin. Med.* **76**:986.

Ehlenberger, A. G., and Nussenzweig, V., 1977, *J. Exp. Med.* **145**:357.

Ellman, L., Green, I., Judge, F., and Frank, M. M., 1971, *J. Exp. Med.* **134**:162.

Erickson, B. W., Tippett, P. S., and Hugli, T. E., 1977, *Fed. Proc.* **36**:2476 (abstr).

Fearon, D. T., 1977, *Fed. Proc.* **36**:1244 (abstr).

Fearon, D. T., and Austen, K. F., 1975a, *Proc. Natl. Acad. Sci. USA* **72**:3220.

Fearon, D. T., and Austen, K. F., 1975b, *Ann. N.Y. Acad. Sci.* **256**:441.

Fearon, D. T., and Austen, K. F., 1975c, *J. Exp. Med.* **142**:856.

Fearon, D. T., and Austen, K. F., 1975d, *J. Immunol.* **115**:1357.

Fearon, D. T., and Austen, K. F., 1977, *Proc. Natl. Acad. Sci. USA* **74**:1683.

Fearon, D. T., Austen, K. F., and Ruddy, S., 1973, *J. Exp. Med.* **138**:1305.

Fearon, D. T., Austen, K. F., and Ruddy, S., 1974a, *J. Exp. Med.* **139**:355.

Fearon, D. T., Austen, K. F., and Ruddy, S., 1974b, *J. Exp. Med.* **140**:426.

Fiedel, B. A., Rent, R., Myhrman, R., and Gewurz, H., 1976, *Immunology* **30**:161.

Fernandez, H. N., and Hugli, T. E., 1976, *J. Immunol.* **117**:1688.

Flexner, S., and Noguchi, H., 1903, *J. Exp. Med.* **6**:277.

Frank, M. M., May, J., Gaither, T., and Ellman, L., 1971, *J. Exp. Med.* **134**:176.

Frank, M. M., Sergent, J. S., Kane, M. A., and Alling, D. W., 1972, *New Engl. J. Med.* **286**:808.

Gewurz, H., Shin, H. S., and Mergenhagen, S. E., 1968, *J. Exp. Med.* **128**:1049.

Gigli, I., and Austen, K. F., 1969a, *J. Exp. Med.* **129**:679.

Gigli, I., and Austen, K. F., 1969b, *J. Exp. Med.* **130**:833.

Gigli, I., Kaplan, A. P., and Austen, K. F., 1971, *J. Exp. Med.* **134**:1446.

Gigli, I., Porter, R. R., and Sim, R. B., 1976, *Biochem. J.* **157**:541.

Gitlin, J. D., Rosen, F. S., and Lachmann, P. J., 1975, *J. Exp. Med.* **141**:1221.

Goldlust, M. B., Shin, H. S., and Mayer, M. M., 1971, *J. Immunol.* **107**:318.

Goldlust, M. B., Shin, H. S., Hammer, C. H., and Mayer, M. M., 1974, *J. Immunol.* **113**:998.

Goldman, J. N., 1974, *Transplant. Proc.* **6**:21.

Goldman, J. N., and Austen, K. F., 1974, *J. Infect. Dis.* **129**:444.

Goldman, J. N., Ruddy, S., and Austen, K. F., 1972, *J. Immunol.* **109**:353.

Goldstein, I. M., and Weissmann, G., 1974, *J. Immunol.* **113**:1583.

Goodkofsky, I., and Lepow, I. H., 1971, *J. Immunol.* **107**:1200.

Götze, O., 1975, in: *Proteases and Biological Control*, Vol. 2 (E. Reich, D. B. Rifkin, and E. Shaw, eds.), 255–272, Cold Spring Harbor Laboratory, Long Island, N.Y.

Götze, O., and Müller-Eberhard, H. J., 1970, *J. Exp. Med.* **132**:898.

Götze, O., and Müller-Eberhard, H. J., 1971, *J. Exp. Med.* **134**:90s.

Götze, O., and Müller-Eberhard, H. J., 1974, *J. Exp. Med.* **139**:44.

Götze, O., and Müller-Eberhard, H. J., 1976, *Adv. Immunol.* **24**:1.

Götze, O., Medicus, R. G., and Müller-Eberhard, H. J., 1977, *J. Immunol.* **118**:525.

Hadding, U., and Müller-Eberhard, H. J., 1969, *Immunology* **16**:719.

Haines, A. L., and Lepow, I. H., 1964, *J. Immunol.* **92**:468.

Hall, R E., and Colten, H. R., 1977, *Proc. Natl. Acad. Sci. USA* **74**:1707.

Hammer, C. H., Nicholson, A., and Mayer, M. M., 1975, *Proc. Natl. Acad. Sci. USA* **72**:5076.

Hammer, C. H., Abramovitz, A. S., and Mayer, M. M., 1976, *J. Immunol.* **117**:830.

Hammer, C. H., Abramovitz, A. S., and Mayer, M. M., 1977, *Fed. Proc.* **36**:743 (abstr).

Harpel, P. C., and Cooper, N. R., 1975, *J. Clin. Invest.* **55**:593.

Harpel, P. C., Hugli, T. E., and Cooper, N. R., 1975, *J. Clin. Invest.* **55**:605.

Haupt, H., and Heide, K., 1965, *Clin. Chim. Acta* **12**:419.

Heusser, C., Boesman, M., Nordin, J. H., and Isliker, H., 1973, *J. Immunol.* **110**:820.

Huber, H., Polley, M. J., Linscott, W. D., Fudenberg, H. H., and Müller-Eberhard, H. J., 1968, *Science* **162**:1281.

Hugli, T. E., 1975, *J. Biol. Chem.* **250**:8293.

Hugli, T. E., Vallota, E. H., and Müller-Eberhard, H. J., 1975*a*, *J. Biol. Chem.* **250**:1472.

Hugli, T. E., Morgan, W. T., and Müller-Eberhard, H. J., 1975*b*, *J. Biol. Chem.* **250**:1479.

Humphrey, J. H., and Dourmashkin, R. R., 1969, *Adv. Immunol.* **11**:75.

Hunsicker, L. G., Ruddy, S., and Austen, K. F., 1973, *J. Immunol.* **110**:128.

Hurst, M. M., Volanakis, J. E., Stroud, R. M., and Bennett, J. C., 1976, *J. Clin. Invest.* **58**:16.

Iida, K., Fujita, T., Inai, S., Sasaki, M., Kato, T., and Kobayashi, K., 1976, *Immunochemistry* **13**:747.

Kay, J., and Kassell, B., 1971, *J. Biol. Chem.* **246**:6661.

Kehoe, J. M., and Fougereau, M., 1969, *Nature (London)* **224**:1212.

Kitamura, H., and Inai, S., 1974, *J. Immunol.* **113**:1992.

Kitamura, H., Itakura, N., and Inai, S., 1976, *Immunochemistry* **13**:771.

Klein, P. G., and Wellensiek, H. J., 1965, *Immunology* **8**:590.

Klemperer, M. R., Austen, K. F., and Rosen, F. S., 1967, *J. Immunol.* **98**:72.

Klemperer, M. R., Donaldson, V. H., and Rosen, F. S., 1968, *J. Clin. Invest.* **47**:604.

Klemperer, M. R., Rosen, F. S., and Donaldson, V. H., 1969, *J. Clin. Invest.* **48**:44a (abstr).

Knobel, H. R., Villiger, W., and Isliker, H., 1975, *Eur. J. Immunol.* **5**:78.

Koethe, S. M., Austen, K. F., and Gigli, I., 1973, *J. Immunol.* **110**:390.

Kohler, P. F., and Müller-Eberhard, H. J., 1967, *J. Immunol.* **99**:1211.

Kolb, W. P., and Müller-Eberhard, H. J., 1973, *J. Exp. Med.* **138**:438.

Kolb, W. P., and Müller-Eberhard, H. J., 1974, *J. Immunol.* **113**:479.

Kolb, W. P., and Müller-Eberhard, H. J., 1975*a*, *Proc. Natl. Acad. Sci. USA* **72**:1687.

Kolb, W. P., and Müller-Eberhard, H. J., 1975*b*, *J. Exp. Med.* **141**:724.

Kolb, W. P., and Müller-Eberhard, H. J., 1976, *J. Exp. Med* **143**:1131.

Kolb, W. P., Haxby, J. A., Arroyave, C. M., and Müller-Eberhard, H. J., 1972, *J. Exp. Med.* **135**:549.

Kolb, W. P., Haxby, J. A., Arroyave, C. M., and Müller-Eberhard, H. J., 1973, *J. Exp. Med.* **138**:428.

Kolb, W. P., Morgan, W. T., and Müller-Eberhard, H. J., 1976, *J. Immunol.* **116**:1738.

Kondo, M. Gigli, I., and Austen, K. F., 1972, *Immunology* **22**:305.

Koopman, W. J., Sandberg, A. L., Wahl, S. M., and Mergenhagen, S. E., 1976, *J. Immunol.* **117**:331.

Lachmann, P. J., and Müller-Eberhard, H. J., 1968, *J. Immunol.* **100**:691.

Lachmann, P. J., and Thompson, R. A., 1970, *J. Exp. Med.* **131**:643.

Lachmann, P. J., Kay, A. B., and Thompson, R. A., 1970*a*, *Immunology* **19**:895.

Lachmann, P. J., Munn, E. A., and Weissmann, G., 1970*b*, *Immunology* **19**:983.

Lachmann, P. J., Bowyer, D. E., Nicol, P., Dawson, R. M. C., and Munn, E. A., 1973*a*, *Immunology* **24**:135.

Lachmann, P. J., Nicol, P., and Aston, W. P., 1973*b*, *Immunochemistry* **10**:695.

Laurell, A. B., and Martensson, U., 1974, *Acta Pathol. Microbiol. Scand.* **82**:585.

Laurell, A. B., Martensson, U., and Sjöholm, A. G., 1976, *Acta Pathol. Microbiol* **84**:455.

Lay, W. H., and Nussenzweig, V., 1968, *J. Exp. Med.* **121**:991.

Leon, M. A., 1965, *Science* **147**:1034.

Lepow, I. H., Naff, G. B., Todd, E. W., Pensky, J., and Hinz, C. F., Jr., 1963, *J. Exp. Med.* **117**:983.

Lepow, I. H., Willms-Kretschmer, K., Patrick, R. A., and Rosen, F. S., 1970, *Am. J. Pathol.* **61**:13.

Levy, L. R., and Lepow, I. H., 1959, *Proc. Soc. Exp. Biol. Med.* **101**:608.
Lint, T. F., Petras, K. A., and Baker, P. J., 1975, *Fed. Proc.* **34**:965 (abstr).
Lint, T. F., Behrends, C. L., Baker, P. J., and Gewurz, H., 1976a, *J. Immunol.* **117**:1440.
Lint, T. F., Osofsky, S. G., Nemerow, G. R., Tausk, K., and Gewurz, H., 1976b, *Clin. Res.* **24**:543A.
Lint, T. F., Behrends, C. L., and Gewurz, H., 1977, *J. Immunol.* **19**:883.
Loos, M., Hill, H. U., Wellek, B., and Heinz, H.-P., 1976a, *FEBS Lett.* **64**:341.
Loos, M., Volanakis, J. E., and Stroud, R. M., 1976b, *Immunochemistry* **13**:789.
Lundh, B., Laurell, A.-B., Wetterquist, H., White, T., and Granerus, G., 1968, *Clin. Exp. Immunol.* **3**:733.
Lynen, R., Brade, V., Wolf, A., and Vogt, W., 1973, *Hoppe-Seyler's Z. Physiol. Chem.* **354**:37.
Marcus, R. L., Shin, H. S., and Mayer, M. M., 1971, *Proc. Natl. Acad. Sci. USA* **68**:1351.
Mayer, M. M., 1972, *Proc. Natl. Acad. Sci. USA* **69**:2954.
Mayer, M. M., 1973, *Sci. Am.* **229**:54.
Mayer, M. M., 1977, *Harvey Lect.* Series 72, 1976–1977.
Mayer, M. M., Miller, J. A., and Shin, H. S., 1970, *J. Immunol.* **105**:327.
McLeod, B., Baker, P., and Gewurz, H., 1974, *Immunology* **26**:1145.
McLeod, B., Baker, P., Behrends C., and Gewurz, H., 1975a, *Immunology* **28**:379.
McLeod, B., Baker, P., and Gewurz, H., 1975b, *Immunology* **28**:133.
McLeod, B., Lint, T. F., Baker, P. Behrends, C., and Gewurz, H., 1975c, *Immunology* **28**:741.
Medicus, R. G., 1977, *Fed. Proc.* **36**:1244 (abstr).
Medicus, R. G., Götze, O., and Müller-Eberhard, H. J., 1976a, *Scand. J. Immunol.* **5**:1049.
Medicus, R. G., Götze, O., and Müller-Eberhard, H. J., 1976b, *J. Exp. Med.* **144**:1076.
Medicus, R. G., Schreiber, R. D., Götze, O., and Müller-Eberhard, H. J., 1976c, *Proc. Natl. Acad. Sci. USA* **73**:612.
Minta, J. O., 1976, *J. Immunol.* **117**:405.
Minta, J. O., and Lepow, I. H., 1974, *Immunochemistry* **11**:361.
Minta, J. O., Goodkofsky, I., and Lepow, I. H., 1973, *Immunochemistry* **10**:341.
Molenar, J. L., Muller, M., and Pondman, K. W., 1973, *J. Immunol.* **110**:1570.
Morgan, P. H., and Nair, I. G., 1975, *Biochem. Biophys. Res. Commun.* **66**:1037.
Morgan, W. T., Vallota, E. H., and Müller-Eberhard, H. J., 1974, *Biochem. Biophys. Res. Commun.* **57**:572.
Müller-Eberhard, H. J., 1971, in: *Progress in Immunology* (B. Amos, ed.), p. 553, Academic Press, New York.
Müller-Eberhard, H. J., 1972, *Harvey Lect.* **66**:75.
Müller-Eberhard, H. J., 1975, *Annu. Rev. Biochem.* **44**:697.
Müller-Eberhard, H. J., and Biro, C. E., 1963, *J. Exp. Med.* **118**:447.
Müller-Eberhard, H. J., and Fjellström, K. E., 1971, *J. Immunol.* **107**:1666.
Müller-Eberhard, H. J., and Götze, O., 1972, *J. Exp. Med.* **135**:1003.
Müller-Eberhard, H.J., and Kunkel, H. G., 1961, *Proc. Soc. Exp. Biol. Med.* **106**:291.
Müller-Eberhard, H. J., and Lepow, I. H., 1965, *J. Exp. Med.* **121**:819.
Müller-Eberhard, H. J., Nilsson, U. R., Dalmasso, A. P., Polley, M. J., and Calcott, M. A., 1966a, *Arch. Pathol.* **82**:205.
Müller-Eberhard, H. J., Dalmasso, A. P., and Calcott, M. A., 1966b, *J. Exp. Med.* **123**:33.
Müller-Eberhard, H. J., Polley, M. J., and Calcott, M. A., 1967, *J. Exp. Med.* **125**:359.
Naff, G. B., and Ratnoff, O. D., 1968, *J. Exp. Med.* **128**:571.
Naff, G. B., Pensky, J., and Lepow, I. H., 1964, *J. Exp. Med.* **119**:593.
Nagaki, K., and Stroud, R. M., 1969, *J. Immunol.* **103**:141.

Nagaki, K., and Strodd, R. M., 1970, *J. Immunol.* **105**:170.
Nagaki, K., Iida, K., and Inai, S., 1974, *Int. Arch. Allerg. Appl. Immunol.* **46**:935.
Nagasawa, S., and Stroud, R. M., 1977a, *Fed. Proc.* **36**:1208 (abstr).
Nagasawa, S., and Stroud, R. M., 1977b, *Proc. Natl. Acad. Sci. USA* **74**:2998.
Nagasawa, S., and Stroud, R. M., 1977c, *Immunochemistry* **14**:749.
Nagasawa, S., Takahashi, K., and Koyama, J., 1974, *FEBS Lett.* **41**:280.
Nagasawa, S., Shiraishi, S., and Stroud, R. M., 1976, *J. Immunol.* **116**:1743.
Nagasawa, S., Volanakis, J. E., Schrohenloher, R. E. and Stroud, R. M., 1977, manuscript in preparation.
Nelson, R. A., Jr., 1953, *Science* **118**:733.
Nelson, R. A., Jr., 1966, *Surv. Ophthalmol.* **11**:498.
Nelson, R. A., Jr., and Biro, C. E., 1968, *Immunology* **14**:527.
Nicholson, A., Brade, V., Lee, G. D., Shin, H. S., and Mayer, M. M., 1974, *J. Immunol.* **112**:1115.
Nicholson, A., Brade, V., Schorlemmer, H.-U., Burger, R., Bitter-Suermann, D., and Hadding, U., 1975, *J. Immunol.* **115**:1108.
Nicol, P. A. E., and Lachmann, P. J., 1973, *Immunology* **24**:259.
Nilsson, I. M., Andersson, L., and Björkman, S. E., 1966, *Acta Med. Scand.* **448**:1 Suppl. 1.
Nilsson, U. R., and Müller-Eberhard, H. J., 1965, *J. Exp. Med.* **122**:277.
Nilsson, U. R., and Müller-Eberhard, H. J., 1967, *Immunology* **13**:101.
Nilsson, U. R., Tomar, R. H., and Taylor, F. B., 1972, *Immunochemistry* **9**:709.
Nilsson, U. R., Mandle, R. J., Jr., and McConnell-Mapes, J. A., 1975, *J. Immunol.* **114**:815.
Osler, A. G., Oliveira, B., Shin, H. S., and Sandberg, A. L., 1969, *J. Immunol.* **102**:269.
Patrick, R. A., Taubman, S. B., and Lepow, I. H., 1970, *Immunochemistry* **7**:217.
Pensky, J., and Schwick, H. G., 1969, *Science* **163**:698.
Pensky, J., Levy, L. R., and Lepow, I. H., 1961, *J. Biol. Chem.* **236**:1674.
Pensky, J., Hinz, C. F., Jr., Todd, E. W., Wedgwood, R. J., Boyer, J. T., and Lepow, I. H., 1968, *J. Immunol.* **100**:142.
Pepys, M. B., Mirjah, D. D., Dash, A. C., and Wansbrough-Jones, M. H., 1976, *Cell. Immunol.* **21**:327.
Pepys, M. B., Dash, A. C., Munn, E. A., Feinstein, A., Skinner, M., Cohen, A. S., Gewurz, H., Osmand, A. P., and Painter, R. H., 1977, *Lancet* **1**:1029.
Pickering, R. J., Gewurz, H., and Good, R. A., 1968, *J. Lab. Clin. Med.* **72**:298.
Pickering, R. J., Naff, G. B., Stroud, R. M., Good, R. A., and Gewurz, H., 1970, *J. Exp. Med.* **131**:803.
Pillemer, L., 1955, *Tr. N.Y. Acad. Sci.* **17**:526.
Pillemer, L., Blum, L., Lepow, I. H., Ross, O. A., Todd, E. W., and Wardlaw, A. C., 1954, *Science* **120**:279.
Pillemer, L., Schoenberg, M. D., Blum, L., and Wurz, L., 1955, *Science* **122**:545.
Podack, E. R., Kolb, W. P., and Müller-Eberhard, H. J., 1976a, *J. Immunol.* **116**:263.
Podack, E. R., Kolb, W. P., and Müller-Eberhard, H. J., 1976b, *J. Immunol.* **116**:1431.
Podack, E. R., Kolb, W. P., and Müller-Eberhard, H. J., 1976c, *Fed. Proc.* **35**:254.
Podack, E. R., Kolb, W. P., and Müller-Eberhard, H. J., 1976d, *J. Immunol.* **116**:1746.
Podack, E. R., Kolb, W. P., and Müller-Eberhard, H. J., 1977, *Fed. Proc.* **36**:1209 (abstr).
Polley, M. J., and Müller-Eberhard, H. J., 1967, *J. Exp. Med.* **126**:1013.
Polley, M. J., and Müller-Eberhard, H. J., 1968, *J. Exp. Med.* **128**:533.
Raepple, E., Hill, H. U., and Loos, M., 1976, *Immunochemistry* **13**:251.
Ratnoff, O. D., and Naff, G. B., 1969, *J. Lab. Clin. Med.* **74**:380.
Ratnoff, O. D., Pensky, J., Ogston, D., and Naff, G. B., 1969, *J. Exp. Med.* **129**:315.

Reid, K. B. M., 1974, *Biochem. J.* **141**:189.

Reid, K. B. M., 1976, *Biochem. J.* **155**:5.

Reid, K. B. M., and Porter, R. R., 1976, *Biochem. J.* **155**:19.

Reid, K. B. M., Lowe, D. M., and Porter, R. R., 1972, *Biochem. J.* **130**:749.

Rent, R., Ertel, N., Eisenstein, R., and Gewurz, H., 1975, *J. Immunol.* **114**:120.

Ritz, H., 1912, *Z. Immunitätsforsch. Exp. Ther.* **13**:62.

Rommel, F. A., and Mayer, M. M., 1973, *J. Immunol.* **110**:637.

Rosenfeld, S. I., Ruddy, S., and Austen, K. F., 1969, *J. Clin. Invest.* **43**:2283.

Ross, G. D., and Polley, M. J., 1974, *Fed. Proc.* **33**:759 (abstr).

Ross, G. D., Polley, M. J., Rabellino, E. M., and Grey, H. M., 1973, *J. Exp. Med.* **138**:798.

Ruddy, S., and Austen, K. F., 1969, *J. Immunol.* **102**:533.

Ruddy, S., and Austen, K. F., 1971, *J. Immunol.* **107**:742.

Ruddy, S., and Whaley, K., 1977, *Fed. Proc.* **36**:1244 (abstr).

Ruddy, S., Widener, H., and Whaley, K., 1977, in: *Clinical Aspects of the Complement System* (N. Opferkuch and K. Rother, eds.), Thieme Verlag, Stuttgart.

Ruley, E. J., Forristal, J., Davis, N. C., Andres, C., and West, C. D., 1973, *J. Clin. Invest.* **52**:896.

Sakai, K., and Stroud, R. M., 1973, *J. Immunol.* **110**:1010.

Sakai, K., and Stroud, R. M., 1974, *Immunochemistry* **11**:191.

Sandberg, A. L., Osler, A. G., Shin, H. S., and Oliveira, B., 1970, *J. Immunol.* **104**:329.

Sandberg, A. L., Snyderman, R., Frank, M. M., and Osler, A. G., 1972, *J. Immunol.* **108**:1227.

Schreiber, R. D., and Müller-Eberhard, H. J., 1974, *J. Exp. Med.* **140**:1324.

Schreiber, R. D., Medicus, R. G., Götze, O., and Müller-Eberhard, H. J., 1975, *J. Exp. Med.* **142**:760.

Schreiber, R. D., Götze, O., and Müller-Eberhard, H. J., 1976a, *J. Exp. Med.* **144**:1062.

Schreiber, R. D., Götze, O., and Müller-Eberhard, H. J., 1976b, *Scand. J. Immunol.* **5**:705.

Schultz, D. R., and Arnold, P. I., 1975, *J. Immunol.* **115**:1558.

Schumaker, V. N., Calcott, M. A., Spiegelberg, H. L., and Müller-Eberhard, H. J., 1976, *Biochemistry* **15**:5175.

Shearer, W. T., Atkinsor, J. P., Frank, M. M. and Parker, C. W., 1975, *J. Exp. Med.* **141**:736.

Sheffer, A. L., Austen, K. F., and Rosen, F. S., 1972, *New Engl. J. Med.* **287**:452.

Shelton, E., Yonemasu, K., and Stroud, R. M., 1972, *Proc. Natl. Acad. Sci. USA* **69**:65.

Shimada, A., and Tamura, N., 1972, *Immunology* **22**:723.

Shin, H., Pickering, R. J., and Mayer, M. M., 1971a, *J. Immunol.* **106**:473.

Shin, H., Pickering, R. J., and Mayer, M. M., 1971b, *J. Immunol.* **106**:480.

Shiraishi, S., and Stroud, R. M., 1975, *Immunochemistry* **12**:935.

Sim, R. B., and Porter, R. R., 1976, *Biochem. Soc. Tr.* **4**:127.

Sim, R. B., Porter, R. R., Reid, K. B. M., and Gigli, I., 1977, *Biochem. J.* **163**:219.

Sissons, J. G. P., West, R. J., Fallows, J., Williams, D. G., Boucher, B. J., Amos, N., and Peters, D. K., 1976, *New Engl. J. Med.* **294**:461.

Sitomer, G., Stroud, R. M., and Mayer, M. M., 1966, *Immunochemistry* **3**:57.

Snyderman, R. Shin, H. S., Phillips, J. K., Gewurz, H., and Mergenhagen, S. E., 1969, *J. Immunol.* **103**:413.

Soter, N. A., Austen, K. F., and Gigli, I., 1975, *J. Immunol.* **114**:928.

Spitzer, R. E., Vallota, E. H., Forristal, J., Sudora, E., Stitzel, A., Davis, N. C., and West, C. D., 1969, *Science* **164**:436.

Spitzer, R. E., Stitzel, A. E., and Urmson, J., 1976, *Immunochemistry* **13**:15.

Stitzel, A. E., and Spitzer, R. E., 1974, *J. Immunol.* **112**:56.

Stolfi, R. L., 1968, *J. Immunol.* **100**:46.

Stolfi, R. L., 1970, *J. Immunol.* **104**:1212.

Stossel, T. P., Field, R. J., Gitlin, J. D., Alper, C. A., and Rosen, F. S., 1975, *J. Exp. Med.* **141**:1329.

Stroud, R. M., Austen, K. F., and Mayer, M. M., 1965, *Immunochemistry* **2**:219.

Stroud, R. M., Mayer, M. M., Miller, J. A., and McKenzie, A. T., 1966, *Immunochemistry* **3**:163.

Strunk, R., and Colten, H. R., 1974, *J. Immunol.* **112**:905.

Tack, B. F., and Prahl, J. W., 1976, *Biochemistry* **15**:4513.

Takahashi, K., Nagasawa, S., and Koyama, J., 1975*a*, *FEBS Lett.* **50**:330.

Takahashi, K., Nagasawa, S., and Koyama, J., 1975*b*, *FEBS Lett.* **55**:156.

Takahashi, K., Nagasawa, S., and Koyama, J., 1976*a*, *FEBS Lett.* **65**:20.

Takahashi, K., Tamoto K., and Koyama, J., 1976*b*, *J. Antibiot.* **29**:983.

Tamura, N., and Baba, A. S., 1976, *Immunology* **31**:151.

Tamura, N., and Nelson, R. A., 1967, *J. Immunol.* **99**:582.

Tamura, N., Shimada, A., and Chang, S., 1972, *Immunology* **22**:131.

Tauber, J. W., Polley, M. J., and Zabriskie, J. B., 1976, *J. Exp. Med.* **143**:1352.

Taubman, S. B., 1975, *Biochim. Biophys. Acta* **393**:542.

Taylor, P. A., Fink, S., Bing, D. H., and Painter, R. H., 1977, *J. Immunol.* **118**:1722.

Teisberg, P., Akesson, I., Olaisen, B., Gedde-Dahl, T., Jr., and Thorsby, E., 1976, *Nature (London)* **264**:253.

Thompson, R. A., 1972*a*, *Immunology* **22**:147.

Thompson, R. A., 1972*b*, *Br. Med. J.* **1**:282.

Thompson, R. A., and Lachmann, P. J., 1970, *J. Exp. Med.* **131**:629.

Thompson, R. A., and Rowe, D. S., 1968, *Immunology* **14**:745.

Valet, G., and Cooper, N. R., 1974*a*, *J. Immunol.* **112**:339.

Valet, G., and Cooper, N. R., 1974*b*, *J. Immunol.* **112**:1667.

Vallota, E. H., Forristal, J. Spitzer, R. E., Davis, N. C., and West, C. D., 1970, *J. Exp. Med.* **131**:1306.

Vallota, E. H., Hugli, T. E., and Müller-Eberhard, H. J., 1973, *J. Immunol.* **111**:294.

Vallota, E. H., Götze, O., Spiegelberg, H. L., Forristal, J., West, C. D., and Müller-Eberhard, H. J., 1974, *J. Exp. Med.* **139**:1249.

Vogt, W., Dieminger, L., Lynen, R., and Schmidt, G., 1974, *Hoppe-Seyler's Z. Physiol. Chem.* **355**:171.

Vogt, W., Schmidt, G., Lynen, R., and Dieminger, L., 1975, *J. Immunol.* **114**:671.

Vogt, W., Dames, W., Schmidt, G., and Dieminger, L., 1977, *Immunochemistry* **14**:201.

Volanakis, J. E., and Kaplan, M. H., 1974, *J. Immunol.* **113**:9.

Volanakis, J., Schrohenloher, R., and Stroud, R., 1977, *J. Immunol.* **119**:337.

Ward, P. A., Cochrane, C. G., and Müller-Eberhard, H. J., 1966, *Immunology* **11**:141.

Weiler, J. M., Daha, M. R., Austen, K. F., and Fearon, D. T., 1976, *Proc. Natl. Acad. Sci. USA* **73**:3268.

Wellek, B., and Opferkuch, W., 1975, *Clin. Exp. Immunol.* **19**:223.

West, C. D., Hinrichs, V., and Hinkle, N. H., 1961, *J. Lab. Clin. Med.* **58**:137.

West, C. D., McAdams, A. J., McConville, J. M., Davis, N. C., and Holland, N. H., 1965, *J. Pediatr.* **67**:1089.

West, C. D., Davis, N. C., Forristal, J., Herbst, J., and Spitzer, R., 1966, *J. Immunol.* **96**:650.

Whaley, K., and Ruddy, S., 1976*a*, *J. Exp. Med.* **144**:1147.

Whaley, K., and Ruddy, S., 1976*b*, *Science* **193**:1011.

WHO Committee on Complement Nomenclature, 1970, *Immunochemistry* **7**:137.

Wissler, J. H., 1972, *Eur. J. Immunol.* **2:**73.

Wuepper, K. D., Bokisch, V. A., Müller-Eberhard, H. J., and Stoughton, R. B., 1972, *Clin. Exp. Immunol.* **11:**13.

Yasmeen, D., Ellerson, J. R., Dorrington, K. J., and Painter, R. H., 1976, *J. Immunol.* **116:**518.

Yonemasu, K., and Stroud, R. M., 1971, *J. Immunol.* **106:**304.

Yonemasu, K., and Stroud, R. M., 1972, *Immunochemistry* **9:**545.

Yonemasu, K., Stroud, R. M., Niedermeier, W., and Butler, W. T., 1971, *Biochem. Biophys. Res. Commun.* **43:**1388.

Ziccardi, R. J., and Cooper, N. R., 1976*a*, *J. Immunol.* **116:**496.

Ziccardi, R. J., and Cooper, N. R., 1976*b*, *J. Immunol.* **116:**504.

Ziccardi, R. J., and Cooper, N. R., 1977, *J. Immunol.* **118:**2047.

Ziegler, J. B., Watson, L., and Alper, C. A., 1975, *J. Immunol.* **114:**1649.

Ziegler, J. B., Watson, L., Goodkofsky, I., Alper, C. A., and Lepow, I. H., 1976, *J. Immunol.* **116:**75.

5

Immunochemistry of Bovine Serum Albumin

A. F. S. A. Habeeb

I. Introduction

The molecular basis of protein antigenicity has been of great interest for over three decades, but only very recently has the entire antigenic structure of a protein been determined. So far the antigenic structures of only sperm whale myoglobin and hen egg-white lysozyme have been entirely and precisely determined. The antigenic structure of myoglobin (Atassi, 1975; for a more comprehensive treatment see Atassi, 1977b) comprises five conformationally distinct antigenic sites each made up of six or seven surface amino acid residues that are in direct peptide bond linkage. The recent completion of the entire antigenic structure of lysozyme (Atassi and Habeeb, 1977; Lee and Atassi, 1977a,b; Atassi and Lee, 1978a,b; Atassi, 1978a,b) has revealed that the three antigenic sites of this protein differ from those of myoglobin in a fundamental and fascinating way. Whereas the antigenic sites of myoglobin are composed of residues that are *directly* linked to one another by peptide bonds, those of lysozyme are each made up of conformationally adjacent surface residues that are *not* linked directly by peptide bonds but are brought into close proximity by the folding of the protein molecule. These sites react with their respective antibodies as if their residues were in direct peptide bond linkage (Atassi *et al.*, 1976a; Lee and Atassi, 1976). This was unequivocally demonstrated by "surface-simulation" synthesis, a novel and unorthodox

A. F. S. A. Habeeb · Department of Biochemistry and Nutrition, University of Puerto Rico, Medical Sciences Campus, San Juan, Puerto Rico 00936.

approach in which the conformationally adjacent residues constructing the site were linked into a single peptide that did *not* exist in the protein but attempted to mimic a surface region of it (Atassi *et al.*, 1976*a;* Lee and Atassi, 1976). It is extremely interesting that the lysozyme antigenic sites, prepared by surface-simulation synthesis, show a directional preference for binding with antibody and have a restricted conformational freedom (Lee and Atassi, 1977*a,b;* Atassi and Lee, 1978*a,b*).

Our recent studies on bovine and human serum albumins reveal a hitherto unusual immunochemical feature, namely that these two proteins carry repeating and equivalent or identical antigenic sites (Atassi *et al.*, 1976*b;* Habeeb and Atassi, 1976*b*, 1977, 1978; Habeeb, 1978*a,b*). This unique immunochemical property of albumin makes the elucidation of its antigenic structure of immense value in furthering our understanding of the immunochemistry of proteins.

Serum albumin is the most abundant plasma protein (3.5–5.5%) and is responsible for the binding and transport of various metabolically and pharmacologically active molecules, e.g., bilirubin, uric acid, vitamin C, acetylcholine, cholinesterase, adenosine, aureomycin, barbiturate, chloromycetin, digitonin, fatty acids, atabrine, neosilversalvarsan, penicillin, salicylate, *p*-aminosalicylate, sulfonamide, streptomycin, acid dyes, histamine, triiodothyronine, and thyroxine (Bennhold, 1962; Putnam, 1975). Moreover, albumin tightly binds various metal ions, e.g., Zn^{2+} (Giroux, 1975), Mn^{2+}, Co^{2+}, and Ni^{2+} (Friedberg, 1975). The remarkable affinity of serum albumin for the binding of these various ligands is accounted for by its unusual ability to exhibit subtle conformational flexibility of the molecule (Karush, 1950; Foster, 1960). Albumin from either human, bovine, or rabbit was shown to be essential and can replace serum or plasma for growth of stimulated lymphocytes (Spieker-Polet and Polet, 1976).

An interesting conformation-dependent catalytic activity of bovine serum albumin (BSA), sheep albumin, and horse albumin has been reported (Taylor and Vatz, 1973), namely the acceleration of decomposition (by a factor of 10^4) of the Meisenheimer complex 1,1-dihydro-2,4,6-trinitrocyclohexadienate. The physiological importance of this activity, however, is presently not known and is not exhibited by human serum albumin.

A great deal of work has been carried out on BSA, and it has been used as the protein of choice for various immunological experiments. In view of the radical hypothesis which has been advanced that BSA has equivalent, repeating antigenic sites (Atassi *et al.*, 1976*b;* Habeeb and Atassi, 1976*b*, 1977), there is a need to bring the relevant information on bovine serum albumin together. The present chapter will summarize the current state of knowledge on the structure of BSA and the work done to delineate the antigenic reactive regions.

II. Structure of Bovine Serum Albumin

A considerable amount of information is available on the reversible, pH-dependent molecular conformational alterations which occur in both bovine and human serum albumins. This work has yielded valuable knowledge regarding the structural organization of the albumin molecule and has been instrumental in devising conditions and procedures for the enzymatic fragmentation of the protein and is therefore pertinent to an immunochemical consideration.

Serum albumin exists in a compact form between pH 4.3 and 10.5 but undergoes conformational expansions below pH 4.3 and above pH 10.5 (Tanford *et al.*, 1955*a,b;* Yang and Foster, 1954; Bro *et al.*, 1955; Weber, 1952). Conformational transitions not accompanied by molecular expansion also occur, namely the N-F transition between pH 4.8 and 3.9 and the neutral transition, N-B, observed between pH 7 and 9 (Leonard *et al.*, 1963).

A. Conformational Transitions of Albumin

1. The Acid Transition

Fluorescence depolarization measurements from pH 5 to 1.9 of solutions of BSA-fluorescent dye conjugates indicated a decrease in the rotational relaxation times. This was attributed to an increase in the freedom of rotational motion within the molecule (Harrington *et al.*, 1956) caused by the presence of subunits held in a compact structure at neutrality. On lowering of the pH, the subunits became loose and were capable of rotation without affecting the internal structure of the subunits. Parallel light-scattering measurements, sedimentation velocity, and diffusion data confirmed that no changes in molecular weight occurred but indicated a swelling or increased asymmetry of the molecule as the pH was lowered from 4 to 2 (Harrington *et al.*, 1956). A study of the electrophoretic mobility of BSA as a function of pH (Aoki and Foster, 1957*a,b*) showed separate, single electrophoretic components below pH 3.5 and above pH 4.6 (termed "F" and "N," respectively) and showed that between pH 3.5 and 4.5 there were two components. The relative amounts of these two components varied with the pH, being equal at pH 4. The difference in mobilities of the N and F forms corresponded to three charge differences. The calculated effective radius of BSA was constant at pH 3.2–4.3, indicating no molecular expansion during the N-F transition (Aoki and Foster, 1957a,b). However, as the pH was lowered to 2.1, an expansion of the molecule was observed. Aoki and Foster (1957b) accredited the N-F transition, and not the acid expansion of the molecule as suggested by Tanford (1950), with causing anomalies in the titration curve of BSA. In the N form the anionic form of the carboxyl groups participated in electrostatic interactions, resulting in the stabilization of the native compact structure of the molecule and a concomitant decrease in their pK to 3.7, whereas in the F form this stabilization was disrupted, resulting in the expected pK of 4.4 for the carboxyl groups.

In order to study further the mechanism of the N-F transition, the reversible conformational changes in bovine serum albumin (BSA) and human serum albumin (HSA) were followed by changes in the specific rotation at 313 nm (which does not reflect changes in the secondary structure) as a function of pH (Leonard and Foster, 1961). In solutions containing chloride ions, isomerization at pH 4 occurred in a single step, was accompanied by a decrease in levorotation, and was sharper than that seen by electrophoresis. In solutions containing strongly binding anions (e.g., thiocyanate or perchlorate), isomerization occurred in two equal steps separated by a plateau (Fig. 1). This plateau was observed only by optical rotation studies. The first step in isomerization was also demonstrated by electrophoresis, while the second step was seen also by difference spectroscopy (not by electrophoresis) and involved exposure of four buried tyrosine residues. Based on the model proposed by Foster (1960), which depicted the albumin molecule to consist of four compact subunits with three intrasurfaces, two of which were hydrophobic in character, it was suggested that the N-F transition is due to intramolecular dissociation of the subunits with small alteration of secondary or tertiary structure within the subunits. The first transition resulted from an opening of one hydrophobic intrasurface and coincided with the isomerization observed in electrophoresis. On the other hand, the second transition was not demonstrable by electrophoresis but was observed spectroscopically by solvent perturbations (Herskovitz and Laskowski, 1960) to result in the exposure of 20% of the tyrosine residues and was a consequence of an opening of the second hydrophobic intrasurface. Therefore, the successive opening of the two hydrophobic inner surfaces of serum albumin subunits contributed to this two-step character of the changes in optical rotation (Leonard and Foster, 1961). The decrease in optical rotation during isomerization was not due to a decrease of helix

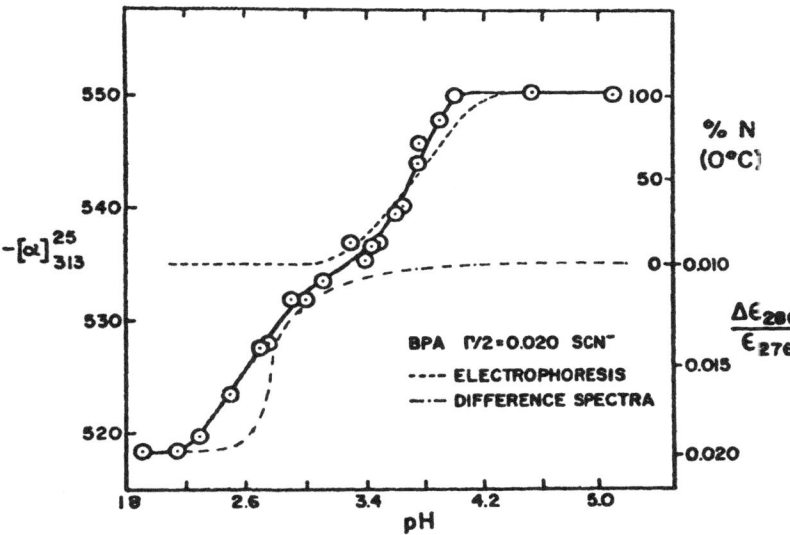

Figure 1. Dependence of specific rotation at 313 nm on pH value, BSA in 0.02 M thiocyanate. Distribution of N and F components as determined by electrophoresis shown in upper dashed line, results of perturbation difference spectra in lower broken line. From Leonard and Foster (1961).

content alone but also to alteration in tertiary structure resulting from changes in hydrogen-bonding patterns, in electrostatic interaction, and in the polarizability of the environment of chromophoric residues (Leonard and Foster, 1961).

As the pH of albumin was lowered beyond the N-F transition, an expansion of the molecule occurred, as demonstrated by an increase in viscosity (Yang and Foster, 1954) as well as by a decrease in the sedimentation coefficient (Bro *et al.*, 1955; Charlwood and Ens, 1957).

2. The Neutral Transition

In the pH range 7–9 a conformational transition occurred in BSA which was manifested by an increase in dye-binding sites (Klotz *et al.*, 1952; Katz and Klotz, 1953), a decrease in levorotation at 365 nm (Jirgensons, 1958), a change in the ultraviolet fluorescence behavior (Steiner and Edelhoch, 1961), and an increase in exchangeability of nonexchangeable hydrogen ions as the pH was raised to pH 8.5 (Benson and Hallaway, 1970). The specific optical rotation at 313.2 nm of BSA or HSA was found to decrease progressively as the pH increased from 7 to 9 and suggested a transition to a conformationally different isomer. An increase in electrolyte concentration as well as the presence of strongly binding anions (e.g., perchlorate or thiocyanate) shifted the transition to lower pH (Leonard *et al.*, 1963). Little if any change in the helix content was associated with these changes in optical rotation, since the Moffit parameter, b_0, remained constant. This decrease in optical rotation has been attributed to the unmasking of hydrophobic regions with a concomitant enhancement of the rotation of side chains which were immobilized in the native structure (Kauzman *et al.*, 1940; Leonard *et al.*, 1963). Similarly, the finding that 150 unexchangeable hydrogens become exchangeable in BSA when the pH was adjusted to 3 or 8.5 (Benson and Hallaway, 1970) may be due to changes in the tertiary structure rather than helical unfolding. Both the conformational changes associated with the neutral transition and those responsible for the N-F transition resulted in all the nonexchangeable hydrogens becoming exchangeable. This behavior may indicate a similarity in the conformation of albumin at both these transitions due to exposure to the solvent of the intersurfaces between the constituent compact domains with concomitant exposure of certain amino acid side chains. Vijai and Foster (1967) suggested that electrostatic interactions occurred between the cationic ε-amino groups and the anionic form of carboxyl groups. Moreover, studies by Harmsen *et al.* (1971) indicated the participation of imidazole groups in salt bridge formation. Zurawski and Foster (1974) followed the changes in the environment of the sulfhydryl group of BSA as a function of pH and temperature in the neutral transition by nuclear magnetic resonance spectra of a fluorinated label. Although the sulfhydryl group was not involved directly in the neutral transition (both the mercaptalbumin and nonmercaptalbumin have the same transition characteristics as monitored by specific rotation at 300 nm), there were some changes in the local environment of the sulfhydryl group as revealed by a change in the chemical shift of the ^{19}F label. It was proposed that in neutral solution electrostatic interactions might bring the sulfhydryl group close to a cationic site composed of one or more histidine residues (Zurawski and Foster, 1974). During the neutral transition, deprotonation of the histidine residues or protonation of a carboxylate anion during the N-F transition resulted in a movement of the sulfhydryl group away from these cationic groups with loss of their perturbing effect on the ^{19}F label. The freedom of mobility of the N-terminal segment of BSA containing the sulfhydryl group may explain the intramolecular sulfhydryl-disulfide interchange between two or more disulfide bonds (Nikkel and Foster, 1971; Stroupe and Foster, 1973). A recent study by Habeeb (1978a) showed that the neutral transitions of BSA, and HSA, are associated with an increase in reducibility

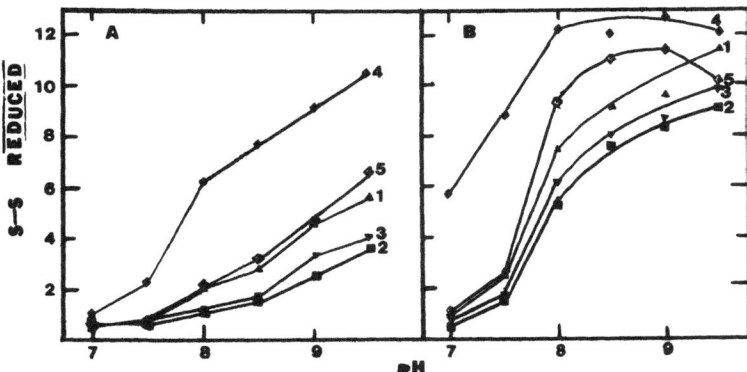

Figure 2.   Number of disulfide bonds (S—S) reduced with β-mercaptoethanol as a function of pH in various batches of Cohn fraction V. A: Reduction at room temperature. B: Reduction at 40°C. From Habeeb (1978a).

of the disulfide bonds by β-mercaptoethanol (Figs. 2 and 3). These results indicated that the alterations in the tertiary structure of BSA were accompanied by a loosening of certain areas in the molecule, thereby exposing the disulfide bonds. However, only a portion of the total disulfide bonds were available for reduction, and variabilities in the reducibility of the disulfide bonds of different preparations of albumin were observed.

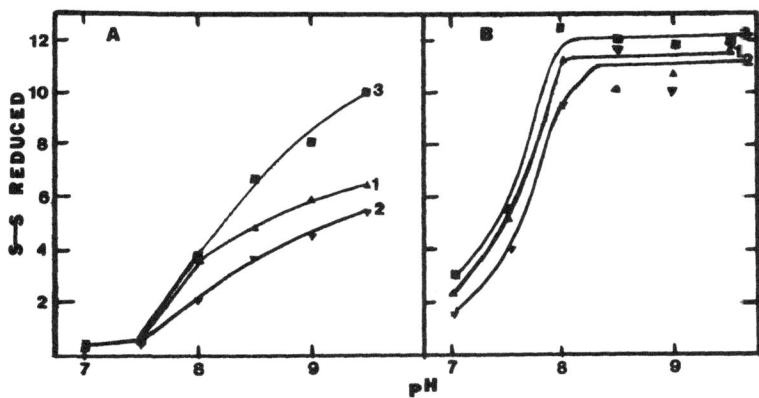

Figure 3.   Number of disulfide bonds (S—S) reduced with β-mercaptoethanol as a function of pH in various batches of human serum albumin. 1, From Cutter Lab; 2, crystalline HSA lot No. 65C-8320 from Sigma; 3, fatty-acid-free lot No. 16C-7281 from Sigma. A: Reduction at room temperature. B: Reduction at 40°C. From Habeeb (1978a).

B. Molecular Organization of Bovine Serum Albumin

Based on the behavior of albumin below pH 4.5, Foster (1960) proposed a model for BSA which consisted of four globular domains held by short randomly coiled polypeptide chains. The molecule was proposed to be compact between pH 4.2 and 7. As the pH decreased from 4.2 to 3.9, a limited expansion of the molecule took place, caused by separation of globular regions due to electrostatic repulsion. This conformation was stable between pH 3.9 and 3.6. On lowering of the pH, further unfolding of the globular domains occurred and the molecule existed in an expanded form, exhibiting an increased Stokes radius, increased intrinsic viscosity, and decreased sedimentation coefficient. Similarly, at pH 7–10, a neutral transition ensued, reflecting a perturbation of the conformation, but was not accompanied by an expansion of the molecule. However, at a pH above 10.5, expansion of the molecule occurred. Similar conformational alterations can be produced at neutral pH by imparting a net negative charge to the albumin molecule by succinylation (Habeeb *et al.*, 1958; Habeeb, 1967*a*).

Other similar models have been suggested. King (1973) proposed that albumin was formed of two globular domains connected by a short, flexible polypeptide chain. Each domain was thought to be composed of two or more compact subregions. The compact structure of the albumin was attributed to intermolecular association of these subregions and between the two domains. Conformational motility was exhibited by the different domains, depending on environmental conditions. The environmentally dictated conformational mobilities led to variations in the sites of enzymatic cleavage. This was manifested by the pattern of digestion with pepsin at different pH values and by the mode of tryptic cleavage. Similarly, Hilak *et al.* (1974) suggested that BSA had a compact conformation in the N form. During the N-F transition, the amino-terminal region remained compact, while the carboxyl terminal region partially unfolded and progressively exposed sites available for peptic cleavage.

From low-angle X-ray scattering, Luzzati *et al.* (1961) proposed an ellipsoid-of-revolution model in which 65% of the protein existed as a compact core and the remaining 35% formed an outer envelope. However, this model did not show a good agreement between calculated and experimental values of low-angle X-ray scattering, diffusion coefficients, and intrinsic viscosity (Bloomfield, 1966). Good agreement between the calculated and experimental values of these parameters was obtained with a model depicting BSA to be formed of a linear trimer, the radius of the central sphere being 26.6 Å and that of the two adjacent and touching spheres being 19Å.

Based on its amino acid sequence (Brown, 1975), BSA consists of three compact domains which have some degree of homology with each other. Each domain contains 190 amino acids residues, and the entire structure is maintained by 17 disulfide bonds (Fig. 4). The homology between domains 1 and 2 is 25%, that between domains 2 and 3 is 21%, and that between domains 1 and 3 is 18% (Brown, 1975). Most of the sequence homologies involve one or two amino acid residues. An exception is a homologous stretch of four amino acid residues (Arg-Arg-His-Pro) at sequences 143–146 and 334–337. The 17 disulfide bonds are arranged in nine loops, eight contain double disulfide bridges, and one loop has a single disulfide bond. Of the eight loops containing double disulfide bridges, seven loops have adjacent half-cystines, each of which is linked to a different half-cystine at different sites on the chain. The other double loop has the two adjacent half-cystines separated by three amino acid residues. Sequence 400–402 has not been resolved. The free sulfhydryl group at position 34 is located in an accessible crevice (Fuller-Noel and Hunter, 1972; Stone et al., 1965; Griffith and McConnell, 1966) which is 9.5 Å in depth as determined by spin-label studies (Hull et al., 1975). At pH 2.3, where the acid expansion of the molecule occurs, the crevice is opened, as shown by the relative freedom of rotation of all spin labels (Hull et al., 1975). A considerable amount of conformational freedom in the amino-terminal sequence carrying the sulfhydryl group exists in BSA. It is this ability of mobility of the sulfhydryl group which may be important in catalyzing the sulfhydryl-disulfide interchange (Zurawski and Foster, 1974). From the amino acid sequence of BSA (Brown, 1975) three disulfide bonds may be partially considered as candidates for participation in the sulfhydryl-disulfide interchange, namely $Cys_{53}-Cys_{62}$, $Cys_{75}-Cys_{91}$, and $Cys_{90}-Cys_{101}$. A tryptophan residue and one or more cystine residues are located in a crevice in the neighborhood of Cys-34 (Fuller-Noel and Hunter, 1972). Although Trp-134 and Trp-212 are farther from Cys-34 in sequence, one of them may be brought into proximity of Cys-34 by the folding of the polypeptide chain.

C. Microheterogeneity

In 1954 Colvin, Smith, and Cook advanced the concept of microheterogeneity of proteins. They concluded that a native protein should be described "as a population of closely related individiuals which may differ either discretely or continuously in a number of properties" and cited plasma albumin as an example.

Serum albumin is commercially available as the following: (1) Cohn

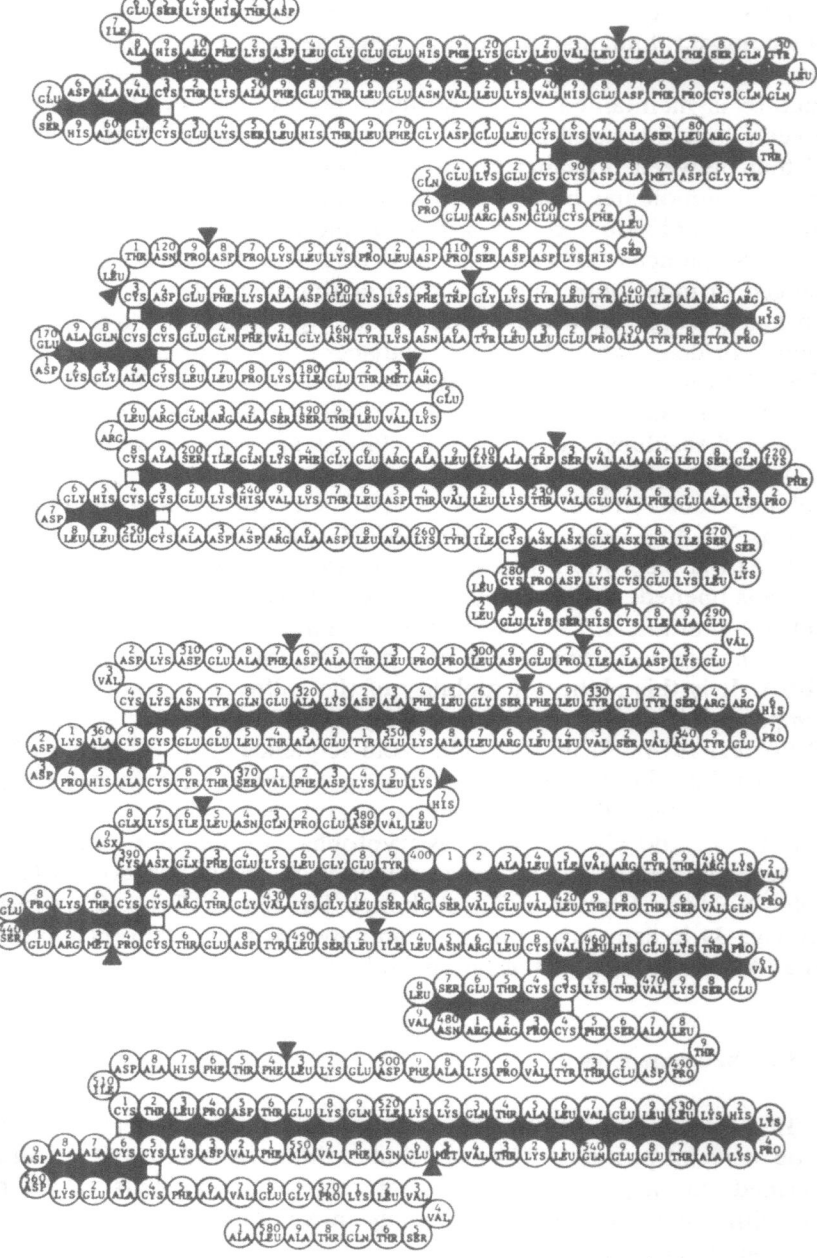

Figure 4.   Amino acid sequence of bovine serum albumin. From Brown (1975).

fraction V, prepared from pooled plasma or serum by a cold ethanol fractionation method (Cohn *et al.*, 1946) which involves the precipitation of proteins by varying the alcohol concentration, ionic strengths, pH, and temperature. This product is to be expected to vary in its free sulfhydryl content, fatty acid content, and the amount of dimer and higher polymers. (2) Crystalline albumin prepared from Cohn fraction V by crystallization from an ethanol-water mixture by decanol or a fatty acid (Cohn *et al.*, 1947). (3) Defatted albumin, prepared from either fraction V or crystalline albumin by defatting with charcoal at low pH (Chen, 1967) or any other procedure. The heterogeneity of albumin has both an extrinsic and an intrinsic origin. The former is the result of binding of fatty acids or other ligands, and the latter is the outcome of variable covalent structures, e.g., sulfhydryl content, differences in charge, or differences in disulfide pairing. Both the extrinsic and intrinsic factors affect the conformation of the molecule. The detection of conformational differences can be used to reveal heterogeneity.

An extensive amount of work has been devoted to an understanding of the origin of the heterogeneity of albumin, which may be summarized as follows:

1. Variation in the free sulfhydryl content.
2. Variation in binding of fatty acids.
3. Variation in the folding as revealed by differences in availability of disulfide bonds to reduction.
4. Differences among various populations of serum albumin in their physicochemical properties.
5. Differences in isoelectric point.

1. Sulfhydryl Content

Fresh serum contains only serum albumin monomers. However, dimers and higher oligomers form on standing and during some fractionation procedures. Monomers can be isolated from contaminating dimers and oligomers by gel filtration on Sephadex G-100 or G-150 (Pedersen, 1962).

Freshly isolated serum albumin monomer consists of 70% mercaptalbumin (containing one sulfhydryl group/mole albumin) and 30% non-mercaptalbumin (where the sulfhydryl group is blocked through mixed disulfide formation with cystine and, to a lesser extent, glutathione). The presence of the free sulfhydryl group in mercaptalbumin causes a pH-dependent increase in heterogeneity from pH 7 to 10. Heterogeneity is also observed after reversible denaturation in 6 M guanidine (Moore and

Foster, 1968; Sogami and Foster, 1968). The observed heterogeneity was
attributed to a sulfhydryl-disulfide interchange (Sogami et al., 1969),
since it was prevented by blocking of the sulfhydryl group.

On chromatography of BSA on DEAE-cellulose (Hartley et al., 1962;
Spencer and King, 1971; Habeeb, 1978a) or on DEAE-Sephadex (Janatova et al., 1968a,b,), mercaptalbumin eluted first, followed by nonmercaptalbumin, then by dimers and higher oligomers (Fig. 5). Both nonmercaptalbumin and dimers were heterogeneous in their chromatographic
patterns as well as in their reducibility by β-mercaptoethanol. Only a
fraction of nonmercaptalbumin was reducible with β-mercaptoethanol
under nondenaturing conditions, while the other required denaturation
for reduction. The former was a mixed disulfide involving the sulfhydryl
group of BSA, whereas in the latter the mixed disulfide involved a buried
nonnative sulfhydryl group (Andersson, 1966). Cohn fraction V and charcoal-defatted BSA showed a similar chromatographic pattern on DEAE-
Sephadex A-50 (Janatova et al., 1968a). Chromatographic patterns both
on DEAE-cellulose (Spencer and King, 1971) and on DEAE-Sephadex
(Janatova et al., 1968b) showed a main asymmetrical peak with considerable tailing. Better fractionation was achieved (Habeeb, 1978b) on
DEAE-cellulose (Fig. 6) using a stepwise elution system (Habeeb and

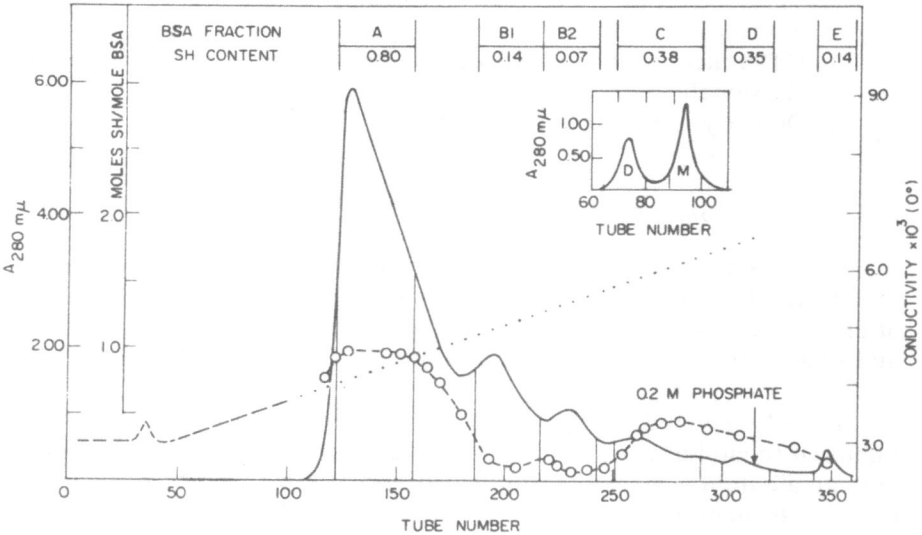

Figure 5. Elution profile of BSA after fractionation on DEAE-Sephadex A-50. —, Absorbance of eluate at 280 nm; O—O, —SH content of eluted albumin; ···, conductivity of
eluate. Insert: Subfraction of BSA fraction C on Sephadex G-150. D, Dimer; M, monomer.
From Janatova et al. (1968b).

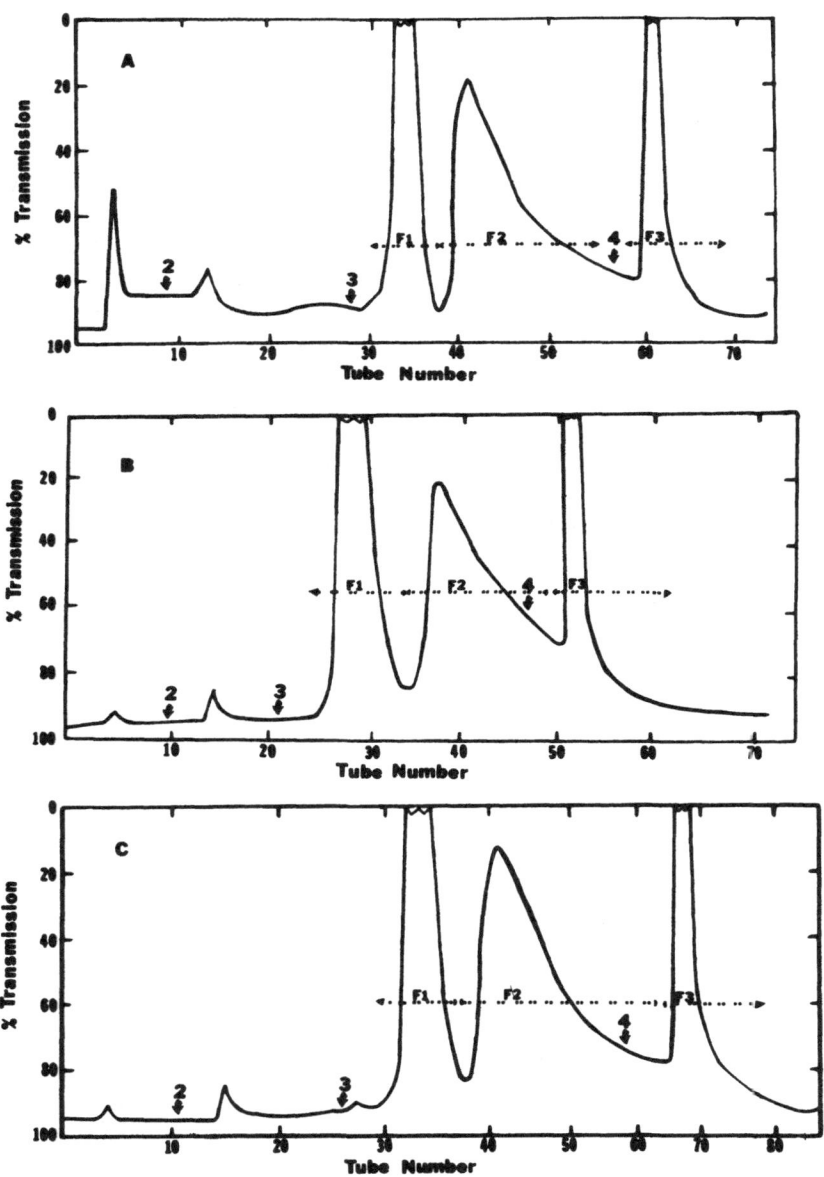

Figure 6.   Chromatography of BSA on DEAE-cellulose using stepwise elution. The starting buffer was 0.005 M sodium phosphate buffer pH 6.2 followed by 2, 0.0175 M sodium phosphate buffer pH 6.2; 3, 0.075 M NaCl in 0.0175 M phosphate buffer pH 6.2; 4, 0.2 M NaCl in 0.0175 M sodium phosphate pH 6.2. A: Cohn fraction V lot No. 4394 from ICN. B: Crystalline BSA, lot No. 46C-8090 from Sigma. C: Fatty-acid-free BSA lot No. 46C-7450 from Sigma. From Habeeb (unpublished work).

Francis, 1976) starting with (1) 0.005 M sodium phosphate buffer pH 6.2 and then (2) 0.0175 M sodium phosphate buffer pH 6.2 followed by (3) 0.075 M NaCl in 0.0175 M phosphate buffer pH 6.2 and finally (4) 0.2 M NaCl in 0.0175 M phosphate buffer pH 6.2. Cohn fraction V, crystalline BSA, and defatted BSA (Fig. 6) had similar elution patterns showing three major components. The first and third peaks were narrow and symmetrical while the second peak was broad with some trailing. Both F1 and F2 were rich in their content of the free sulfhydryl group whereas the reverse was true for F3 (Table I). Components eluted with the low ionic strength buffer 1 or 2 (Fig. 6) represented plasma contaminants. After blocking of the sulfhydryl group of BSA with iodoacetamide, the modified BSA gave the same elution pattern on DEAE-cellulose as unmodified BSA (Habeeb, 1978b). Therefore, the elution pattern is not dependent on the presence or absence of the free sulfhydryl group but rather on the charge of the population of BSA. In contrast to DEAE-cellulose, sulfoethyl Sephadex C-50 was reported to fractionate BSA into fatty-acid-bound mercaptalbumin, fatty-acid-free mercaptalbumin, and nonmercaptalbumin (Hagenmaier and Foster, 1971).

Although pure bovine mercaptalbumin prepared by chromatography on sulfoethyl Sephadex C-50 was found to be more homogeneous than parent BSA as shown by its solubility-pH profile and solubility behavior in concentrated ammonium sulfate solutions, it did not yield separate N and F boundaries on electrophoresis; however, it exhibited heterogeneity with respect to binding with detergents, and two components were resolvable by electrophoresis (Hagenmaier and Foster, 1971).

A reversible "aging" of mercaptalbumin (in salt-free water at pH 9

Table I. Free Sulfhydryl Content of Fractions Obtained by Chromatography of Bovine Serum Albumin on DEAE-Cellulose (mol/mol BSA)[a]

Bovine serum albumin	Unfractionated	F1	F2	F3
Cohn fraction V				
3	0.50	0.80	0.67	0.32
4	0.56	0.72	0.74	0.34
5	0.25	0.74	0.87	0.25
Crystalline BSA				
6	0.78	0.91	0.85	0.48
8	0.68	0.96	0.78	0.40
Defatted BSA				
4	0.65	0.79	0.93	0.65

[a] From Habeeb (unpublished work).

for 96 hr under N_2) resulted in the appearance of a discrete new component which was more cationic than mercaptalbumin at pH 4.82 but not at higher pH. This aging was prevented by blocking the free sulfhydryl group (Nikkel and Foster, 1971). However, in sulfhydrylblocked mercaptalbumin, aging can be initiated by the presence of an externally added mercaptan. The isoelectric point of mercaptalbumin was 4.83 while that of the aged derivative was 5.23. Aged mercaptalbumin was estimated to carry a charge 6 units more positive than mercaptalbumin. There was no loss in free sulfhydryl group on aging, indicating that the process is catalyzed by the free sulfhydryl of albumin. Moreover, the sulfhydryl group was recovered at the same position in the aged derivative as shown by peptide maps. It was suggested that at least two disulfide bonds were involved in the sulfhydryl-disulfide interchange which accompanied a conformational reorganization (Nikkel and Foster, 1971). The work clearly showed that, under these conditions of aging, the free sulfhydryl group served a catalytic function (in re-forming two new disulfide bonds) and was recovered at the same position as in the native molecule. However, it should be recognized that other sulfhydryl-disulfide exchanges can occur without recovery of the sulfhydryl group in the same position as native BSA. In these cases, denaturing conditions were required to reveal the free sulfhydryl group (Hartley et al., 1962; Andersson, 1966; Janatova et al., 1968b). Moreover, oxidation of the sulfhydryl group of BSA may occur during freeze-drying and is accelerated in the presence of peroxidizable fatty acids such as linoleic acid (Fuller-Noel and Hunter, 1972). Under these conditions, the sulfhydryl group was not recovered completely on reduction.

Although DEAE-cellulose apparently fractionated BSA with respect to its sulfhydryl content, the separation of mercaptalbumin and nonmercaptalbumin was achieved on the basis of their isoelectric points. The different components were stable and not interconvertible on reversible denaturation with 6 M urea but differed in their thermal and acid denaturation properties (Spencer and King, 1971). Fractions with higher isoelectric points had higher solubility-pH profiles and were more susceptible to heat denaturation. However, only 1 unit charge difference between the major components was observed, and it is hard to visualize how such a small difference can contribute so perceptibly to the stability of the molecule. Other unknown factors may have been superimposed on the isoelectric point differences and may have led to the observed effects.

Despite the fractionation of BSA on DEAE-cellulose (irrespective whether it was Cohn fraction V, defatted BSA, crystalline BSA, or sulfhydryl blocked-BSA) into three components with different isoelectric points and sulfhydryl contents, all the components exhibited identical immunochemical reactivities (Habeeb, 1978*b*) with anti-BSA antisera, as demonstrated by their precipitin curves shown in Fig. 7. It is therefore evident that the antigenic reactive sites in BSA were not affected by the heterogeneity which was manifested by DEAE-cellulose chromatography and sulfhydryl content (Habeeb, 1978*b*).

2. Binding of Fatty Acids

Commercially available serum albumins (whether Cohn fraction V or crystalline BSA) contain variable and inconsistent amounts of free fatty acids (0.08–2.4 mol/mol albumin). These fatty acids are entirely (99%) removed by charcoal defatting (Chen, 1967). Differences in free fatty acids in serum albumin have been attributed to variations in the levels of free fatty acids in plasma. Analysis of free fatty acids in human serum (Saifer *et al.*, 1961) showed a complex composition of 43 different fatty acids, 26 of which were identified. Eight fatty acids—namely oleic, palmitic, linoleic, arachidonic, palmitoleic, myristic, linolenic, and stearic acids—constituted 90% of the total. A similar fatty acid distribution was shown in BSA (Fuller-Noel and Hunter, 1972). The presence of fatty acids in BSA imparts a conformational stability to the molecule, which assumes a more compact conformation as shown by a decreased reactivity of amino groups with fluorodinitrobenzene (Green, 1963) or with trinitrobenzene sulfonic acid (Andersson *et al.*, 1971) and a decrease in the availability of the disulfide bonds to reduction with β-mercaptoetha-

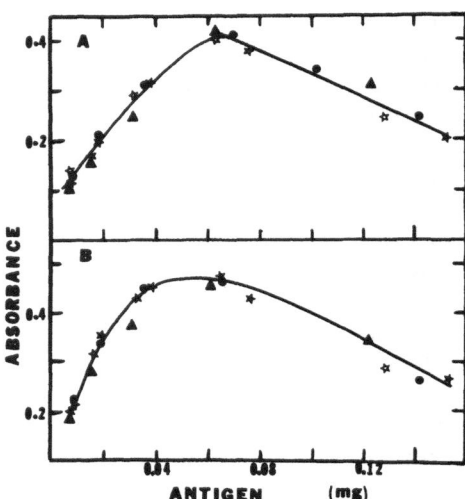

Figure 7. Precipitin curves of fractions of BSA isolated by DEAE-cellulose chromatography with anti-BSA. Absorbance at 280 nm: ●, BSA; ★, F1; ☆, F2; ▲, F3. A: Anti-BSA No. 535. B: IgG fraction of anti-BSA No. P. From Habeeb (unpublished work).

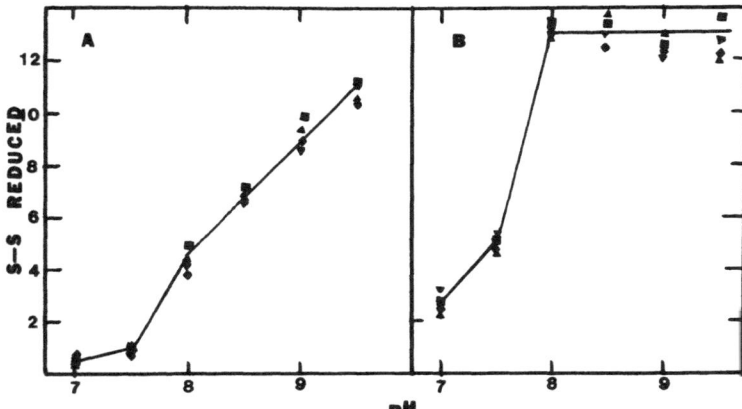

Figure 8.   Number of disulfide bonds (S—S) reduced with β-mercaptoethanol as a function of pH in various batches of defatted BSA. ▼, ▲, ◆, and ■ represent samples 1, 2, 3, and 4, respectively. A: Reduction at room temperature. B: Reduction at 40°C. From Habeeb (1978*a*).

nol (Habeeb, 1978*a*). A decrease in stability of serum albumin accompanied the process of defatting, as shown by increased sulfhydryl-disulfide interchange (Sogami and Foster, 1968; Sogami *et al.,* 1969), resulting in aggregation and increased heterogeneity. This reaction was prevented by blocking the free sulfhydryl group with iodoacetamide or *N*-ethylmaleimide. The conformational heterogeneity observed in various batches of Cohn fraction V, as revealed by the availability of the disulfide bonds to reduction, was eliminated by charcoal defatting. The resultant albumin preparations showed 11 disulfide bonds available for reduction at pH 9.5 at room temperature, and 13 disulfide bonds were reducible at 40°C (Fig. 8). It is remarkable that, despite the conformational heterogeneity, Cohn fraction V, fatty-acid-free BSA, and crystalline BSA precipitated the same amount of antibody from anti-BSA serum at equivalence (Fig. 9). However, the shapes of the precipitin curves were not identical (Habeeb, unpublished work).

3. Folding as Revealed by Reactivity of the Disulfide Bonds

Disulfide bonds play an important role in stabilizing the conformation of proteins and in bringing amino acid residues that are distant in sequence into close proximity. The availability of disulfide bonds for reaction with β-mercaptoethanol, sodium sulfite, or peracetic acid has been used as a sensitive probe for conformational changes accompanying

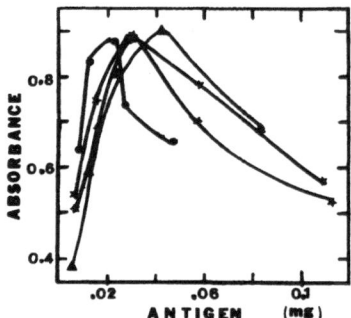

Figure 9. Precipitin curves of various batches of BSA with anti-BSA. Absorbance at 750 nm: ▲, Cohn fraction V No. 1; ☆, defatted BSA No. 1; ★, crystalline BSA No. 8; ●, crystalline BSA No. 6. From Habeeb (unpublished work).

chemical modification of proteins (Habeeb, 1966*a*). A progressive increase in reactivity of the disulfide bonds in BSA with sodium sulfite was demonstrated in solutions of urea as the concentration of urea increased from 0 to 5 M at room temperature or 40°C (Table II). Each sample after reaction with iodoacetamide showed two components (Comp 1 and Comp 2) which were separable on Sephadex G-200 or by electrophoresis on

Table II. Susceptibility of the Disulfide Bonds to Reaction in Bovine Serum Albumin[a] and Human Serum Albumin[b]

	Conditions of reaction[c]				Relative amount (%)	
	Temperature (°C)	Time (hr)	Urea (M)	S—S cleaved	Comp 1	Comp 2
Sulfitolysis						
BSA-1	RT	½	3	2.3	—	—
2	RT	1	3	3.8	24	76
3	RT	2	3	4.2	31	69
4	RT	3	3	5.4	36	64
5	40	5	3	7.6	82	18
6	40	5	4	15.4	N.D.	N.D.
7	40	5	5	16.4	N.D.	N.D.
Reduction						
HSA	RT	6	3	4.5	44	56
F1	RT	6	3	7.0	57	43
F2	RT	6	3	6.0	47	53
F3	RT	6	3	4.5	38	62
HSA	RT	6	6	13.0	85	15
F2	RT	6	6	15.5	99	1

[a] From Habeeb and Borella (1966).
[b] From Habeeb (1968*b*).
[c] RT, room temperature.

agar in barbital buffer (Habeeb and Borella, 1966). The earlier-eluting component (Comp 1) had a Stokes radius of > 20.2 nm and had more disulfide bonds cleaved. It consisted of two populations of molecules, an expanded form and an aggregated form, having sedimentation coefficients, $s_{20,w}$, of 1.85 S and 15.9 S, respectively. The later-eluting component (Comp 2) had a Stokes radius of 3.7 nm, an $s_{20,w}$ of 4.6 S, and a mobility on agar electrophoresis similar to that of native BSA. It was remarkable that the amount of Comp 1 relative to Comp 2 increased as conditions of sulfitolysis promoted more disulfide bond cleavage. Therefore, the data indicated that BSA was heterogeneous insofar as the availability of its disulfide bonds to sulfitolysis was concerned. Under a given set of conditions, the disulfide bonds of only a fraction of the molecules were available for reaction, and the remainder of the molecules were resistant to sulfitolysis. The resistant molecules became progressively reactive as conditions promoted more unfolding of the protein molecule. Similar results were obtained with HSA (Habeeb, 1968b), where HSA in 3 M KCl was fractionated into subfractions F1, F2, and F3 by stepwise lowering of the pH (pH 4.7, 4.5, and 3.75, respectively). Subfractions showed variability in the disulfide bonds to reduction with β-mercaptoethanol. The first fraction, F1, was more susceptible to reduction in 3M urea than F2 and F3. Each of the subfractions was reduced with β-mercaptoethanol in 3 M urea, and the liberated sulfhydryl groups were blocked with iodoacetamide. The reaction product consisted of two components separable on Sephadex G-200 corresponding to a fast-eluting component (an expanded molecule) and a slow-eluting component (similar to HSA). The relative proportions of the fast- and slow-eluting forms varied in the subfractions (Table II). It is significant that F3, which was less susceptible to reduction than F 1, showed a lower proportion of the fast-eluting component. Moreover, even under conditions which promoted complete unfolding (6 M urea, 6 hr) about 1% of the molecules were resistant to reduction. The results with both BSA and HSA demonstrated that these proteins consist of different populations of molecules which vary in the availability of their disulfide bonds to either sulfitolysis or reduction. This may suggest differences in pairing of the disulfide bonds. Other unknown structural or environmental differences in the vicinity of the disulfide bonds may influence their reactivity. Despite the conformational differences demonstrated in subfractions from HSA, their immunochemical reactivities with anti-HSA antiserum (by quantitative precipitin curves) were identical, indicating that the antigenic reactive sites were not affected by these conformational variations (Habeeb, 1968b).

4. Heterogeneity Revealed by Physicochemical Methods

Serum albumin consisted of a population of molecules which, while having some similarities in their properties, differed in the pH of N-F transition (Foster *et al.*, 1965). The different species underwent the N-F transformation at a slightly but definitely different pH value. At a given pH value (within the N-F transition) most of the molecules were in either the N or the F form. Partial separation of BSA or human mercaptalbumin into three narrow subfractions (Fig. 10) was achieved by a stepwise lowering of the pH (from pH 5 to 3.8) of a solution of serum albumin in 3 M KCl (Petersen and Foster, 1965*a*). Each subfraction had a distinct solubility-pH profile (Fig. 11), the midpoint of the pH-solubility profile for subfraction I> subfraction II> subfraction III indicating that each subfraction contained a population of molecules which had distinct properties and were quite different from one another. A number of other differences existed among these subfractions. The hydrogen ion titration behavior of the subfractions differed in the regions of carboxyl, ϵ-amino, and phenolic groups, but not in the region of imidazole and α-amino groups (Petersen and Foster, 1965*a*). Moreover, the subfractions were found to vary in their susceptibility to heat denaturation, as detected by an increase in viscosity (Fig. 12) as well as by ultracentrifugal analyses. Thus subfractions having a high midpoint in their solubility-pH profile were more denaturable (Petersen and Foster, 1965*a*) than those with lower solubility-pH profiles (FI> FII> FIII). Albumin was shown to

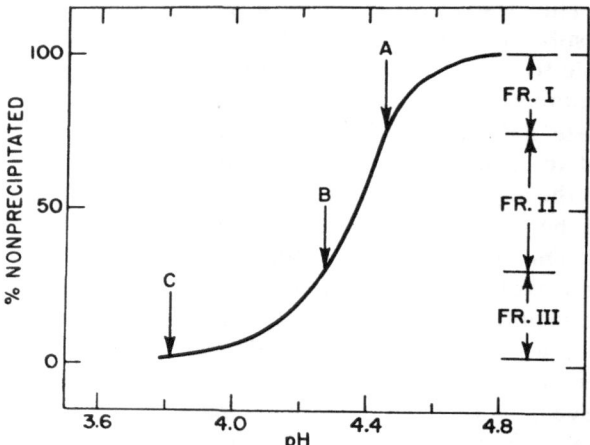

Figure 10.   Solubility of human mercaptalbumin in 3.0 M KCl as a function of pH, showing stepwise precipitation into three subfractions. From Petersen and Foster (1965*a*).

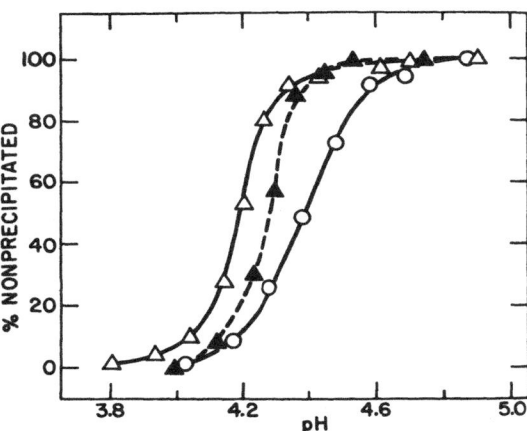

Figure 11. Solubility as a function of pH in 3.0 M KCl, after 15 min, for subfractions of human mercaptalbumin (HMA). The HMA was chromatographed on Sephadex G-200 prior to subfractionation. ○, Subfraction I; ▲, subfraction II; △, subfraction III. From Petersen and Foster (1965a).

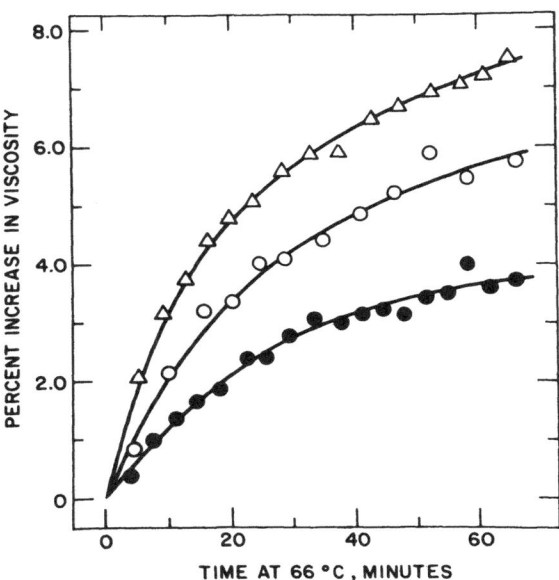

Figure 12. Increase in viscosity during heating of Pentex lot 9 BSA and two subfractions at 66°C. △, Subfraction II; ○, control BSA; ●, subfraction IV. From Petersen and Foster (1965b).

exhibit heterogeneity during heat denaturation (Stokrova and Sponar, 1963) in that it contained molecules of differing heat stabilities, which was attributed to structural differences among this population of molecules. The availability of disulfide bonds to reduction in HSA subfractions (Habeeb, 1968*b*) was also found to parallel their susceptibility to denaturation. While these various differences in physicochemical properties were detected, they could not be assigned to any definite structural property.

Microheterogeneity was also demonstrated by a membrane equilibrium solubility method which was insensitive to fatty acid contaminants (Wong and Foster, 1969*a*). Fractional precipitation of serum albumin by ammonium sulfate yielded fractions which exhibited distinct solubility-Σ profiles (Σ being the concentration of salt in the dialysate) (Fig. 13). Each fraction also demonstrated different solubility-pH profiles (Fig. 14). That the solubility-Σ and solubility-pH profiles were related was revealed by the finding that the least soluble fraction in ammonium sulfate precipitated at a higher pH (Fig. 14). Charcoal-defatted BSA whose sulfhydryl group was blocked by cystine or iodoacetamide and fractions obtained by precipitation with ammonium sulfate showed distinct solubility-Σ profiles, which were unaltered in the renatured proteins after denaturation in 6 M guanidine HC1 (Wong and Foster, 1969*b*). Similarly, charcoal-defatted and sulfhydryl-blocked BSA recovered its native conformation (after denaturation in 6 M guanidine HC1 and renaturation) as shown by

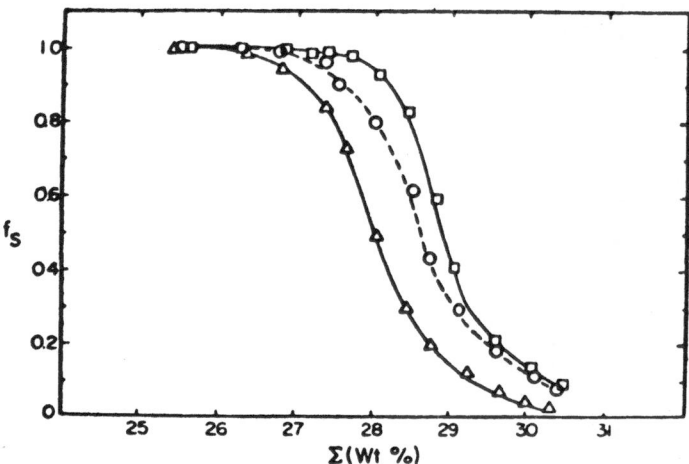

Figure 13. Solubility-Σ profiles of subfractions of charcoal-defatted BSA. $\bigcirc$, Control BSA; $\triangle$, least-soluble fraction; $\square$, most-soluble fraction. Each subfraction constituted approximately one-third of the protein. From Wong and Foster (1969*a*).

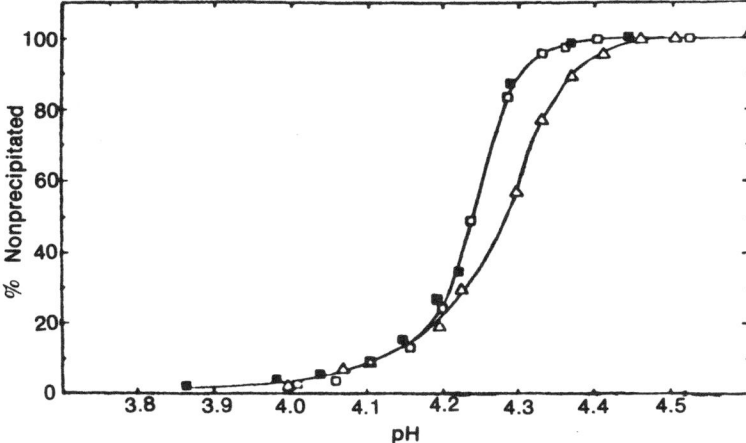

Figure 14.   Solubility-pH profiles of Σ subfractions of charcoal-defatted crystallized BSA.
△, Least-soluble subfraction; ■, □, two separate experiments on the most-soluble fraction.
Each subfraction constituted approximately one-third of the sample. From Wong and Foster
(1969a).

its solubility-pH profile in 3 M KCl and optical rotatory dispersion
(Moore and Foster, 1968). However, unless the sulfhydryl group was
blocked, an increase in heterogeneity, attributed to sulfhydryl-disulfide
interchange, was observed following denaturation in 6 M guanidine HCl
and renaturation (Moore and Foster, 1968; Wong and Foster, 1969b).
Therefore, the observed microheterogeneity was not due to differences
in the three-dimensional structure among the population of the albumin
molecules but rather resided in differences in their covalent structures
(Wong and Foster, 1969b). This is in agreement with the conclusions
derived from the elution pattern of reversibly denatured fractions from
BSA on DEAE-cellulose (Spencer and King, 1971) and also from iso-
lectric focusing experiments (Spencer and King, 1971; Salaman and Williamson, 1971).

5. Differences in Isoelectric Point

Bovine serum albumin (Spencer and King, 1971; Salaman and Williamson, 1971; Wallevik, 1973, 1976) or human serum albumin (Ui, 1971)
showed two or three major components in isoelectric focusing. The fact
that heterogeneity persisted in defatted BSA after reversible denaturation
in 6 M guanidine HCl or 6 M urea eliminated bound ligands as the only
cause of heterogeneity. Also, the finding that serum albumin from six

individual calves, eight individual humans, and four mice was heterogeneous by isoelectric focusing (Spencer and King, 1971) excluded sequence variation arising from heterozygosity of the structural gene. Heterogeneity was also observed in urea-denatured albumin (Spencer and King, 1971) and in reduced and alkylated albumin (Salaman and Williamson, 1971), thus establishing that heterogeneity was not due to conformational differences but was the outcome of charge differences in the covalent structure of the albumin molecule. Indeed, Spencer and King (1971) found that the two major components of albumin comprising 76% and 20% of the total differed by 1 unit of charge. The isoelectric point of the major component of albumin in 6 M urea agreed with the calculated value and was 1 pH unit higher than in the absence of 6 M urea (Salaman and Williamson, 1971; Ui, 1971). The shift in the isoelectric point of albumin in urea was attributed to exposure of hidden uncharged amino groups due to unfolding in urea (Salaman and Williamson, 1971) rather than the normalization of carboxylic groups on unfolding (Ui, 1971). Salaman and Williamson (1971) calculated that the isoelectric point would increase by 0.07 pH unit when 50 hidden carboxyl groups in the anionic form became protonated after exposure to 6 M urea, whereas if seven un-ionized amino groups buried in hydrophobic regions became exposed the isoelectric point approached the experimental value.

D. Fragmentation of Bovine Serum Albumin by Proteolytic Enzymes

Bovine serum albumin exists as a compact molecule at pH 4.2–10.5. In the pH range of the N-F transition (pH 4.2–3.6) the compact regions are separated from each other, thus exposing a limited number of flexible segments of the molecule (which hold the compact domains together) to peptic digestion. As the pH is lowered further, to pH 3.0, unfolding occurs enabling the molecule to be hydrolyzed by pepsin at various sites. Various investigators have made use of this behavior to obtain a variety of peptides from BSA. Similarly, in the neutral transition, the amino-terminal region is unfolded but the carboxyl-terminal region maintains its compact structure. Therefore, tryptic digestions in the pH range of the neutral transition have yielded large fragments comprising the last third of the molecule.

1. Cleavage by Pepsin

At pH 3 the product from peptic hydrolysis of BSA was complex (Weber and Young, 1964a,b; Peters and Hawn, 1967; Pearlman and Fong,

1972; Braam *et al.*, 1971, 1974), consisting of several fragments. The complexity of the mixture was demonstrated by variations in the fragments isolated by different investigators employing peptic digestion performed under very similar conditions. This may be due to differences in the pH of peptic cleavage, incomplete isolation of all the constituent fragments, heterogeneity of some of the isolated fragments, and preferential isolation of a given fragment or fragments due to the method of fractionation. Although Weber and Young (1964b) isolated three fragments of molecular weights 12,500, 29,000, and 34,000, heterogeneity in physical properties and amino acid composition was shown in the first fragment. From similar peptic digest Peters and Hawn (1967) isolated two fragments whose locations were established by Feldhoff and Peters (1975) within the sequence of BSA reported by Brown (1975) on the basis of molecular weight, amino acid analysis, and amino- and carboxyl-terminal sequences. One fragment corresponded to the sequence Asp_1–Leu_{24} (molecular weight 2800) and the other to Phe_{504}–Ala_{581} (molecular weight 8500). The remainder of the cleavage product was heterogeneous by electrophoresis and was not studied further. A fragment (molecular weight 10,000, denoted "KL") with strong steroid-binding activity was isolated from a peptic digest of BSA (Pearlman and Fong, 1972). In addition, a complex mixture of peptides with molecular weights of 14,000, 27,000, and 34,000 was identified. The fragment KL was assigned the location Phe_{307}–Leu_{385} by Feldhoff and Peters (1975). In the presence of 0.0032 M octanoic acid, brief cleavage of BSA with pepsin at pH 3.7 gave a number of fragments, two of which were the main product and were recovered in about 16% yield (King, 1973). In addition to the above two fragments, which corresponded to Asp_1–Asp_{306} and Phe_{307}–Leu_{585}, several other fragments corresponding to sequences Ile_{453}–Leu_{503}, Phe_{307}–Leu_{385}, Phe_{49}–Glu_{185}, and Lys_{186}–Asp_{306} were isolated and identified (Feldhoff and Peters, 1975). Fragments Leu_{453}–Leu_{503} and Phe_{307}–Leu_{385} were degradation products of Phe_{307}–Ala_{581}. Also, Phe_{41}–Glu_{185} and Lys_{186}–Asp_{306} were cleavage products of Asp_1–Asp_{306} (Feldhoff and Peters, 1975). Only fragment Phe_{307}–Ala_{581} bound octanoic acid. However, the binding constant was double in the presence of the amino-terminal fragment Asp_1–Asp_{306}. Braam *et al.* (1971, 1974) carried out a systematic study on the peptic digestion of BSA at pH 3.6–3.9 and were able to isolate, characterize, and localize a number of these fragments within the albumin molecule. They determined the molecular weights, amino acid composition, amino-terminal residues, copper binding, and sulfhydryl content. Ten components were identified, one of which corresponded to uncleaved BSA. Fragments 2, 3, 4, and 5 were derived from the amino terminus and had molecular weights of 54,000, 47,000, 40,000, and 31,000, respectively. Fragments 6 and 7, 8, 9, and 10 were derived from the carboxyl terminus and had molecular weights of 24,000, 16,000, 12,000, and 4000, respectively. Fragment 4 may correspond to the region Asp_1–Leu_{385}, fragment 5 to Asp_1–Asp_{306}, and fragment 10 to Phe_{504}–Ala_{581} (Feldhoff and Peters, 1975). Braam *et al.* (1974) concluded that the first peptic cleavages occur near the COOH terminus, at the NH_2 terminus of fragment 8. Further cleavage occurred toward the NH_2 terminus, thus liberating fragments 3, 4, and 5.

A summary of the fragmentation of BSA by pepsin is given in Table III.

2. Cleavage by Trypsin

Commercially available BSA has been found to vary in its susceptibility to tryptic digestion (King and Spencer, 1970; Habeeb, 1977a). Some batches were resistant to trypsin, and the susceptibility to tryptic digestion paralleled the availability of disulfide bonds to reduction in the

Table III.   Peptic Fragments from Bovine Serum Albumin

Conditions	Fragments	Comments
pH 3 for 35–60 min at 25°C[a]	a. 12,500 b. 29,000 c. 34,000	Purity was not established Amino acid composition of b and c was identical but differed from that of a
pH 3 for 30 min at 25°C[b]	Asp_1–Leu_{24} (mol. wt. 2800) Phe_{504}–Ala_{581} (mol. wt. 8500)	Fragments were homogeneous and their alignment within BSA molecule was established by Feldhoff and Peters (1975)
pH 3 for 2 hr at 25°C[c]	Complex mixture a. 14,000 b. 27,000 c. 34,000 d. Asp_1–Leu_{24} e. KL Phe_{307}–Leu_{385} (mol. wt. 10,050)	Fragment KL has strong binding activity for steroids; its location in BSA has been assigned by Feldhoff and Peters (1975)
pH 3.7 in presence of 0.0032 M octanoic acid for 20 min at 25°C[d]	Fragment A Phe_{307}–Ala_{581} (mol. wt. 28,000) Fragment B Asp_1–Asp_{306} (mol. wt. 34,000)	In absence of octanoic acid, fragment A was degraded further; the alignment of these fragments was established by Feldhoff and Peters (1975); only fragment A binds octanoic acid and the binding constant is doubled in presence of fragment B

(Continued)

Table III.   (Continued)

Conditions	Fragments	Comments
pH 3.7 at 25°C for 30–40 min[e]	1. Mol. wt. 69,000 2. Mol. wt. 54,000 3. Mol. wt. 47,000 4. Asp_1–Leu_{385} mol. wt. 40,000 (binds Cu^{2+}) 5. Asp_1–Asp_{306} mol. wt. 31,000 (binds Cu^{2+}) 6. and 7. Mol. wt. 24,000 8. Mol. wt. 16,000 9. Mol. wt. 12,000 10. Phe_{504}–Ala_{581} mol. wt. 4000 or less	Fragments 2, 3, 4, and 5 all contain Asp as NH_2-terminal residue, suggesting that they are derived from NH_2-terminal end; the positions of 6 and 7 are not clear, they may be derived from COOH-terminal; fragment 8 is part of COOH-terminal end and it generates fragments of 9 and 10 by further cleavage; the alignments of fragments 4, 5, and 10 inside BSA were suggested by Feldhoff and Peters (1975)
pH 3.7 at 25°C for 20 min in presence of 0.0032 M octanoic acid[f]	1. Asp_1–Asp_{306} 2. Phe_{307}–Ala_{581} 3. Ile_{453}–Leu_{503} 4. Phe_{307}–Leu_{385} 5. Phe_{49}–Glu_{185} 6. Lys_{186}–Asp_{306}	All fragments were pure with no internal scissions; fragments 5 and 6 are derived from adjacent regions at the NH_2-terminal half; similarly, fragments 3 and 4 are derived from the COOH-terminal half
pH 3.7 at 25°C for 20 min in absence of octanoic acid[f]	Asp_1–Leu_{385}	

[a] Weber and Young (1964a,b).
[b] Peters and Hawn (1967).
[c] Pearlman and Fong (1972).
[d] King (1973).
[e] Braam et al. (1971, 1974).
[f] Feldhoff and Peters (1975).

pH range of the neutral transition (Habeeb, 1977a). The restriction in both the tryptic digestion and the reducibility of disulfide bonds was due to bound fatty acids. In fact, on removal of fatty acids, BSA exhibited increased reactivity of the disulfide bonds to reduction, as well as an enhanced susceptibility to tryptic digestion (Habeeb, 1977a). Therefore, variation in the cleavage products with trypsin has been reported and is dependent on the conditions of tryptic hydrolysis. Limited tryptic hydrolysis of defatted BSA (pH 8.8 at 0°C for 29 min) gave a complex mixture of peptides (molecular weights 20,000 and 40,000) from which a fragment derived from the COOH-terminal end (King and Spencer, 1970) with a molecular weight 40,000 was isolated in pure form, and had valine as its NH_2-terminal residue. Two other fragments having similar molecular weights were isolated but with leucine and tyrosine as NH_2-terminal residues. The components of molecular weight 20,000 were neither fractionated nor identified, and the elution pattern showed still other low molecular weight fragments. Tryptic hydrolysis (at 37°C for several hours) of BSA which was bound on a column of palmitylaminoethylaminoagarose yielded two fragments having sequences Leu_{115}–Arg_{184} and His_{377}–Ala_{581}. However, in aqueous solution two fragments were identified as cleavage product of BSA by trypsin, corresponding to sequences Leu_{115}–Arg_{184} and Cys_{198}–Ala_{581} (less Phe_{204}–Lys_{238}) (Peters and Feldhoff, 1975). In aqueous solution at pH 8.2 and 40°C, trypsin gave complex cleavage products of which two fragments of molecular weights 22,500 and 8000 were isolated in a pure form and in high yield (Habeeb and Atassi, 1976a,b). The larger fragment was assigned sequence His_{377}–Lys_{571} and was found to be immunochemically active. On the other hand, the specific fragmentation at arginine residues by trypsin (after reversible protection of free amino groups by citraconylation) gave a complex mixture of peptides from which a large fragment was isolated in a pure form and was assigned sequence Phe_{11}–Arg_{193} (less Arg_{144}) (Atassi et al., 1976b). It is noteworthy that citraconylation of BSA induced drastic conformational changes and cleavage occurred at a susceptible bond, which resulted in the liberation of a compact fragment from the NH_2-terminal third of the BSA molecule (Atassi et al., 1976b). In a similar way, fragmentation of BSA with pepsin at pH 3.7 released fragments from the NH_2-terminal end. A summary of the tryptic fragmentation of BSA is given in Table IV.

3. Cleavages by Subtilisin

Serum albumin or iodoacetamide-blocked defatted BSA (in the presence of 100 mol SDS/mol albumin) showed limited susceptibility to subtilisin cleavage (Pederson and Foster, 1969; Adkins and Foster, 1966). Two fragments were recovered of molecular weights 31,000 (F1) and 38,000 (F2). Their amino acid compositions were different, suggesting that they were derived from different segments of the molecule. Together the amino acid composition of the two fragments accounted for the amino acid composition of the albumin molecule. Another fragment of molecular weight 21,000 was isolated, and it was suggested to be the product of further cleavage of one of the larger fragments, F1. At equimolar concentrations and neutral pH the two large fragments associated to form one molecular species which sedimented as albumin. Amino-terminal

Table IV. Tryptic Fragments from Bovine Serum Albumin

Conditions	Fragments	Comments
pH 8.8 at 0°C[a]	1. Fragment 20,000 mol. wt. derived from N terminal 2. Fragment 40,000 mol. wt. derived from C terminal	Fragment 2 binds octanoic acid and L-tryptophan, binding constant for the fragment was one-third that for albumin
pH 8.15 at 25°C for 60 min[b]	1. $Leu_{115}-Arg_{184}$ 2. $Cys_{198}-Ala_{581}$ (less $Phe_{204}-Lys_{238}$)	
On a column of palmityl-aminoethylaminoaga-rose at 37°C, pH 7.4[b]	1. $Leu_{115}-Arg_{184}$ 2. $His_{377}-Ala_{581}$	
pH 8.2 at 40°C for 1 hr[c]	1. $His_{377}-Lys_{571}$ 2. Fragment mol. wt. 8000	Fragment 2 has not been localized within BSA molecule but is different from fragment 1 of Peters and Feldhoff (1975)
pH 8.2 at 40°C of citraconyl-BSA[d]	1. $Phe_{11}-Arg_{193}$ (less Arg_{144})	

[a] King and Spencer (1970).
[b] Peters and Feldhoff (1975).
[c] Habeeb and Atassi (1976a,b).
[d] Atassi et al. (1976b).

studies revealed that F2 was derived from the NH$_2$-terminal half of the albumin molecule (Pederson and Foster, 1969), while F1 had phenylalanine as its NH$_2$-terminal residue.

4. Cleavage by Chymotrypsin

Chymotryptic digestion of an expanded form of BSA (60–80% of the amino groups citraconylated) gave several fragments of molecular weights 35,000, 25,000, 20,000, 19,000, 8000, and 2000 or less (Jonas and Weber, 1970). The isolated fragments were contaminated with minor components of nearby bands. Variations in basic, acidic, and nonpolar amino acid residues existed among the different fractions, indicating that these amino acids were not evenly distributed within the molecule. Some fractions—for example, those of molecular weights 8000 and 19,000—did not show conformational changes at pH 2–8 while those of molecular weights 35,000, 25,000, and 20,000 unfolded at pH 2–4. It was proposed (Jonas and Weber, 1970) that, in the initial chymotryptic attack on citraconyl-BSA, fragments of molecular weights 35,000, 20,000, and 2000 or less were formed. Other fragments were then liberated by secondary attack on vulnerable peptide bonds as in the following scheme:

$$\text{citraconyl-BSA} \rightarrow 35,000 + 20,000 + 2000 \text{ or less}$$

$$\begin{array}{ccc} \swarrow & \searrow & \searrow \\ 25,000 & 19,000 & 8000 \end{array}$$

Based on the amino acid composition and by comparison with fragments obtained by other workers (Pederson and Foster, 1969; Weber and Young, 1964a,b; Peters and Hawn, 1967), an alignment of the different fragments within the BSA molecule was made (Jonas and Weber, 1970). This alignment is shown in the following scheme:

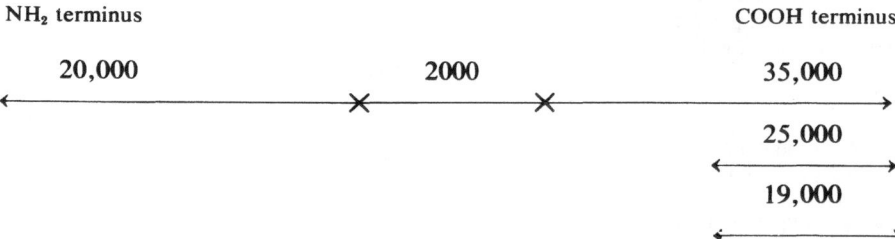

However, this assignment can be considered as tentative since the amino acid sequence of BSA was not available at that time. This mode of fragmentation of citraconylated BSA by chymotrypsin is in contrast to the fragmentation of citraconyl-BSA by trypsin (Atassi et al., 1976b), in which the main fragment corresponded to sequence $Phe_{11}-Arg_{193}$ (derived from the amino-terminal region).

E. Conformational Studies on Fragments from Bovine Serum Albumin and on Modified Albumin

1. Conformational Studies on Fragments

Various studies on the conformation of fragments obtained by either peptic or tryptic hydrolysis of BSA have indicated that the fragments maintain their compact structure. Hilak et al. (1974) examined the effect of pH on the conformation of fragments 3 (molecular weight 47,000 derived from the NH_2-terminal end of BSA), Asp_1-Leu_{385}, and Asp_1-Asp_{306} obtained by peptic cleavage (Braam et al., 1974), and also fragment T_{23} (King and Spencer, 1970) (derived from the COOH-terminal end of BSA) by tryptic hydrolysis. A change in conformation (specific rotations at 233 and 313 nm) occurred, and its extent increased (from BSA to the fragment of molecular weight 47,000 to Asp_1-Leu_{385}) as the pH was lowered from 5.7 to 2.5. No loss in α-helical content of fragment Asp_1-Leu_{385} was observed as the pH decreased from 6 to 4, whereas fragment T_{23} showed a decrease in α-helical content from 42% to 36% due to partial unfolding as the pH was lowered from 6 to 3. Based on these data, Hilak *et al* (1974) concluded that the change in $[\alpha]_{313}$ during the N-F transition was localized in the NH_2-terminal region and was not due to a loss of α-helix, while the change in $[\alpha]_{233}$ was localized in the COOH-terminal segment. Hilak *et al.* (1974) proposed that the loose structure of the COOH terminus was stabilized by interacting with the NH_2-terminal segment of the molecule. During the N-F transition, the COOH-terminal fragment unfolded while the NH_2-terminal fragment underwent an isomerization without loss of α helix. During the neutral transition, changes in $[\alpha]_{313}$ vs. pH were also detected in fragments 3, Asp_1-Leu_{385}, and partially in Asp_1-Asp_{306} but not in fragment T_{23}. The stability of the fragments increased with an increase in the molecular weight, indicating that the increased length of the peptide chain from Asp_1-Asp_{306} to Asp_1-Leu_{385} to the 47,000 molecular weight fragment to BSA had a stabilizing effect on the conformation, which is to be expected. The primary binding site of pyridoxal-5'-phosphate was localized in fragments Asp_1-Leu_{385} and Asp_1-Asp_{306} (Hilak *et al.*, 1975). While the environment of the primary binding site was apolar with BSA and Asp_1-Leu_{385}, it was exposed to the solvent in Asp_1-Asp_{306}, indicating that sequence 307–385 had a stabilizing effect on the conformation.

Fragments of BSA (obtained from peptic or tryptic digests) corresponding to the sequences 1–385, 198–581, 1–306, 307–581, 377–581, 49–185, 186–306, 307–385, 504–581, and 115–184 showed CD spectra similar to the spectrum of BSA, indicating very little conformational variations (Reed *et al.*, 1975).

Each of the fragments had helical contents of 50–70% and less than 22% β structure. It is to be cautioned, however, that whereas the CD spectra may indicate very little changes in the secondary structures of these fragments, their stabilities may be compromised under certain environmental conditions, as was shown by Hilak *et al* (1974, 1975) under condtions of the N-F and neutral transitions. Moreover, sensitive techniques may reveal subtle conformational alteration. Such a case was shown with fragment 1–306, which had no catalytic activity in decomposing a Meisenheimer complex (Taylor and Silver, 1976). The loss of catalytic activity was the outcome of a conformational alteration which damaged the active site (Taylor, 1976). It is noteworthy that mixing fragments 1–306 and 307–581 resulted in a recovery of 35% of the catalytic activity relative to BSA (Taylor and Silver, 1976), demonstrating partial reformation of the active site.

On the other hand, the shorter fragments 455–503 and 1–24 showed considerably altered conformations (Reed *et al.*, 1975). Several fragments retained their binding activities; for example, fragments 1–385, 1–306, and 186–306 bound bilirubin; fragments 377–581, 307–581, and 198–581 (less 204–238) contained the strong binding site for palmitate; while fragments 198–581, 1–385, and 1–306 contained a second binding site for palmitate. Both bromocresol green and 8-anilino 1-naphthalenesulfonate were bound by these fragments, and the binding was dependent on the size of the fragment.

2. Conformational Studies of Bovine Serum Albumin Modified by Proteinase Contaminants

Proteolytic enzyme contaminants were detected in commercial preparations of BSA fraction V and to a lesser extent in crystalline BSA (Wilson and Foster, 1971; Aoki and Foster, 1975). These contaminants caused scission of BSA peptide bonds on handling. Two different enzymes were present. One was active at pH 9 and cleaved BSA near residue 230 (Aoki and Foster, 1975) to yield two fragments (molecular weight 27,000 and 42,000). The second cleaved BSA at pH 3.8, resulting in a slightly expanded molecule. Initially with the acid proteinase cleavage occurred within a disulfide loop at a site close to residue 400 (Aoki and Foster, 1975), and after reduction and alkylation two fragments were separated. One fragment was derived from the NH_2-terminal end (molecular weight 46,000) and the second was derived from the COOH-terminal region (molecular weight 24,000). Further cleavage produced a fragment derived from the COOH-terminal which had a molecular weight of 21,000 (Wilson and Foster, 1971).

The site of cleavage by the acid proteinase occurred within the disulfide loop between Cys-390 and Cys-434 at X-Phe in the region of residues 400–403, which has not yet been sequenced (Zurawski *et al.*, 1975). It is noteworthy that the cleavage of one peptide bond in BSA resulted in a modified molecule which acquired an increased Stokes radius and a 15% decrease in helicity (from ORD and CD data). On the other hand, the tertiary structure was only slightly affected, judged by fluorescence emission spectra and binding of 8-anilino-2-naphthalenesulfonic acid. The cleaved albumin showed both the N-F and the neutral transitions, but at a pH closer to the isoionic point, indicating a somewhat weakened stability.

3. Conformation of Reduced-Reoxidized Bovine Serum Albumin and Fragments

Bovine serum albumin contains 17 disulfide bonds. The amino acid sequence (Brown, 1975) shows that the disulfide bonds are arranged in nine loops (see Fig. 4), seven of which are in double loops involving adjacent half-cystines and one double loop where the half-cystines are separated by three amino acid residues. This particular arrangement of the disulfide bonds may impart certain characteristic features to the albumin molecule. Only one disulfide bond was available for reaction with β-mercaptoethanol at pH 7 in aqueous buffer (Habeeb, 1966a), while the remaining disulfide bonds became progressively unmasked in urea as the urea concentration increased from 2 to 6 M. Moreover, the conformational changes associated with the neutral transition resulted in partial exposure of the disulfide bonds to reduction with β-mercaptoethanol (Habeeb, 1977a). Different batches of BSA demonstrated variations in their reducibility. However, on defatting this apparent variability was eliminated. A number of studies were performed to ascertain the recovery of the native conformation after reduction and reoxidation. Such studies have shown that stable isomers were formed which differed from the native albumin in a number of physicochemical properties but still retained some biological activity. Air reoxidation of reduced BSA (with β-mercaptoethanol in 8 M urea or 6 M guanidine hydrochloride) yielded a mixture of polymers and a monomer (Andersson, 1969). Although the monomer had the same elution volume on Sephadex and sedimentation coefficient as native BSA, it differed from it in optical rotation, solubility-pH profile in 3 M KCl, and tryptophan fluorescence (indicating a relocation of the tryptophan in a more hydrophobic environment). The yield of monomer was improved if the sulfhydryl group was free (Taylor *et al.*, 1975). The monomer was heterogeneous and contained less than 10% of native albumin (Andersson, 1969). It is significant that the reoxidation of reduced BSA in the presence of 3×10^{-5} M sodium caprylate or in 2×10^{-5} M sodium palmitate yielded a monomer which contained 80% native albumin as shown by optical rotation and tryptophan fluorescence. Also, binding studies with fluorescein or methyl orange indicated an impurity of 5-10% which did not have the native conformation. That fatty acids were necessary to recover the native conformation on reoxidation of reduced BSA may indicate that fatty acids participate in inducing the correct folding of the native conformation during its biosynthesis. At least in the case of BSA, the recovery of the native conformation is dependent on the presence of fatty acids. Peters and Goetzl (1969) also observed that reduced and reoxidized BSA yielded six components which differed in the elution volume on Sephadex and also in their electro-phoretic mobility. However, a monomer was formed (in 40–50% yield) which was partially unfolded as shown by optical rotatory dispersion measurments. The unfolded protein may represent a derivative with mis-matched disulfide bonds. Distribution of the disulfide bonds of BSA in the nine loops, which contain half-cystines in close proximity, may favor this incorrect pairing. It is remarkable that this nonnative BSA was able to react equally as well as BSA with antisera to BSA (Peters and Goetzl, 1969) and also to recover 61–72% of its catalytic activity of decomposing a Meisenheimer complex (Taylor *et al.*, 1975). Such behavior is rather unusual and may be due to certain characteristic structural features of BSA. Most notable is the possibilty that the mismatched disulfide bonds occur within the two disulfide bonds of a given loop and not between the disulfide bonds from different loops. It is likely that the antigenic sites as well as the catalytic site are regenerated despite the unfolding at regions outside the antigenic or catalytic sites.

Refolding of reduced BSA is accelerated by glutathione or rat liver disulfide interchange enzyme (Teale and Benjamin, 1976a). The degree of refolding was assessed from the regain of immunochemical reactivity. From its ability to inhibit the reaction of [^{125}I]-BSA with anti-BSA, the refolded monomer was assumed to represent the native structure since it inhibited the reaction of [^{125}I]-BSA–anti-BSA by 100%, irrespective of whether it was derived from glutathione reoxidation or air reoxidation. Moreover, all the monomers showed similar tryptophan fluorescence emission maxima. The results of Teale and Benjamin (1976a) are in contrast to those reported by Andersson (1969), and also by Peters and Goetzl (1969) in which various physicochemical studies indicated that the recovered monomer was nonnative in conformation. However, in the case of BSA, the recovered "nonnative" albumin reacted as well as native albumin with anti-BSA (Peters and Goetzl, 1969). Therefore, the inhibition of [^{125}I]-BSA–anti-BSA by refolded BSA shown by Teale and Benjamin (1976a) cannot be considered as proof of its native structure. At the moment, the two sets of results cannot be reconciled. Catalyzed reoxidation of reduced BSA and fragments 377–581, 198–581, 115–184, 1–183, 184–581, 1–306, and 184–306 (by the microsomal enzyme or glu-tathione system) was studied by Teale and Benjamin (1976b). They pre-pared "restricted antibodies" against given fragments by passing anti-BSA on an immunoadsorbent of the respective fragment. These "re-stricted" antibodies were used with [^{125}I]-BSA as a probe to determine the extent of re-formation of the native antigenic sites on reoxidation of reduced BSA or its fragments, and also the re-formation of a given domain on reoxidation of reduced BSA. It was shown by this immunochemical method that certain regions of BSA folded faster than others. The extent of folding of various segments within the albumin molecule followed the sequence 115–184 (75%) > 377–581 (60%) > albumin (47%) > 1–183, 184–581, 184–306 (33%). Regions 115–184 and 377–581 refolded faster, while sequence 1–306 (NH_2-terminal) was slightly slower than sequence 184–581 (COOH-terminal). The results show that smaller peptides folded faster than larger ones; for example, compare sequences 377–581 and 184–581, 115–184 and 1–183, and 184–581 and 184–306. Both fragments 198–581 and 377–581 regained their native structures after reduction and reoxidation when tested immunochemically using [^{125}I]-BSA and the restricted antibody. Using fragments 377–581, 198–581, and 1–581, and anti-377–581, it was reported that the degrees of refolding of the reduced and reoxidized fragments were 377–581 > 198–581 > 1–581. These results indicated that refolding of fragment 377–581 (third domain) was slowed by the presence of the second domain and still more by the presence of both the second and first domains.

Several comments are in order concerning the results of Teale and Benjamin (1976a,b): (1) The validity of obtaining restricted antibodies against fragments 1–183, 184–581, 377–581, 184–306, and 115–184 by adsorption on immunoadsorbents of these fragments is unresolved. This is especially so in light of the concept that BSA has repeating, identical antigenic sites (Atassi et al., 1976b; Habeeb and Atassi, 1976b, 1977), which was derived from studies where it was demonstrated that while neither fragment 11–193 nor fragment 377–571 precipitated with anti-BSA, each by itself inhibited the reaction of BSA–anti-BSA almost completely (89–93%). Also, each fragment on an immunoadsorbent removed almost all (89–95%) of the BSA antibodies. Antibodies to each fragment cross-reacted and were completely removed by immunoadsorbents of the homologous or heterologous fragments and with BSA. (2) The validity of using anti-BSA to measure the recovery of the native structure is in doubt in light of the work of Peters and Goetzl (1969), where it was shown that despite the absence of the native structure after reduction and reoxidation of BSA the immunochemical reactivity was undiminished. Moreover, the recovery of the catalytic activity toward the Meisenheimer complex was 73% (Taylor et al., 1975). In other words, the experiments of Peters and Goetzl (1969) and Taylor et al. (1975) demonstrated that the antigenic reactive sites and the catalytic site, respectively, were recovered despite the absence of native structure (less than 10%, by Andersson, 1969). (3) The impediment of the folding of a given segment by the presence of a larger fragment (e.g., 115–184 compared to 1–183 and 377–581 compared to 198–581 and 1–581) is rather unusual, since it has been shown that at least with ribonuclease, lysozyme, myoglobin, and staphylococcal nuclease the entire polypeptide chain is essential for the native folding of the molecule. Moreover, Hilak *et al.* (1974) showed that the stability of fragments of BSA increased with an increase in chain length. At least in the case of BSA and its fragments, the immunochemical method is incapable of differentiating between the native and nonnative structure. (4) The degree of cross-reactivity of these "restricted" antibodies was not determined, and the possibility exists that they represent anti-BSA antibodies with different affinities. (5) The purity or homogeneity of the product of reduction and reoxidation of BSA fragments was not established, and therefore the accuracy of the results will be overshadowed by the presence of inactive contaminants such as aggregates, monomers with mismatched disulfide bonds.

    The recovery of the native conformation of fragment 1–306 or 307–581 on reduction and reoxidation was estimated from the catalytic activity of reduced and reoxidized fragment in the presence of the native complementary fragment (Taylor and Silver, 1976) and was compared to the activity of a mixture of native fragments 1–306 and 307–581. The activity recovered when refolded fragment 307–581 was added to native complementary fragment was 45% compared to 15% with refolded fragment 1–306. Based on recovery of catalytic activity (Taylor and Silver 1976), these results demonstrate that fragment 307–581 showed a greater tendency to recover the native conformation than did fragment 1–306. However, the results may only mean the partial recovery of the catalytic site, which may be insensitive to various conformational perturbations at other parts of the albumin molecule (as shown by Andersson, 1969; Peters and Goetzl, 1969).

III. Immunochemistry of Chemical Derivatives of Bovine Serum Albumin

    In order to identify the amino acid residues in the antigenic reactive sites, the following three approaches have so far been pursued in BSA: (1) studies on the immunochemistry and conformation of chemical derivatives of BSA specifically modified at particular amino acid residues, (2) the isolation of immunochemically reactive fragments liberated by proteolytic digestion of the protein, and (3) studies of the effects of chemical modification of selected amino acid residues on the immunochemistry and conformation of these immunochemically reactive peptides.

    The chemical modification approach for probing the nature of a protein active site is extremely valuable, especially if the specificity of the reagent is well documented, the derivative is purified and character-ized, and any resultant conformational changes are determined. When a modification gives rise to a conformational change, interpretations of the alteration in activity will be difficult. However, the absence of both a conformational alteration (by several parameters) and a change in activity may suggest nonparticipation of the modified residues in a reactive site. In this latter case, the nature of the modification must be considered since it has been shown (Atassi and Habeeb, 1969; Habeeb and Atassi, 1971) that the nature of the modification determines its influence on the biological activity. The modification may not, in fact, be chemically or sterically sufficient to impair the participation of the side chain in the biological role in which it is normally involved (Atassi and Habeeb, 1969). It is therefore advantageous to modify a given amino acid side chain by more than one reagent.

The amount of work on the effect of chemical modification on the immunochemical reactivity of BSA is rather limited, and the role of several amino acid residues on the antigenic reactive site has not yet been established. Notwithstanding, the studies that were accomplished to date will be reviewed.

A. Modification of the Cystine Residues in Bovine Serum Albumin

Bovine serum albumin has 17 disulfide bonds of which only one is available to reduction at pH 7 in aqueous buffers (Habeeb, 1966a, 1977a); the remaining disulfide bonds become progressively unmasked in the presence of urea as the urea concentration increases from 2 to 6 M. Moreover, in the region of the neutral transition (pH 7.5–9.5), a progres-sive increase in availability of the disulfide bonds to reduction is obtained with considerable variation from batch to batch whether albumin used is Cohn fraction V, crystallized, or defatted. It is shown that the number of reducible disulfide bonds varied between 3.5 and 10.5 in five batches of Cohn fraction V, and between 5 and 11 in three batches of crystalline BSA, but was remarkably constant at 11 disulfide bonds in four batches of defatted BSA (Habeeb, 1977a). This number of reducible disulfide bonds is an average number, and heterogeneity of the reaction product is to be considered as a possibility. A number of studies were performed to ascertain the role played by the disulfide bonds on the immunochemical reactivity of BSA.

Under conditions of partial or even complete sulfitolysis of BSA, a heterogeneous reaction product was obtained (Habeeb and Borella, 1966). Two components were separated by Sephadex G-200 chromatography. The first component was eluted at the void volume and represented unfolded molecules with cleaved disulfide bonds (S-BSA), and the second eluted as BSA and had two disulfide bonds cleaved. With progressive sulfitolysis, the proportion of the first component increased and was accompanied by an increase in the number of cleaved disulfide bonds. Bovine serum albumin derivative (with two disulfide bonds cleaved) had about 88% ability to react with anti-BSA while S-BSA showed complete loss of activity by the Farr technique (Farr, 1958) on scission of nine or more disulfide bonds (Habeeb and Borella, 1966; Goetzl and Peters, 1972). Completely reduced and alkylated BSA showed a highly disordered structure; the helical content dropped to 16–23% compared to 36–47% for BSA with one reduced disulfide bond and 52–58% for native BSA (Goetzl and Peters, 1972). The results would indicate that some of the disulfide bonds are important for maintaining the conformation of (or are part of) the antigenic sites.

Reduction and reoxidation of BSA yielded six components which differed in their elution volume on Sephadex G-100 and their electrophoretic mobility on starch gel (Peters and Goetzl, 1969). A monomer was recovered in 40–50% yield whose conformation was stable and was significantly different from that of native BSA (values for b_0 and $[m']_{233}$ were 50–60% lower than those for native BSA). It was remarkable that several reduced and reoxidized BSA preparations which demonstrated variation in the relative amount of polymers and monomer were capable of precipitating with anti-BSA (92% compared to native BSA). However, the monomer of reduced and reoxidized albumin had equal reactivity (107%) to that of BSA with antisera to the native protein despite the marked conformational alteration, which may be due to generation of a molecule with erroneous disulfide pairing. Such behavior is rather unusual and may be due to certain characteristic structural features of BSA and its antigenic sites. Most notable is the possibility that mismatched disulfide bonds occur within the two contiguous disulfide bonds at the ends of a loop and not between the disulfide bonds from different loops. Such restriction in the reformation of the disulfide bonds may lead to the generation of the antigenic sites despite the unfolding at regions outside the antigenic reactive sites. At least in this case, the immunochemical reactivity cannot be used as a criterion for recovery of the native conformation.

B. Modification of Amino Groups

Modification of the amino groups by acetylation with acetic anhydride and deamination by nitrous acid yielded derivatives which showed decreased cross-reactivity with anti-BSA (Maurer *et al.*, 1957). The cross-reactivity amounted to 41–50% with various acetylated derivatives and 66–74% with deaminated BSA. Guanidination resulted in retention of the immunochemical reactivity. Neither the specificity of the reaction nor the resultant conformational changes brought about by the modification were evaluated. The acetylation and deamination reactions are known to be extremely nonselective (for review, see Atassi, 1977*b*).

An extensive study on the role of the amino groups on the immunochemical reactivity of bovine serum albumin was performed (Habeeb, 1967*a,b*, 1968*a*). Several derivatives of bovine serum albumin were prepared by succinylation (Habeeb, 1967*a*), guanidination, amidination, and nitroguanidination (Habeeb, 1967*b*) and by paired modification via succinylation followed by guanidination or nitroguanidination (Habeeb, 1967*b*) or via succinylation followed by amidination. The conformational changes were assessed by (1) determination of the Stokes radius on a calibrated Sephadex G-200 column (Habeeb, 1966*b*), which provides a workable parameter for comparing the overall shape of the molecule, and (2) the availability of the disulfide bonds for reaction with β-mercaptoethanol or sodium sulfite as a probe for conformational changes which affect the vicinity of the disulfide bonds (Habeeb, 1966*a*).

On succinylation of bovine serum albumin, a progressive increase in the Stokes radius of the protein with increased modification was observed. The initial increase in the Stokes radius was gradual up to a modification of 34 amino groups, and then it was followed by a steeper increase on further modification (Fig. 15). However, the availability of the disulfide bonds to sulfitolysis remained unchanged up to succinylation of about 30 amino groups, and then it was followed by a pronounced increase in the reactivity of disulfide bonds with further succinylation. A sharp increase in the electrophoretic mobility (from -5 to -9.3 cm²/V/sec $\times$ 10^{-5}) accompanied the succinylation of up to 30 amino groups, and then it reached -9.8 cm²/V/sec $\times$ 10^{-5} with complete succinylation (Cherry, 1964). These results indicated that the first 30–34 amino groups occupied surface positions on bovine serum albumin domains and that their succinylation was accompanied by minor shape changes (probably as a result of separation of the globular domains) despite the considerable increase in net negative charge. Moreover, the availability of the disulfide bonds to reaction was unchanged, indicating retention of the native compact structures of the domains. This phenomenon is analogous to that observed for BSA at the N-F transition. On further succinylation of more than 34 amino groups (which probably occupy internal positions), the native conformation was disrupted, possibly because of introduction of short-range repulsive forces in place of short-range attractive forces in the native molecule. This conformational disruption was shown by the steep increase in both the Stokes radius and accessibility of the disulfide bonds to reaction. The ability of various succinylated derivatives of BSA to react with antisera to BSA was investigated (Habeeb, 1967a) as a function of the number of modified amino groups and also of the Stokes radius as a conformational parameter. It was shown (Habeeb, 1967a) that the amount of precipitated antibody decreased slowly, followed by a sharper decrease with increase in the number of amino groups modified (Fig. 16). The initial region corresponded to minimal conformational alteration of the antigen, while the latter part was associated with significant conformational changes due to modification. Immunochemical reactivity was most likely influenced by conformational changes rather than charge effects, since the initial region where the change in the net charge was maximal exhibited minimal decrease in immunochemical reactivity. On the other hand, the second stage, where the change in net charge was

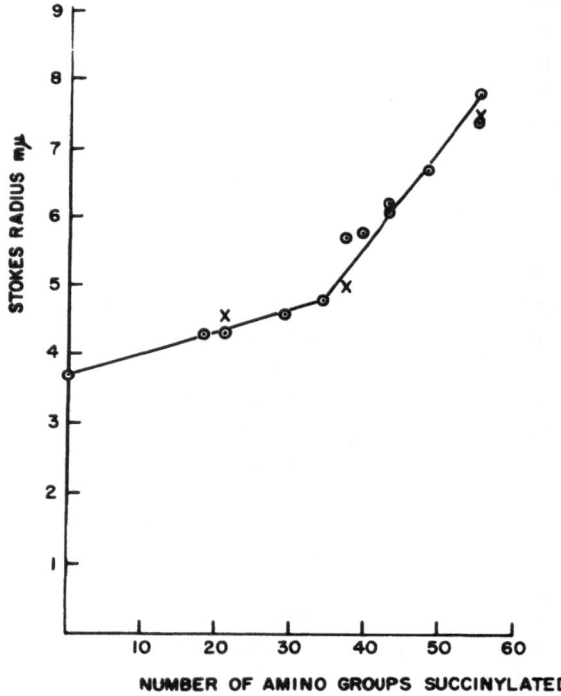

Figure 15. Relationship between the Stokes radius and the number of amino groups succinylated in bovine serum albumin. $\bigcirc$, Values obtained from a calibrated Sephadex G-200 column; $\times$, values calculated from diffusion coefficient determined with the ultracentrifuge. From Habeeb (1967a).

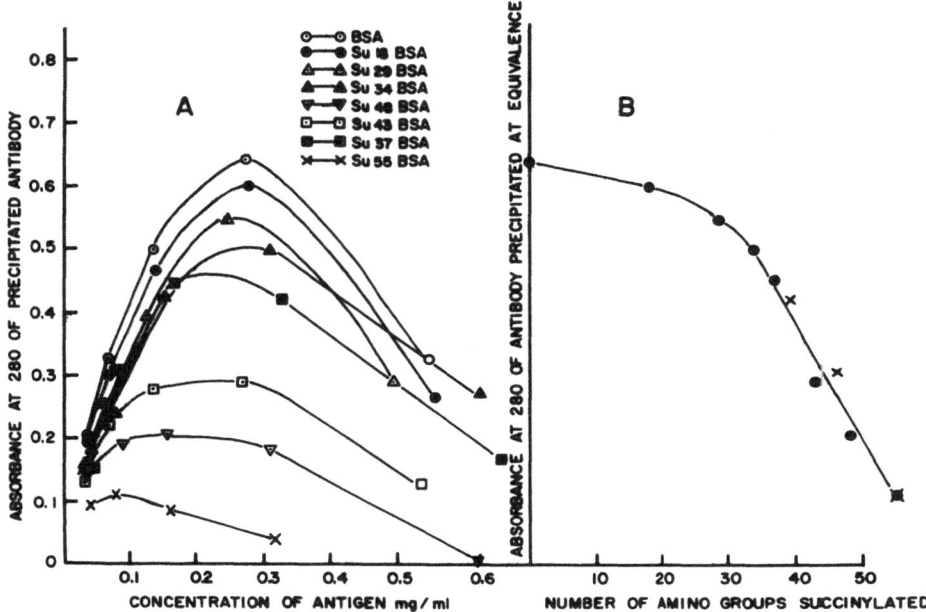

Figure 16. A: Quantitative precipitin curves obtained with various succinylated bovine serum albumin (Su-BSA) and anti-bovine serum albumin. The subscript indicates the number of amino groups modified. B: Amount of anti-BSA antibodies precipitated with various Su-BSA at equivalence as a function of amino groups succinylated. ●, Monomer; ×, aggregate. From Habeeb (1967a).

minimal but showed major conformational alteration, exhibited considerable loss in immunochemical reactivity. A recovery of about 50% of the native precipitation capacity for fully succinylated BSA was achieved by performing the precipitin reaction at pH 5.3 (Cherry, 1964), a pH at which renaturation was 72% as revealed from optical rotation.

Various succinylated BSA (Su-BSA) derivatives, e.g., Su_{32}-BSA and Su_{57}-BSA (partially and extensively modified), were found to be antigenic in rabbits. When a group of succinylated BSA preparations representing different degrees of modification was tested by quantitative precipitin reaction with anti-BSA, anti-Su-$_{32}$-BSA, and anti-Su$_{57}$-BSA, maximum precipitation occurred with the homologous antigen. A relationship was found between the amount of antibody precipitated and the Stokes radius of the antigen (Habeeb, 1967a). Initially a small decrease in the precipitated antibody occurred as the Stokes radius of the antigen either increased or decreased (Fig. 17) compared to the homologous antigen and was then followed by a sharp reduction in the precipitated antibody.

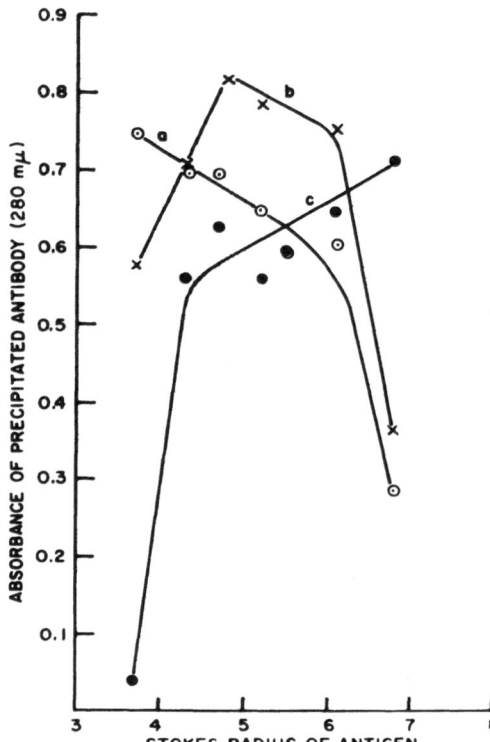

Figure 17. Relationship between the antibody precipitated at equivalence and the Stokes radius of different preparations of succinylated BSA by using (a) anti-BSA, (b) anti-Su_{32}-BSA, and (c) anti-Su_{57}-BSA. From Habeeb (1967a).

This behavior was attributed to the extensive unfolding of the antigen, which would drastically disrupt the antigenic reactive sites and diminish the complementarity of the antigen-antibody binding sites. The above results indicated that the conformational changes accompanying succinylation interfered in the unambiguous interpretation of the role of amino groups in the antigenic active sites of BSA.

Therefore, in order to limit the conformational changes that accompany the modification of the amino groups, several modifications were performed, as well as combinations of these modifications. Guanidination (using 1-guanyl-3,5-dimethylpyrazole nitrate, Habeeb, 1959, 1960, 1972), amidination (by ethyl acetamidate, Wofsy and Singer, 1963), and nitroguanidination (by nitroguanyl-3,5-dimethylpyrazole, Habeeb, 1964) effected 90% modification of the amino groups. Amidination and guanidination of BSA did not affect its net electric charge or its overall shape, the latter being determined from the Stokes radius or intrinsic viscosity. In contrast, nitroguanidinated BSA was more electronegative than Su-

BSA, yet it exhibited limited unfolding compared to the latter as shown by determinations of the Stokes radius and the availability of the disulfide bonds to reaction (Table V). The immunochemical reactivity of guanidinated (Gu-), amidinated (Am-), and nitroguanidinated (NG-) BSA with anti-BSA was 84–91% that of BSA (Habeeb, 1967b), indicating that the amino groups were not part of the antigenic reactive sites in BSA, despite the variety of size and charge of the substituents at the amino groups of albumin. Paired modifications of BSA at the amino groups were performed to effect derivatization of the amino groups which were situated in different parts of the molecule by a variety of reagents. The initial modification was by introducing 21 succinyl groups, which resulted in a slight increase of the Stokes radius and a significant increase in the net negative charge. The latter was probably just enough to cause a slight shift between the globular domains of the albumin molecule, thereby resulting in a 7% decrease in the immunochemical reactivity. After the initial succinylation, the remaining amino groups were exhaustively modified by guanidination or nitroguanidination. It was shown that a slight decrease in immunochemical reactivity accompanied the second modification in $Su_{21}Gu_{33}$-BSA (from 93% to 88%) and more with $Su_{21}NG_{34}$-BSA (from 93% to 80%). In the latter, there was marked conformational al-

Table V.   Properties of Modified Bovine Serum Albumin and Their Immunochemical Reactivity with Anti-Bovine Serum Albumin[a]

Antigen[b]	Stokes radius (nm)	Number of disulfide groups reacted	Percent reactivity with anti-BSA
Bovine serum albumin (BSA)	3.7	1.2	100
Su_{12}-BSA	4.3	1.0	93
Su_{32}-BSA	4.7	1.2	93
Su_{37}-BSA	5.2	2.1	87
Su_{39}-BSA	5.5	2.6	80
Su_{43}-BSA	6.1	3.1	81
Su_{57}-BSA	6.8	9.6	38
$Su_{21}Gu_{33}$-BSA	4.3	1.0	88
$Su_{21}NG_{34}$-BSA	5.7	6.5	80
Am_{58}-BSA	3.9	1.9	84
Gu_{54}-BSA	3.8	2.7	91
NG_{54}-BSA	4.5	1.9	84

[a] From Habeeb (1967b).
[b] Su, succinyl; Gu, guanyl; NG, nitroguanyl; Am, amidinated. The numerical subscript denotes the number of amino groups modified.

teration (Table V), which may account for the decrease. These results with paired modification extended and confirmed the data obtained with guanidinated, amidinated, and nitroguanidinated albumin that the amino groups were not part of the antigenic reactive sites.

Although guanidinated, nitroguanidinated, and amidinated, bovine serum albumin ($Su_{21}Gu_{33}$-, $Su_{21}NG_{34}$-, and $Su_{21}Am_{35}$-BSA) showed strong immunochemical reactivity (80–91%) with anti-bovine serum albumin (indicating that almost all the antigenic reactive sites were retained), the response of the injected rabbits to these immunogens was dramatically altered (Habeeb, 1967b, 1968a). Each antigen was recognized by the injected animal in a distinct way; for example, new sites appeared as immunodominant and others became silent. These results demonstrated that, in two cross-reacting proteins, reciprocal cross-reactivity did not coincide with cross-reactivity and the specificity of the antibody in each case was distinctly different.

The specificity of the antibody depended on the groups introduced. Antibodies to BSA constituted 60% of the specificity in antisera to amidinated BSA, 42% of antisera to guanidinated BSA (Habeeb, 1968a), 76% of antisera to Su_{32}-BSA, 8% of antisera to Su_{57}-BSA, 71% of anti-$Su_{21}Gu_{33}$-BSA, and 23% of anti-$Su_{21}NG_{34}$-BSA. The introduction of nitroguanyl groups dramatically modified the specificity of the antibody in such a way that the major specificity was directed against the nitroguanyl group either as nitrohomoarginine or at antigenic sites with carrier specificity (Habeeb, 1967b). Antibodies directed against each specificity were sequentially adsorbed by the appropriate antigen. Thus anti-$Su_{21}NG_{34}$-BSA was sequentially adsorbed with BSA, Su_{21}-BSA, and $Su_{21}NG_{34}$-BSA to quantitatively determine antibodies of each specificity. It was observed that in antisera to a derivative of BSA the proportion of antibodies with a specificity directed against BSA increased progressively with immunization (Habeeb, 1967b, 1968a, 1969) (Table VI).

Soluble aggregates of bovine serum albumin prepared by glutaraldehyde-induced intermolecular cross-links retained the ability to precipitate all the antibodies from anti-BSA (Habeeb and Hiramoto, 1968). However, distinct quantitative differences were apparent, reflected by a decrease in antibody molar ratio from 6 in the BSA–anti-BSA system to 3 in aggregated BSA–anti-BSA, which indicated that 50% of antigenic sites were masked by polymerization. Glutaraldehyde-aggregated bovine serum albumin elicited the production of antibodies in rabbits. Antibodies with specificity directed to BSA amounted to 50%, and the remainder were directed against new antigenic determinants generated by the modification (Habeeb, 1969).

Table VI. Percentage of Precipitating
Antibodies with Specificity against Bovine
Serum Albumin in Antiserum against
Modified Albumin in Early and Late
Bleeding[a,b]

Antibody against the following antigen	Anti-bovine serum albumin	
	5- to 7-wk bleeding (%)	13- to 15-wk bleeding (%)
Am_{58}-BSA	60	85
Gu_{54}-BSA	42	67
$Su_{21}Am_{35}$-BSA	67	70
GL_{54}-BSA	47	67

[a] From Habeeb (1968a, 1969).
[b] Am, amidinated; Gu, guanidinated; Su, succinylated; GL, glutaraldehyde cross-linked. The numerical subscript denotes the number of amino groups modified.

C. Modification of Carboxylic Groups of Bovine Serum Albumin

Esterification of the carboxyl groups of BSA with methanol HCl resulted in modified derivatives which suffered conformational changes reflected by an increased negative specific rotation, increased susceptibility to tryptic hydrolysis, and reduced peptic hydrolysis (Sri Ram and Maurer, 1959b). Although complete loss of precipitation (with anti-BSA) on 50% esterification was observed (Sri Ram and Maurer, 1959a), soluble complexes were formed between esterified BSA and anti-BSA shown by complement fixation. The presence of conformational alteration as a result of chemical modification together with the poor selectivity of the esterification reaction and the instability of the ester group (for review, see Atassi, 1977a) complicated the interpretation of the data in an unambiguous way.

IV. Immunochemistry of Fragments of Bovine Serum Albumin

The isolation of a large number of immunochemically reactive fragments with a variety of overlaps and representing various parts of the molecule affords a very effective approach to localizing the antigenic

reactive sites of proteins (Atassi, 1972, 1975; Habeeb and Atassi, 1976b).
The success of this approach depends on isolating fragments with little
disruption of the conformation so that the antigenic site remains intact.
In the case of BSA, the fragmentation has to be invariably effected on
the native protein without cleavage of the disulfide bonds.

A. Cleavage by Chymotrypsin

Early studies by Porter (1957) utilizing chymotrypsin, papain, trypsin, mold protease, and pepsin to cleave BSA indicated that digestion
with either trypsin or chymotrypsin yielded immunochemically reactive
fragments. However, the immunochemical activity of the fragments was
greater with chymotrypsin. A pure fragment was isolated from a chymotryptic hydrolysate (pH 8, 14 days, 25°C) of BSA. The fragment had
a molecular weight of about 12,000 but rapidly dimerized. Its amino acid
analysis revealed a free sulfhydryl, one disulfide bond, one tyrosine,
and an absence of tryptophan. However, from its composition and the
presently known amino acid sequence of BSA, this fragment cannot be
placed within the structure of the protein (Brown, 1975). Antisera to BSA
from different rabbits and from the same rabbit after different periods of
immunizations showed considerable variation in reaction with the fragment. The reason for this variability is unknown and remains unex-
plained. With one rabbit antiserum, the fragment gave 25% precipitation
relative to BSA. However, serum from the same animal (late bleeding)
was inhibited completely from reaction with BSA by the fragment at a
molar ratio of fragment to BSA of as low as 1.8:1 (Porter, 1957). The
significance of this observation was overlooked and may be explainable
by the concept that BSA contains repeating identical antigenic sites
(Atassi *et al.*, 1976b; Habeeb and Atassi, 1976a,b, 1977). The inhibitory
activity of the fragment was lost by heating or reduction of the disulfide
bond, thus demonstrating the dependence of the immunochemical reactivity of the fragment on its conformation.

B. Cleavage by Cyanogen Bromide

Cleavage of BSA by cyanogen bromide (King and Spencer, 1968,
1970) generated two fragments, an N fragment (molecular weight 22,000)
corresponding to sequence Asp_1–Met_{183} with one scission at Met_{87}–Ala_{88}
and a C fragment (molecular weight 44,000) corresponding to sequence
Arg_{184}–Ala_{581} with two scissions at Met_{443}–Pro_{444} and Met_{545}–Glu_{546}. The

C fragment inhibited the reaction of [^{131}I]-BSA–anti-BSA by 65%, while the N fragment inhibited the reaction by 40%, indicating no loss in antigenic sites on cleavage (Benjamin and Weigle, 1971). Moreover, the fragments did not cross-react. These results are not in accord with Porter's (1957) observation and more recent work (Atassi *et al.*, 1976*b*; Habeeb and Atassi, 1976*b*) that BSA contains repeating identical or related determinant.

C. Cleavage of Citraconyl-BSA by Trypsin

Based on the observation that reversible masking of the amino groups by citraconylation induced conformational changes in a protein which rendered it accessible to tryptic cleavage at arginine residues (Habeeb and Atassi, 1970; Singhal and Atassi, 1971; Atassi and Habeeb, 1972), we introduced a novel cleavage approach (Atassi *et al.*, 1973) for obtaining fragments with intact disulfide bonds from "tight" proteins. After unmasking of the amino groups, cleavage at the lysyl residues can be achieved, if desired, thus yielding the tryptic peptides with intact disulfide bonds. Bovine serum albumin was subjected, by this procedure, to cleavage at arginine residues (giving the Arg-peptides) or at the arginine as well as the lysine residues (giving Arg,Lys-peptides) (Habeeb *et al.*, 1974). The Arg-peptides did not precipitate with antisera to BSA but inhibited by 83% the reaction of BSA with its antisera and by 97% its reaction with the IgG fraction of the antisera. The IgG fraction accounted for 96% of the total antibody activity in the antisera. The Arg,Lys-peptides had no inhibitory activity. Following this work, a homogeneous fragment was isolated from Arg-peptides by gel filtration on Sephadex G-100 (Atassi *et al.*, 1976*b*). Its purity was established by disk electrophoresis, and its molecular weight was 25,000 by gel filtration on a calibrated Sephadex G-100 column and 23,000 by sodium dodecylsulfate (SDS) gel electrophoresis. From its amino acid composition and NH$_2$-terminal sequence determination of the first 14 residues, it was possible to locate this fragment at sequence 11–193 (less Arg-144) of BSA (Fig. 18). Its molecular weight calculated from its sequence was 20,947. The immunochemistry of the fragment was studied in detail (Atassi *et al.*, 1976*b*). This fragment had an inhibitory activity of 80% toward the precipitin reaction of BSA with its antisera and 88% toward the reaction of BSA with the IgG fraction of the antisera. An immunoadsorbent of the peptide held 84–89% of the total anti-BSA antibody. The fragment was reacted with fluorescein isothiocyanate, and the derivative was found to bind and coelute with antibody to BSA on gel filtration on Sephadex G-

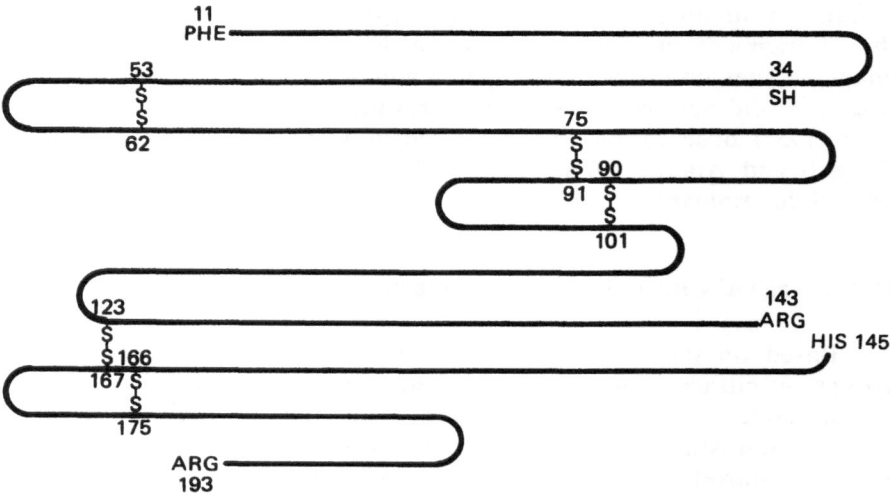

Figure 18.   Position of the disulfide bonds in fragment Phe$_{11}$–Arg$_{193}$ which enable the pieces to remain covalently attached after scission at Arg$_{143}$ and Arg$_{144}$ and removal of the latter. From Atassi *et al.* (1976*b*).

75 column. Two molecules of antibody were bound per mole of peptide. Intactness of the disulfide bonds was essential for maintenance of the inhibitory activity of the peptide. Its immunochemical reactivity was completely destroyed on rupture of the disulfide bonds by performic acid oxidation or by reduction followed by carboxymethylation. Also, cleavage at lysyl peptide bonds, without rupture of the disulfide bonds, destroyed the inhibitory activity of the peptide, because of scission of the polypeptide chain at (or in proximity of) the antigenic reactive sites. Since the peptide comprised less than a third of BSA molecule but accounted for almost all the BSA antigenic reactivity, it was concluded that native BSA carried equivalent antigenic reactive sites (Atassi *et al.*, 1976*b*).

D. Cleavage by Trypsin

A further support to this view has been afforded from our isolation of another fragment from a tryptic digest of bovine serum albumin (Habeeb and Atassi, 1976*a,b*). The fragmentation pattern of crystalline native BSA by trypsin was studied (Habeeb and Atassi, 1976*a,b*) in aqueous solution under various conditions with regard to the yield and size of the fragments obtained. From a partial tryptic hydrolysate of BSA at pH 8.2 (40°C, 1 hr), a homogeneous fragment was isolated in high yield by gel filtration on Sephadex G-100 followed by chromatography on DEAE-cellulose (Fig. 19). The molecular weight of the fragment as determined by gel filtration on a calibrated Sephadex G-100 column and by SDS gel electrophoresis was 22,500. After reduction of the disulfide bonds followed by alkylation with iodoacetamide, the fragment retained its homogeneity by disk electrophoresis and its molecular weight was unchanged, indicating that it was composed of a single peptide chain. From its amino acid composition, sequence of the first 20 residues, and action of carboxypeptidase A or B, it was assigned to sequence 377–571 of BSA (Habeeb and Atassi, 1976a,b). The immunochemistry of the fragment was studied in detail. The inhibitory activity of the fragment was 90–93% toward the immune reaction of BSA with the IgG fraction of antisera to BSA (Fig. 20). An immunoadsorbent of fragment 377–571 removed 89–95% of the antibody to BSA. A fluorescent derivative of the fragment, which retained full immunochemical reactivity, was found to bind and was recovered in the antibody fraction by gel filtration on Sephadex G-75 (Fig. 21). Two moles of antibody was found to bind to 1 mol of fragment 377–571. The disulfide bonds in the peptide were essential for

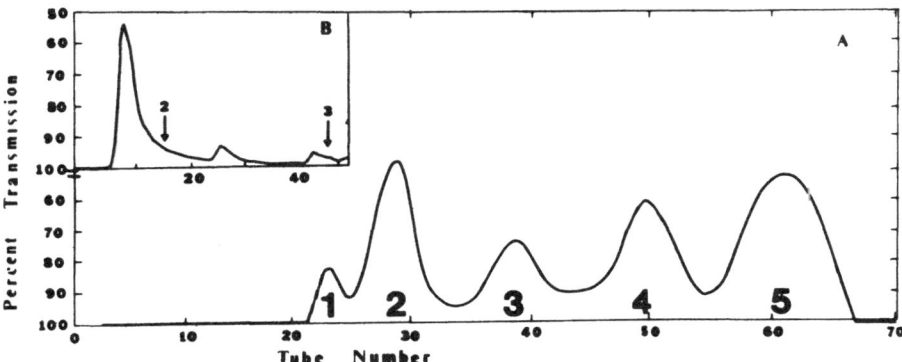

Figure 19.   A: Gel filtration pattern of a 40°C tryptic hydrolysate (1 hr) of bovine serum albumin. The hydrolysate (0.3 g) was applied onto a column (2.7 × 80 cm) of Sephadex G-100 which was eluted with 0.01 M NH_4HCO_3. Fractions (7.5 ml each) were analyzed continuously by an ultraviolet monitor. B: Chromatographic pattern on DEAE-cellulose of peak 3 from A. The material (100 mg) was applied on a column (1.5 × 20 cm) which was subjected to stepwise elution. Initial elution was with 0.005 M sodium phosphate buffer at pH 6.2. At position 2 the column was eluted with 0.0175 M phosphate buffer pH 6.2, and at position 3 the eluent was changed to 0.0175 M phosphate pH 6.2 plus 0.077 M NaCl. Fractions (3 ml) were read continuously by an ultraviolet monitor. From Habeeb and Atassi (1976b).

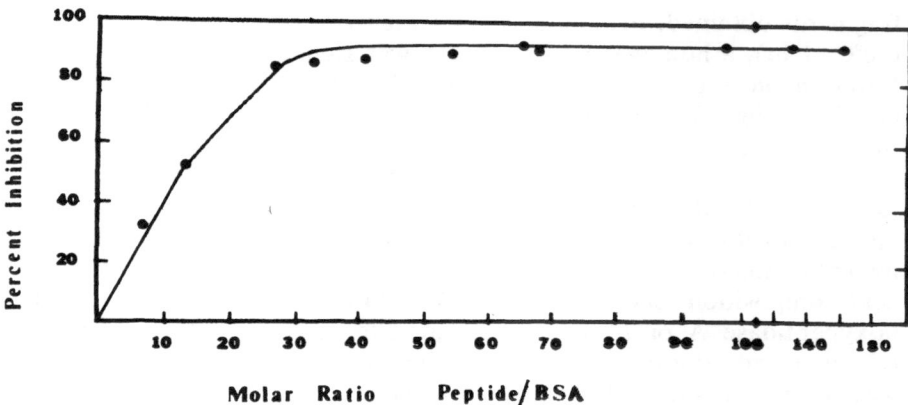

Figure 20.   Inhibition of precipitin reaction of native bovine serum albumin with the IgG fraction of its homologous antiserum by fragment 377–571. The IgG fraction accounted for 95% of the total antibody activity in the antiserum. From Habeeb and Atassi (1976b).

its immunochemical reactivity because the reactivity was abolished on reduction and S-alkylation of the disulfide bonds. Since this fragment comprised only the last third of the BSA molecule, but accounted for 90–95% of its immunochemical reactivity, and since the first third of the BSA molecule also accounted for about 89% of the antigenic reaction of

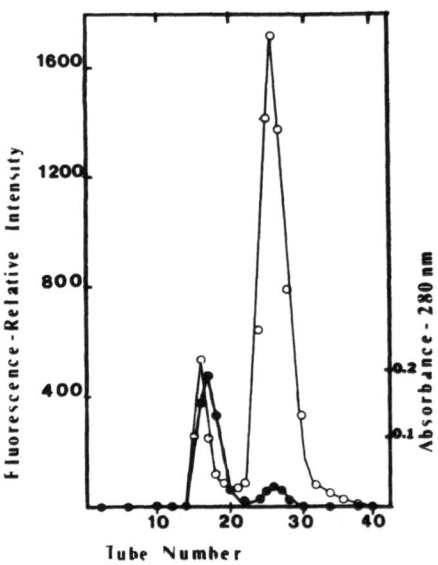

Figure 21.   Elution pattern of a mixture of the IgG fraction of anti-bovine serum albumin and the fluorescent derivative of fragment 377–571 on Sephadex G-100 (1.5 × 86 cm). Fractions (3.3 ml) were monitored for absorbance at 280 nm (●) and for fluorescence at 520 nm (○). From Habeeb and Atassi (1976b).

BSA (Atassi *et al.*, 1976*b*), the immunochemical results can be explained (Atassi *et al.*, 1976*b;* Habeeb and Atassi, 1976*a,b*) only by the concept that BSA carries repeating and immunochemically equivalent or similar antigenic reactive sites.

E. Immunochemical Cross-Reaction of Fragments 11–193 and 377–571

The immunochemical cross-reactions of the fragments were recently studied (Habeeb and Atassi, 1977) in great detail. Both fragments 11–193 and 377–571 were antigenic in rabbits; however, the latter was invariably more immunogenic than the former. Antisera to fragment 377–571 showed substantial cross-reactivity (which increased with time) with BSA and with fragment 11–193 (Table VII and Fig. 22). This cross-reactivity (Habeeb and Atassi, 1977) indicated that antibodies against fragment 377–571 recognized antigenic sites on both BSA and fragment 11–193, the latter was derived from a distant part of BSA, and that its structure was significantly different. It is pertinent to note that the sequence homology between these two fragments is only 18% (Brown, 1976) and involves only one or two amino acid residues. In addition, adsorption of anti-377–571 with BSA removed reactivity with fragment 11–193 and conversely adsorption with fragment 11–193 eliminated reaction with BSA (Table VIII). This finding demonstrated that both BSA and fragment

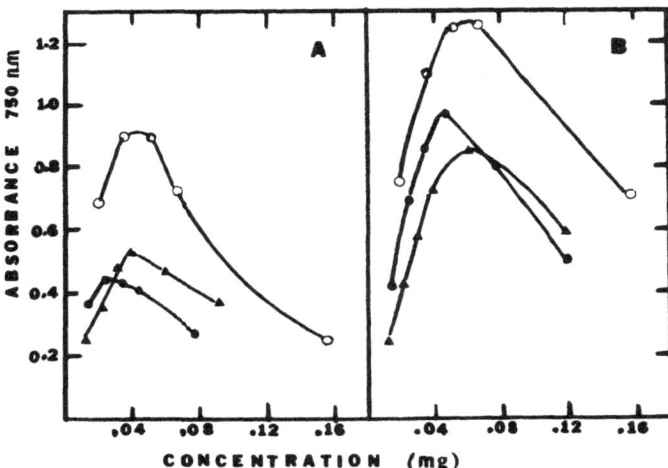

Figure 22. Quantitative precipitin reactions with antisera (489) to fragment 377–571. A: Antiserum from the pool 7- to 10-week bleedings. B: Antiserum from the 11- to 13-week pool. ○, Fragment 377–571; ●, BSA; ▲, fragment 11–193. From Habeeb and Atassi (1977).

Table VII. Quantitative Precipitin Reactions with Antisera to Fragment 377–571[a]

Protein or fragment	Antiserum B5[b]		Antiserum B7[b]		Antiserum 487[c]			Antiserum 488[c]	Antiserum 489[c]	
	18-day bleeding	10-wk bleeding	18-day bleeding	10-wk bleeding	7- to 10-wk pool	11- to 13-wk pool	14- to 16-wk pool	7- to 8-wk pool	7- to 10-wk pool	11- to 13-wk pool
377–571	100	100	100	100	100	100	100	100	100	100
11–193	62.3	93.6	59.0	75.8	17.8	30.9	39.1	47.9	46.4	60.1
BSA	37.1	59.8	62.5	84.5	24.6	60.0	61.1	36.6	38.4	72.0

[a] From Habeeb and Atassi (1977). Values are given in percent precipitation at equivalence relative to reaction of fragment 377–571 with the respective antiserum as 100%. Results represent the average of three to six replicate determinations which varied ±1.2% or less. The percent cross-reaction is based on mg of antibody precipitated at equivalence by each antigen as determined by the Folin reaction and comparison with a standard curve of rabbit IgG run simultaneously.
[b] Single bleedings of these antisera, at the indicated periods after the first injections, were studied.
[c] Antisera from weekly bleedings of the indicated periods after the first injection were pooled in groups, and these pools were studied.

Table VIII.   Reactions of Antisera to Fragment 377–571 after Quantitative
Adsorption with Fragment 11–193

| | Reactions of adsorbed antiserum relative to unadsorbed antiserum[a] | | | | |
| | Antiserum 487[c] | | | Antiserum 489[c] | |
Protein or fragment	7- to 10-wk pool	11- to 13-wk pool	14- to 16-wk pool	7- to 10-wk pool	11- to 13-wk pool
Fragment 11–193[b]	0	0	0	0	0
BSA[b]	6.9	6.3	6.9	5.6	3.1
Fragment 377–571[b]	86.4	60.9	58.8	45.0	34.0
Ab adsorbed by 11–193[d]	21.5	38.7	44.8	38.1	66.1
Total Ab recovery[e]	107.9	99.6	103.6	83.1	100.1

[a] From Habeeb and Atassi (1977). Values are in percent reaction with the adsorbed antiserum relative to the reaction of the unadsorbed antiserum (similarly diluted) with fragment 377–571 as 100%. Results are based on mg antibody precipitated.
[b] Values were determined at equivalence from precipitin curves on each antigen with the adsorbed antiserum, and each represents the average of three or six replicate determinations which varied ±1.2% or less.
[c] See footnote c in Table VII.
[d] This represents the amount of antibody removed on adsorption of the whole antiserum by fragment 11–193 at equivalence.
[e] Value represents the sum of antibody removed by fragment 11–193 and the residual reaction of the supernatant (adsorbed antiserum) with fragment 377–571.

11–193 recognized the same population of antibodies in anti-377–571, which then should be directed against distinct antigenic sites shared by fragments 11–193 and 377–571 and BSA.

Similarly, antisera to fragment 11–193 cross-reacted with both fragment 377–571 and BSA. Furthermore, adsorption of anti-11–193 with fragment 377–571 abolished reaction with BSA, and the reverse was true. These results indicated that antibodies against the antigenic sites on fragment 11–193 recognized the same sites on both BSA and fragment 377–571. It is therefore evident that BSA carries no new antigenic sites that are not expressed on fragment 377–571 despite the fact that the immune response was directed against the NH_2-terminal part 11–193. If this were the case, then both BSA and fragment 11–193 should have equal immunochemical reactivity to that of fragment 377–571 with antisera to the latter. Although with some antisera the cross-reaction was 85–90%, generally it was 50–70% and adsorption neither with BSA nor with fragment 11–193 diminished all immunochemical reactivity with fragment 377–571. This apparent inconsistency was attributed to the presence of soluble immune complex (Habeeb and Atassi, 1977), which was verified to be the case by specific immunoadsorption studies. That an immunoadsorbent carrying BSA or fragment 11–193 was capable of quantitatively removing all antibodies to anti-377–571 (Table IX) clearly demonstrated that no new immunochemical specificity was revealed when fragment 377–571 was used as an immunogen. The behavior of the eluted antibody in quantitative precipitin curves paralleled that of the original antisera. These studies clearly indicated the presence of nonprecipitating antibodies whose precipitating capacity was best manifested with the homologous antigen. Even when they did not precipitate efficiently with BSA or fragment 11–193, they were removable on their respective immunoadsorbent and still showed the same reactivity (in precipitin analysis) as found in the original antisera (i.e., when isolated on the immunoadsorbent they reacted best with the protein or fragment originally used as an immunogen and not with that used for their isolation). It is remarkable that antibodies formed against fragment 377–571 were formed against distinct antigenic sites shared by fragment 11–193 or BSA and conversely antibodies against fragment 11–193 were formed against antigenic sites shared by BSA or fragment 377–571. No new sites other than those on native BSA were able to elicit antibody production on injection of fragment 377–571 or fragment 11–193 representing distant and nonoverlapping parts of the BSA molecule. These results strongly establish that BSA has repeating immunochemically identical or similar antigenic sites. It is not implied that one site is repeating six times, but at least two sites are repeating three times each.

F. Immunochemistry of Chemical Derivatives of Peptide Fragments

The conformations and immunochemical activities of chemical derivatives of fragment 377–571, selectively modified at particular amino acid residues, have been studied (Kazim et al., 1977, 1979) with several antisera prepared against the native fragment as well as against BSA and taken at different times after immunization.

The modification of all four tyrosine residues (Tyr-399, 408, 449, and 494) of fragment 377–571 by nitration with tetranitromethane yielded a homogeneous derivative which, by circular dichroism and optical rotatory dispersion measurements, had suffered no conformational alterations. Disulfide availability studies, however, indicated a slight increase in the reducibility of its disulfide bonds. The nitrated derivative behaved in an identical manner to unmodified peptide 377–571 in precipitin reactions with antisera to 377–571, and was also equally as effective in inhibiting the precipitin reaction of BSA with antisera to BSA. Also, with each of the antisera tested in immunoadsorbent studies, the derivative

Table IX. Immunoadsorbent Studies on Antisera (489) to Fragment 377–571

Immunoadsorbent, antibody recovered and its reactions[a]

Antigen	Whole antiserum	Immunoadsorbent of fragment 377–571		BSA immunoadsorbent		Immunoadsorbent of fragment 11–193	
		Effluent[c]	Ab eluted[d]	Effluent[c]	Ab eluted[d]	Effluent[c]	Ab eluted[d]
I. Antiserum of the 7- to 10-wk pool							
Ab recovered (mg)[b]		0	7.8	0	7.9	0	7.7
BSA	39	0	40	0	49	0	29
Fragment 377–571	100	0	100	0	100	0	100
II. Antiserum of the 11- to 13-wk pool							
Ab recovered (mg)[b]		0	11.7	0	11.9	0	11.3
BSA	72	0	75.4	0	77	0	n.d.
Fragment 377–571	100	0	100	0	100	0	n.d.

[a] From Habeeb and Atassi (1977). Values are given in percent quantitative precipitin reaction at equivalence relative to reaction of fragment 377–571 as 100%. Results represent the average of triplicate analyses which varied ±1.5% or less.

[b] Amount of antibody recovered from 1 ml of whole antiserum applied on the immunoadsorbent.

[c] This fraction represents the amount and reactivity of any antibody that is *not* bound on the immunoadsorbent.

[d] This represents the amount and reactivity of the antibody fraction that was displaced from the immunoadsorbent by 5 M guanidine hydrochloride. After dialysis against 0.01 M phosphate buffer at pH 7.4 containing 0.15 M NaCl, its quantitative precipitin reactions with BSA and fragment 377–571 were determined.

and unmodified peptide 377–571 adsorbed identical amounts of antibodies from antisera to peptide 377–571 and antisera to BSA. The absence of changes in the immunochemical reactivity of this derivative, which was accompanied by a preservation of the native conformation on modification, indicates that Tyr-399, 408, 449, and 494 do not contribute to the antigenic reactivity of this fragment (Kazim *et al.*, 1977, 1979).

Another derivative carboxyethylated at both methionine (Met-443 and -545) residues with β-propiolactone [a reagent possessing remarkable specificity for methionine residues (Taubman and Atassi, 1968; Atassi, 1969)] was prepared (Kazim *et al.*, 1979). No other amino acids were modified, and the homogeneous derivative showed no conformational changes by ORD and CD measurments. The derivative, however, showed a slightly higher reducibility of its disulfide bonds. With antisera to peptide 377–571, the derivative precipitated 12–36% less than unmodified 377–571 at the equivalence point, and in immunoadsorbent studies with these antisera the derivative adsorbed only 71% of the total antibodies bound by the parent peptide. Furthermore, the derivative inhibited the precipitin reaction of BSA with antisera to BSA by only 59%, compared to 92% for peptide 377–571. In view of the absence of conformational changes, this decrease in the immunochemical reactivity as a result of carboxyethylation of the two methionine residues implicates either one or both of methionines-443 and -545 as being at or near an antigenic site (Kazim *et al.*, 1979).

V. Immunochemical Studies on Human Serum Albumin

Human serum albumin (HSA) is very similar to BSA in physical properties (Foster, 1960) and also in the N–F transition near pH 4 (Clark *et al.*, 1962). Therefore, most of the information discussed in Sections I and II will also pertain to HSA. The amino acid sequence of HSA has recently been established (Behrens *et al.*, 1975; Meloun *et al.*, 1975) and shows that the three-domain feature that prevailed in BSA is also evident in the structure of HSA (Fig. 23). However, there were some differences between the data of the two groups. Sequences reported by Meloun *et al* (1975) included phenylalanine at position 157, which was deleted in the original sequence of Behrens *et al.* (1975). However, the latter group (Behrens, private communication, 1977) included a phenylalanine at position 157. Other differences occurred in the assignment of acid/amide states of the acidic amino acids and also in the identity of residues at 16 positions.

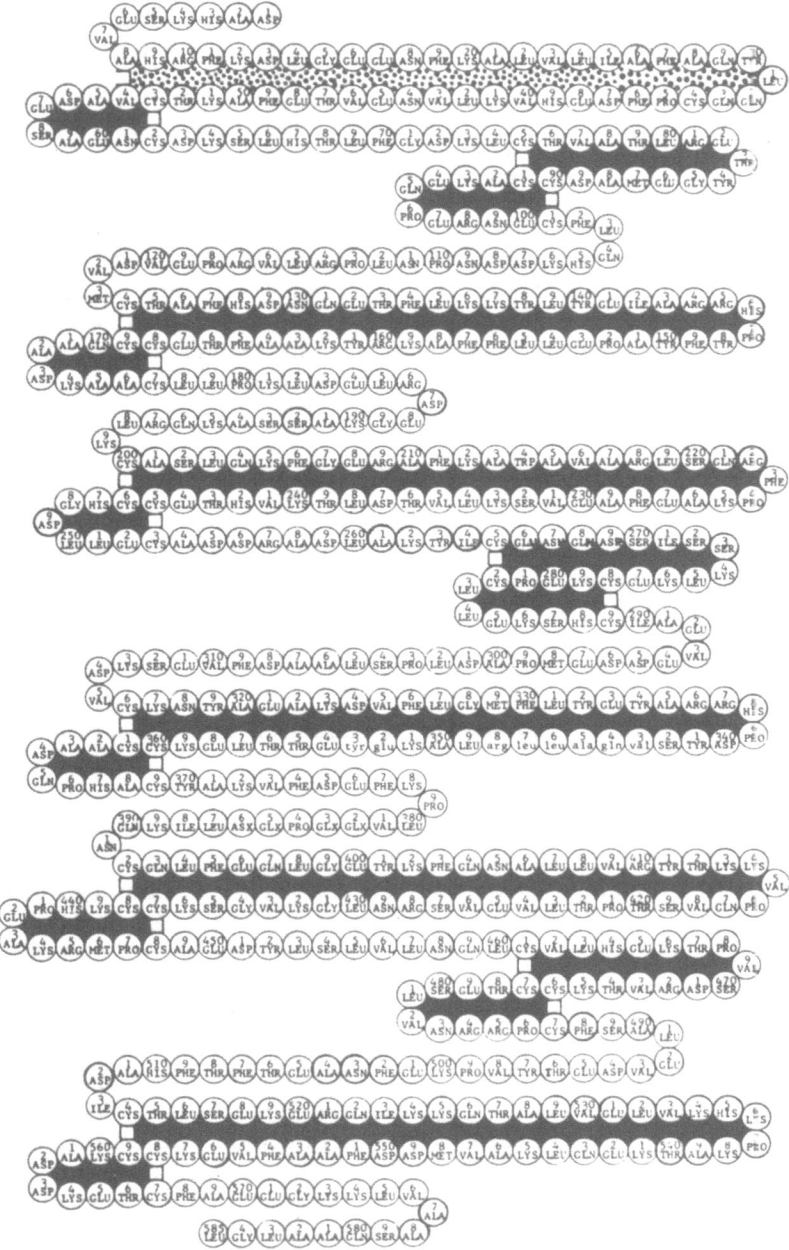

Figure 23. Amino acid sequence of human serum albumin. From Behrens *et al.* (1975).

	37	38	279	281	282	344	345	352
Behrens *et al.* (1975)	Asp	Glu	Lys	Pro	Cys	Gln	Ala	Glu
Meloun *et al.* (1975)	Glu	Asp	Cys	Lys	Pro	Val	Leu	Thr

	364	365	367	368	370	455	464	465
Behrens *et al.* (1975)	Asp	Glu	His	Ala	Tyr	Leu	His	Glu
Meloun *et al.* (1975)	His	Asp	Tyr	Glu	Ala	Val	Glu	His

It is not apparent whether the differences in the sequence of HSA reported by the two groups were the outcome of microheterogeneity, which was often demonstrated, or whether they were due to experimental errors. At the moment, the only strong evidence for microheterogeneity of albumin as a result of the primary structure comes from the work by Lapresle and Doyen (1975), who showed, by cyanogen bromide cleavage of HSA, that about 16% of the molecules lacked methionine at position 123.

Studies on the immunochemistry of HSA have followed two approaches:

1. The effect of chemical modification on the immunochemical reactivity, data for which are very limited.
2. Isolation of immunochemically reactive peptides. A good deal of progress has resulted from this approach.

A. Effect of Chemical Modification on Immunochemical Reactivity of Human Serum Albumin

Various chemically modified derivatives of HSA were evaluated for their immunochemical reactivity with anti-HSA (Jacobsen *et al.*, 1972). Conformational changes accompanying the chemical modification were assessed by ORD studies and from determination of the Stokes radius on a calibrated Sephadex column (Jacobsen *et al.*, 1972). Table X summarizes the results and shows that in some modifications changes in the secondary and tertiary structures revealed by rotatory behavior and the Stokes radius, respectively, were independent. A decreased immunochemical reactivity accompanied the modification of the amino groups which was dependent on the degree of the modification. This behavior was in contrast to that of BSA, where modification of the amino groups by a variety of reagents indicated that lysine residues were not part of the antigenic reactive sites (Habeeb, 1967a,b). Whereas tryptophan, acidic amino acids, and tyrosine residues played a minor role, histidine residues appeared unimportant to the immunochemical reactivity. The immunochemical reactivity was found to correlate best with the Stokes

Table X. Physicochemical Properties and Immunochemical Reactivity of
Modified Human Serum Albumin[a,b]

Reagent	Percent residues modified	$b_0{}^{216}$	Helix from $[M]_{233}$ (%)	Stokes radius (nm)	Immuno- chemical reactivity
Native		−283	44	3.6	100
N-Acetylimidazole	42% Lys; 17% Tyr	−272	40	4.2	46
Acetic anhydride	96% Lys; 41% Try	−154	28	5.3	6
Methylacetimidate	51% Lys	−205	37	3.8	53
Methylacetimidate	90% Lys	−128	42	3.9	39
Succinic anhydride	54% Lys	−257	36	4.7	31
Diethylpyrocarbonate	10% Lys; 12% His	−270	42	3.7	100
Diethylpyrocarbonate	40% Lys; 38% His	−258	40	4.0	44
Diethylpyrocarbonate	55% Lys; 58% His	−285	45	4.2	37
2-Nitrophenylsulfenyl- chloride	100% Trp	−274	38	3.6	94
Ethyl diazoacetate	11% Asp + Glu	−257	48	3.6	91
Tetranitromethane	51% Tyr; 100% Trp	−121	36	3.8	85
Taurine and	9% carboxyl groups	−124	—	3.9	66
carbodiimide	29% carboxyl groups	−127	—	4.2	26
	66% carboxyl groups	−138	—	4.6	5
Glycine amide and	18% carboxyl groups	−196	—	3.7	30
carbodiimide	33% carboxyl groups	−170	—	4.1	0
	59% carboxyl groups	−128	—	4.3	0
	60% carboxyl groups	−8	—	4.7	—

[a] From Jacobsen et al. (1972).
[b] From Funding et al. (1974).

radius of derivatives of HSA (Jacobsen et al., 1972). A similar relationship was reported previously for BSA (Habeeb, 1967a,b). Seven derivatives with modified carboxyl groups (Funding et al., 1974) were prepared
by reaction of HSA with taurine or glycine amide after activation by
carbodiimide. The modification was accompanied by profound changes
in secondary and tertiary structures and a concomitant decrease in immunochemical reactivity. Thus the role of the carboxyl groups in the
antigenic reactive sites has not yet been unambiguously established and
needs further careful study.

B. Immunochemistry of Fragments from Human Serum Albumin

Several immunochemically reactive fragments were isolated from
HSA by chymotryptic hydrolysis (Press and Porter, 1962), by tryptic

fragmentation (Lapresle *et al.*, 1959), or by action of cathepsin D (Lapresle and Webb, 1960; Webb and Lapresle, 1964).

Three fragments (a, b, and c) were isolated from a chymotryptic hydrolysate (pH 10, 9 days, room temperature) of HSA and had molecular weights of (a) 23,400, (b) 19,000, and (c) 7100 (Press and Porter, 1962). Fragment a precipitated 13–18% of anti-HSA and completely inhibited precipitation of the remaining antibody with HSA. Fragment b precipitated (0–10%) with anti-HSA and partially inhibited (28–40%) the precipitation of the remaining antibody with HSA. However, the small fragment c failed to precipitate with anti-HSA but inhibited the reaction of anti-HSA with HSA by 15–30%. The antigenic site of fragment c was considered part of the site of fragment b as addition of fragment c to fragment b did not increase its inhibitory ability with the HSA–anti-HSA system. Fragments a and b showed a reaction of partial identity by double diffusion in agar where spurring was observed. Threfore, fragments a, b, and c incorporated common antigenic sites derived from the same segment of the albumin molecule.

Trypsin hydrolyzed HSA less efficiently (pH 8, 37°C, 24 hr), yielding a mixture of fragments of molecular weights 12,000–30,000 (Lapresle *et al.*, 1959). These fragments gave 65% precipitation with anti-HSA relative to HSA. The mixture was not fractionated, and no peptides possessing inhibitory activity toward HSA–anti-HSA were reported.

However, recently it was found that fatty acid-free HSA was conformationally susceptible to tryptic hydrolysis, yielding an immunochemically active fragment of molecular weight 23,000 (Habeeb, 1978a). The fragment inhibited the reaction of HSA–anti-HSA by 79% and 94% with two immune antisera (see Table XIV). Moreover, an immunoabsorbant of the fragment trapped 93% of antibody to HSA (see Table XV). These results are significant since they point out to the fact that the isolated fragment (molecular weight 23,000) has almost all the antigenic reactive sites (Habeeb, 1978a), a situation analogous to that found with BSA (Atassi *et al.*, 1976b, Habeeb and Atassi, 1976b). From amino acid analysis and sequence determination, the fragment was assigned sequence Leu_{198}–Lys_{389} of HSA and represents the middle third of the molecule.

Human serum albumin was conveniently fragmented by rabbit cathepsin D (1 hr, pH 3.5, 45°C) to yield among the hydrolysis products a fragment (molecular weight 11,000) termed "inhibitor" which inhibited by 15–40% the precipitin reaction of HSA–anti-HSA (Lapresle and Webb, 1960, 1964; Webb and Lapresle, 1964). With two rabbit antisera, the fragment precipitated about 5% of anti-HSA. Antibodies directed against the fragment termed "inhibitor" were isolated from anti-HSA on an immunoadsorbent of the fragment and did not precipitate with the fragment or with HSA (Webb and Lapresle, 1964). Analysis of the ultracentrifugal patterns of a mixture of HSA and pure antifragment antibodies and also of the fragment and pure antifragment antibody indicated that the isolated antibodies were capable of reacting with two sites on either the fragment or the HSA molecule (Webb and Lapresle, 1964). Bellon and Lapresle (1975) have shown that this fragment consists of one polypeptide chain held together by two disulfide bonds. However, it is formed of a mixture of two molecular species since two NH_2-terminal residues (threonine and glutamic acid) are identified. The two components which apparently comprised the last 92 or 89 residues of HSA were not separated, but their existence was confirmed by tryptic cleavage of succinylated derivatives (Bellon and Lapresle, 1975). The complete amino acid sequence of the inhibitor was established by Walker (1976). It differed from the corresponding part of HSA determined by Behrens *et al.* (1975) and by Kostka *et al.* (1975) but agreed well with that reported by Meloun *et al.* (1975). Minor differences involved Glu at position 501 and Asn at 550 reported by Walker (1976) instead of Gln 501 and Asp 550 (Meloun *et al.*, 1975). The two components corresponded to Glu_{495}–Leu_{585} and Thr_{496}–Leu_{585} and are shown schematically in Fig. 24.

An immunochemically reactive fragment designated "F1" (molecular weight 6600) was prepared from the inhibitor by tryptic cleavage (2 hr, pH 8, 37°C) (Lapresle and Webb, 1964). Fragment F1 did not precipitate with anti-HSA, nor did it inhibit the reaction of HSA with anti-HSA. However, 1% of anti-HSA antibodies was recovered on an immunoadsorbent of F1. Analysis of eight rabbit anti-HSA sera indicated that antibodies with a specificity against F1 varied from 1.8% to 7.6% of the total (Oliveira and Lapresle, 1966) and accounted for 3% of the total anti-HSA in a mixture of anti-HSA from 11 rabbits. The isolated specific antibodies (anti-F1) agglutinated red cells sensitized by HSA but not by fragment F1. However, F1 inhibited the agglutination of anti-F1 with red cells sensitized with HSA, indicating that F1 reacted with anti-F1 antibodies. Ultracentrifugal analysis of complexes formed between albumin or F1 and anti F1 antibodies indicated that anti-F1 reacted with one site on either HSA or fragment F1. Recent work (Bellon and Lapresle, 1975; Bellon *et al.*, 1975) has shown that F1 is composed of two parts of the inhibitor fragment. F1 was heterogeneous, being formed of different molecular species (two were major and one was in trace amounts). Each component consisted of two polypeptides held by one interchain disulfide bond (Bellon and Lapresle, 1975). All molecules had one peptide (sequence Ala_{547}–Lys_{573}) with one intrachain disulfide bond Cys_{559}–Cys_{567} in common but differed in the second peptide, which was held to the first

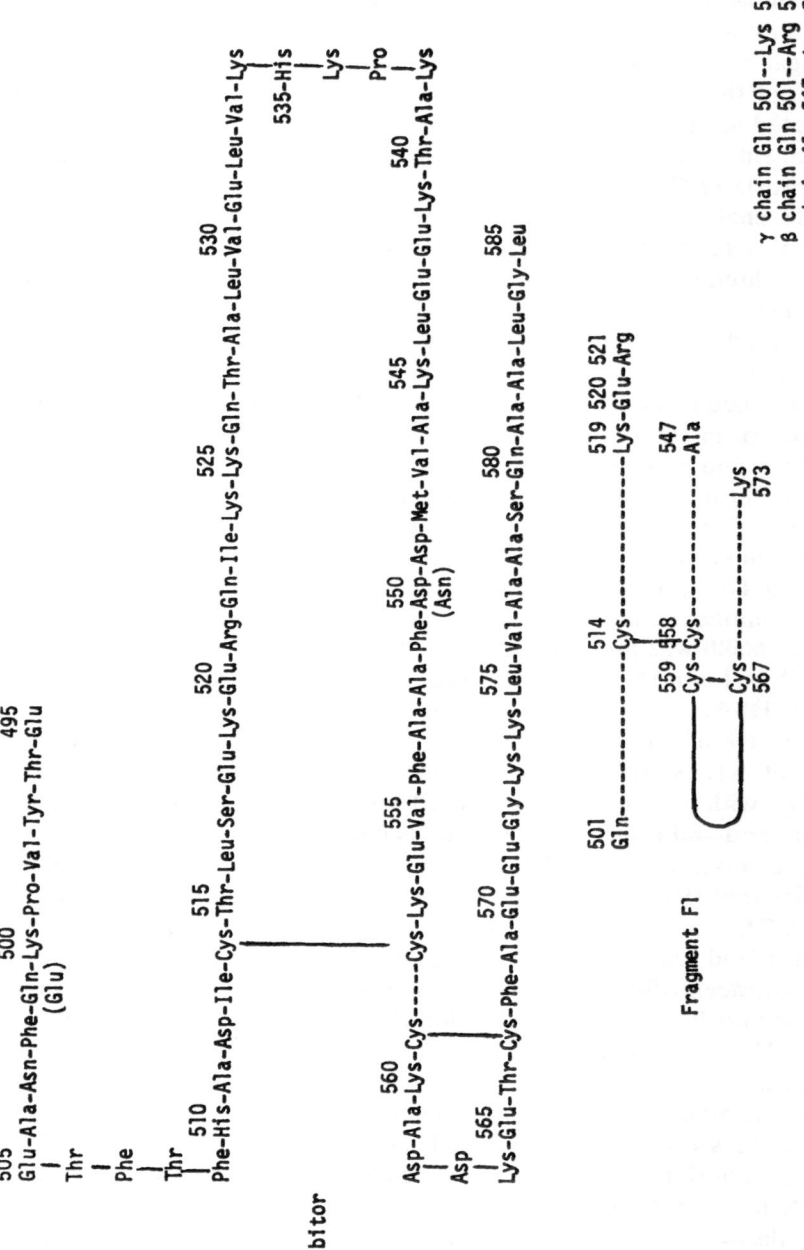

Figure 24. Amino acid sequence of the inhibitor and fragment F1 derived from it. The sequence is derived from the sequence of HSA determined by Meloun *et al.* (1975). Amino acid residues in parentheses are according to sequence obtained by Walker (1976).

peptide by a disulfide bond at Cys_{514}–Cys_{558} (Fig. 24). The variable peptides (in the two major components of F1) comprised sequences Gln_{501}–Lys_{519} and Gln_{501}–Arg_{521}. These sequences were constructed from the data of Bellon and Lapresle (1975) and the amino acid sequence data of Meloun et al. (1975) and Walker (1976). The two peptides were formed of 21 and 19 amino acid residues, respectively, and not of 25 and 23 residues as reported by Bellon and Lapresle (1975). It is remarkable that Lys-557, Lys-560, and Lys-564 were not susceptible to tryptic hydrolysis during conversion of inhibitor to F1. Clearly, the covalent structural changes (Fig. 24) and the concomitant conformational changes that accompanied the liberation of F1 from the inhibitor did contribute greatly to the marked diminution of the immunochemical reactivity, which dropped from 15–40% (in inhibitor) to 3% (in F1). The removal of the connecting peptide Gln_{522}–Leu_{544} seems to have destroyed one antigenic site and drastically impaired the second antigenic site. The small F1 was antigenic in rabbits (Lapresle and Goldstein, 1969), eliciting the production of antibodies which precipitated slightly with the fragment but not with HSA, indicating that new antigenic determinants were recognized by the rabbits on the fragment. Antisera to F1 agglutinated sheep red blood cells sensitized with either HSA or F1 and also cross-reacted with BSA. This cross-reactivity indicated that F1 was derived from a region of the molecule involved in the cross-reactivity between bovine and human albumins. Pure anti-F1 antibody (isolated on F1 immunoadsorbent from anti-F1 antisera) was found to agglutinate red cells sensitized with HSA or F1, and the agglutination was inhibited by both HSA and F1. The inhibition was 10 times greater (on molar basis) with HSA than with F1. Reduction of F1 with β-mercaptoethanol liberated the three constituent peptides (termed "α," "β," and "γ" chains) (Fig. 24). The α chain existed as a polymer and the β and γ as dimers (Bellon et al., 1975). Both the α and β chains independently completely inhibited the agglutination of red blood cells sensitized with F1 by anti-HSA serum. However, α chain displaced 90% of anti-F1 from an F1 immunoadsorbent saturated with anti-F1 whereas β chain displaced 45% of anti-F1. This behavior may indicate the retention of the antigenic structure in the α chain through the disulfide bond, whereas with the β chain the antigenic structure was perturbed. It was remarkable that α chain was antigenic in rabbits, eliciting antibodies which agglutinated red cells sensitized with either HSA or F1. On the other hand, the β chain was a weak antigen. Reduction and carboxymethylation of α chain or β chain abolished their immunochemical reactivity, indicating the essential role played by the disulfide bond in maintaining the conformation of the antigenic reactive site (Bellon et al., 1975).

So far two immunochemically reactive fragments have been isolated from HSA, one corresponding to sequence Glu_{495}–Leu_{585} which accounted for 15–40% inhibition of HSA–anti-HSA (Lapresle and Webb, 1960) and another having sequence Leu_{198}–Lys_{389}, which completely inhibited the reaction of HSA–anti-HSA (Habeeb, 1978a). Further work is being performed to clarify these seemingly different observations.

VI. Structural and Immunochemical Studies on Serum Albumin from Various Species

A. Structural Studies

Partial amino acid sequences of pig serum albumin (Brown et al., 1971) and equine serum albumin (Chincarini and Brown, 1976) are available. The amino acid analyses of bovine, sheep, pig, equine, human, and guinea pig serum albumins (Benjamin and Weigle, 1971) showed that the sheep albumin differed from BSA in about 29 amino acid residues involving 14 amino acids, pig albumin differed in 61 amino acid residues involving 16 amino acids, human albumin in 71 residues involving 17 amino acids, horse albumin in 60 residues involving 17 amino acids, and guinea pig albumin in 54 residues involving 15 amino acids.

Serum albumins from goat, pig, horse, and human showed heterogeneity reflected in charge differences by chromatography on DEAE-cellulose. Each albumin was separated into three fractions using the stepwise elution system as that for BSA (Habeeb, 1978b). All the albumins revealed the same elution pattern, showing three main components of which the first and third components eluted in a symmetrical peak while the second component trailed (Fig. 25).

Serum albumins from goat, horse, and pig exhibited a neutral transition at pH 7.5–9.5 (at room temperature) characterized by increased activity of the disulfide bonds to reduction (Habeeb, 1978b). Further increase in reactivity of the disulfide bonds was exhibited at 40°C. Albumins from goat, horse, and pig had a remarkable tendency to unfold (resulting in exposure of the disulfide bonds); thus a plateau of disulfide reducibility was reached at pH 8 and 40°C, whereas with BSA or HSA a higher pH was required to reach maximal exposure of the disulfide bonds to reduction (Fig. 26).

Amino acid sequence studies of BSA (Brown, 1975) and HSA (Behrens et al., 1975; Meloun et al., 1975) revealed the albumin molecule to consist of three compact domains held by 17 disulfide bonds arranged in

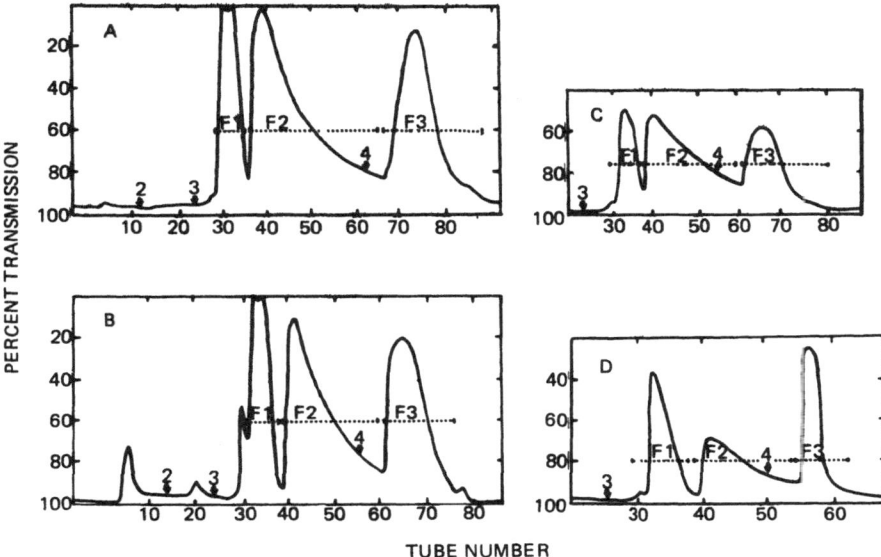

Figure 25. Chromatography of serum albumins on DEAE-cellulose using stepwise elution. The starting buffer was 0.005 M sodium phosphate buffer pH 6 2 followed by 2, 0.0175 M sodium phosphate pH 6.2; 3, 0.075 M NaCl in 0.0715 M phosphate buffer pH 6.2; 4, 0.2 M NaCl in 0.0175 M sodium phosphate pH 6.2. A: Goat serum albumin. B: Horse serum albumin. C: Pig serum albumin. D: Human serum albumin. From Habeeb (unpublished work).

nine loops. The compact domains were connected by short polypeptide segments. Proteolytic enzymes were found to cleave BSA at these loose regions, thus releasing compact fragments. The cleavage of BSA and HSA with trypsin was highly dependent and was inhibited by bound fatty acids. Indeed, with HSA meaningful cleavage was obtained only with fatty-acid-free preparations (Habeeb, 1978a,b). Albumins from goat, horse, pig, and human were cleaved by trypsin (at pH 8.7 for 1 hr at 40°C) to yield a fragmentation pattern (Fig. 27) reminiscent of BSA when chromatographed on Sephadex G-100 or G-75 (Habeeb, 1978a,b). Several large fragments were isolated in addition to the last-eluted peak. The latter consisted of small peptides which were revealed on a peptide map. A large fragment (molecular weight about 23,000) was isolated in a pure form from all tryptic hydrolysates of goat, horse, pig, and human serum albumins. This fragment was immunochemically reactive in the homologous system. The immunochemical reactivity of these fragments will be discussed later.

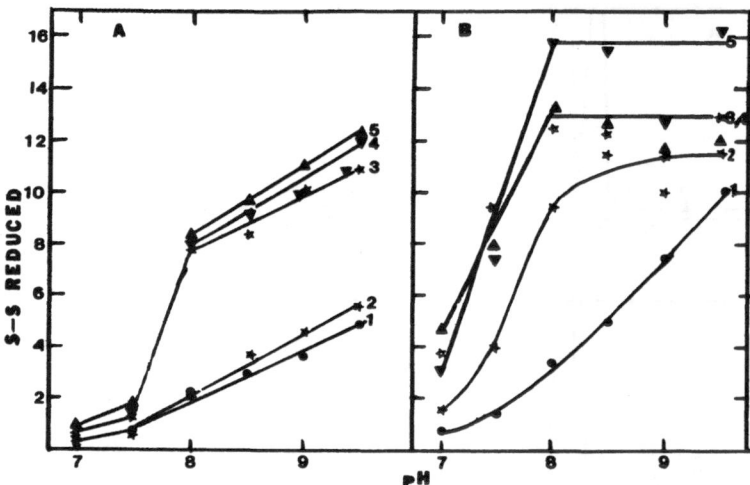

Figure 26.   Number of disulfide bonds (S—S) reduced with β-mercaptoethanol as a function of pH of various serum albumins. 1, Crystalline BSA lot No. 5423 from ICN Pharmaceutical; 2, crystalline HSA lot No. 65C-8320 from Sigma; 3, porcine serum albumin as Cohn fraction V; 4, horse serum albumin as Cohn fraction V; 5, goat serum albumin as Cohn fraction V. A: Reduction at room temperature. B: Reduction at 40°C. From Habeeb (unpublished work).

Cyanogen bromide cleavage of BSA (King and Spencer, 1968) yielded two fragments of molecular weights 44,000 and 22,000. Sheep but not pig serum albumin gave a similar fragmentation pattern (Benjamin and Weigle, 1971; Kamiyama, 1977b). The large fragment was derived from the COOH-terminal end while the fragment having the molecular weight of 22,000 originated from the NH$_2$-terminal segment.

B. Immunochemical Cross-Reactivity of Serum Albumins

Immunochemical cross-reactivity of homologous proteins from different species has been utilized to determine the phylogenetic relationships among the proteins. The cross-reactivity of proteins does not reflect only sequence homology, but is dependent on both sequence and conformational homologies (Atassi, 1970; Atassi et al., 1970a,b; Habeeb, 1977b). Indeed, the low avidity of anti-BSA with horse serum albumin (ESA) (Rangel, 1965) and of anti-BSA with sheep serum albumin (SSA), pig serum albumin (PSA), HSA, and guinea pig serum albumin (GPSA) (Benjamin and Weigle, 1971), which indicated that the antigenic reactive sites were similar rather than identical, may be the result of sequence as well as conformational divergence among homologous proteins from different species. Homologous antigen (BSA) displaced heterologous antigen (ESA) from soluble complexes of ESA–anti-BSA, but heterologous antigen (ESA) did not displace BSA from soluble complexes of BSA–anti-BSA (Rangel, 1965).

The immunochemical cross-reactivity revealed by quantitative precipitin reaction of 22 primate serum albumins with anti-HSA was consistent with the presumed phylogenetic relationships to man on the assumption that the evolutionary modification of protein structure has been

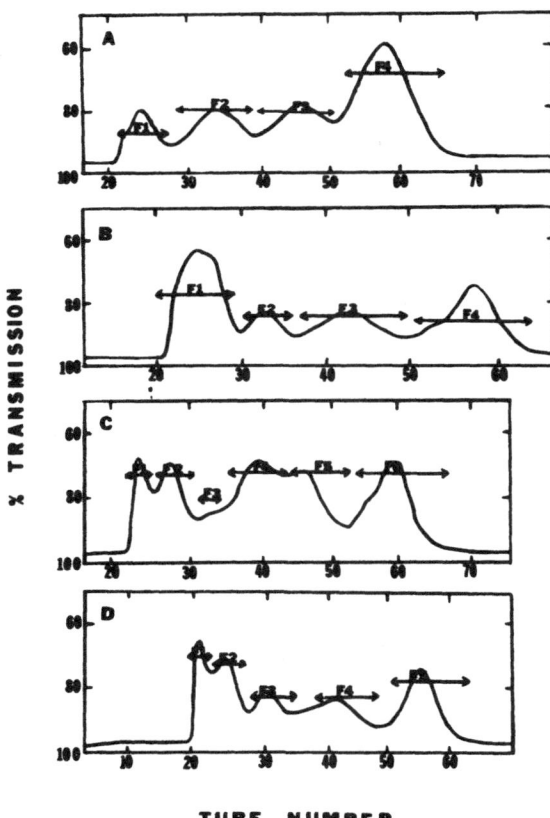

TUBE NUMBER

Figure 27.   Gel filtration of tryptic hydrolysates of various serum albumins. The hydrolysate (0.3 g) was applied onto a column (2.7 × 80 cm) of Sephadex G-75 and eluted with 0.01 M HN₄HCO₃. Fractions (7.5 ml) were analyzed continuously by an ultraviolet monitor. Tryptic hydrolysates of (A) goat serum albumin, (B) horse serum albumin, (C) pig serum albumin, and (D) human serum albumin. From Habeeb (1978a).

Table XI.   Immunochemical Cross-Reactivity of Serum Albumins by Precipitin Reaction[a,b]

	Anti-BSA	Anti-GSA	Anti-PSA	Anti-HSA
Bovine serum albumin	100	40.8	0	4.7
Goat serum albumin	63.9	100	0	2.8
Horse serum albumin	9.0	6.4	0	7.5
Porcine serum albumin	19.4	6.0	100	5.5
Human serum albumin	10.4	5.6	0	100

[a] From Habeeb (unpublished work).
[b] Results are expressed as percent precipitation by each albumin, at equivalence, relative to the homologous reaction.

progressive and divergent (Hafleigh and Williams, 1966). Results of studies utilizing quantitative microcomplement fixation to compare human serum albumin with the serum albumins of apes, monkeys, and prosimians were consistent with the accepted phylogenetic position of these groups (Sarich and Wilson, 1966).

Cross-reactivity between various serum albumins (bovine, deer, sheep, goat, pig, horse, and rat) was investigated by precipitation, gel diffusion, and passive hemagglutination (Timpl et al., 1967). With quantitative precipitation, cross-reactivity of anti-BSA with heterologous albumins (compared to the homologous system) was 70% for deer, 66% for SSA, 60% for GSA, 23% for PSA, 19% for HSA, 12% for ESA, and 11% for rat albumin. Whereas about six antigenic determinants were calculated for BSA (from precipitin curves), the combined results of passive hemagglutination and gel diffusion gave a higher value (13 antigenic determinants on BSA). The discrepancy between the two values was attributed to steric hindrance during the precipitin reaction. Similar extents of cross-reactivity as determined by the antigen-binding capacities were also found (Benjamin and Weigle, 1971; Kamiyama, 1977a). In a recent study (Habeeb, 1978a,b) the immunochemical cross-reactivity of BSA, GSA, PSA, ESA, and HSA with homologous and heterologous antisera was investigated both by the precipitin reaction (Table XI) and by immunoadsorbents (Habeeb, 1978a,b) (Tables XII and XIII). With anti-BSA, GSA showed considerable cross-reactivity (64%) followed by PSA (19.4%), HSA (10.4%), and ESA (9%). On the other hand, with anti-GSA, with the exception of BSA (40.8%) other heterologous albumins gave a weak precipitin reaction (5.6–6%). With anti-PSA, no precipitation occurred with the heterologous albumins, and with anti-HSA weak precipitation was apparent with heterologous albumins. These results indicated that reciprocal cross-reactivity was not identical to cross-reactivity.

Table XII.   Immunochemical Cross-Reaction of Anti-Bovine Serum Albumin and Heterologous Serum Albumins Determined on Immunoadsorbents[a]

Anti-BSA	Seph-GSA (%)	Seph-ESA (%)	Seph-PSA (%)	Seph-HSA (%)
Adsorbed[b]	71	35.7	66.4	39
Antibody precipitating with BSA	83.7	51.7	71.8	43
Antibody precipitating with homologous antigens as that of immunoadsorbent	67	13.9	24.4	14.5
Unadsorbed[c]	29	64.3	33.6	61
Antibody precipitating with BSA	67.3	86.8	88	92.4

[a] From Habeeb (1978a).
[b] Antibody absorbed was eluted from immunoadsorbent by 5 M guanidine HCl pH 7 and then dialyzed vs. water followed by phosphate/saline buffer pH 7.2. The amount of total antibody was computed from absorbance at 280 nm using a factor of 1.38 for absorbance of 1 mg antibody/ml. Precipitin curves were done on the antibody using BSA and also the homologous native antigen as that on immunoadsorbent.
[c] The unadsorbed antibody was adsorbed on Sepharose BSA immunoadsorbent, and after elution with 5 M guanidine HCl and dialysis its concentration was calculated from its absorbance at 280 nm. Precipitin curves were done using BSA as antigen and percent of precipitating antibody was estimated.

This is to be expected since cross-reacting albumins have similar rather than identical antigenic determinants and an animal will respond differently to the two sets of antigenic determinants. Of significance is the high level of cross-reactivity when immunoadsorbents were utilized to trap the cross-reacting antibodies (Table XII). Thus when anti-BSA was passed over an immunoabsorbant of Sepharose-GSA, 71% of the antibody was adsorbed (compared to 64% by precipitin reaction). Of the eluted antibody, 83.7% precipitated with BSA and 67% precipitated with

Table XIII.   Immunochemical Cross-Reaction of Antialbumins with Bovine Serum Albumin Immunoadsorbent[a]

	Anti-GSA (%)	Anti-PSA (%)	Anti-HSA (%)
Adsorbed on Seph-BSA[b]	56.6	30.2	27.3
Antibody precipitating with BSA	67	22.3	19
Unadsorbed on Seph-BSA	43.4	69.2	72.7
Antibody precipitating with homologous antigen as an immunoadsorbent[c]	55	46.4	78.3

[a] From Habeeb (unpublished results).
[b] Antibody adsorbed on immunoadsorbent was eluted with 5 M guanidine HCl, and after dialysis precipitin curves were performed with anti-BSA.
[c] The unadsorbed antibody was adsorbed on a homologous immunoadsorbent and the pure antibody was eluted, dialyzed, and used for a precipitin reaction with the homologous albumin.

GSA. A high proportion of anti-BSA—35.7%—was adsorbed by ESA immunoadsorbent, 66.4% by Sepharose-PSA, and 39% by Sepharose-HSA. The cross-reacting antibodies were found to precipitate more with BSA than with the homologous albumin that is in the immunoadsorbent. The high cross-reactivity shown by immunoadsorbent is the result of the presence of high proportions of nonprecipitating antibodies which escaped detection in the quantitative precipitin reaction and were trapped by the immunoadsorbent. Therefore, in determination of cross-reactivity, special precaution has to be exercised to account for the presence of nonprecipitating antibodies.

Similarly when anti-GSA, anti-PSA, and anti-HSA were adsorbed on an immunoadsorbent of BSA, a higher degree of cross-reactivity was shown than with quantitative precipitin reaction (Table XIII). Significantly, 30.2% of anti-PSA was adsorbed on Sepharose-BSA immunoadsorbent compared to 0% by precipitation and 27.3% of anti-HSA was trapped by HSA immunoadsorbent compared to 4.7% by precipitation. The adsorbed antibodies were found to show a low degree of precipitation with BSA. The unadsorbed antibody on Sepharose-BSA varied in its ability to precipitate with the homologous albumin, but it was higher than the precipitating ability of the adsorbed antibodies with BSA. The data presented here are in contrast to results reported by Kamiyama (1977a) on a limited number of albumins where cross-reactivity obtained by immunoadsorbents agreed with that by quantitative precipitin reaction with anti-BSA and GSA, anti-GSA and BSA, and anti-SSA and BSA.

C. Immunochemical Reactivity of Fragments of Albumins

Cleavage of BSA, SSA (Benajamin and Weigle, 1971; Kamiyama, 1977b), and GSA (Kamiyama, 1977b) with cyanogen bromide yielded an NH_2–terminal fragment (molecular weight 22,000) and a COOH-terminal fragment (molecular weight 44,000). The two fragments were non-cross-reacting (Benjamin and Weigle, 1971; Kamiyama, 1977b). Inhibition of the homologous reaction by the NH_2-terminal fragment was about 40% and by the COOH-terminal fragment was about 70%. The homologous reactions were more effectively inhibited by the homologous antigen and its fragments than by the heterologous antigen and its fragments. Moreover, the heterologous reactions were inhibited to the same extent by either albumin, but the albumin or its fragments against which the antibody was directed reached a maximum inhibition at a lower concentration than did the other albumin or its fragments (Benjamin and Weigle, 1971).

The NH$_2$-terminal fragments or the COOH-terminal fragments of GSA and SSA showed antigenic identity (Kamiyama, 1977b) but partial identities between NH$_2$- and COOH-terminal fragments of BSA and GSA, and BSA and SSA. Immunoadsorbents prepared with the NH$_2$-terminal fragments of BSA, GSA, or SSA bound 25-35% of the antibodies to intact homologous albumin, and the remainder bound to immunoadsorbents containing the homologous COOH-terminal fragments (Kamiyama, 1977b). The lack of cross-reaction between the NH$_2$-terminal fragment of BSA and the COOH-terminal fragment is in contrast to results by Habeeb and Atassi (1977) where cross-reaction was found between fragments 11-193 and 377-571 and albumin.

An immunochemically reactive fragment of molecular weight 21,000-23,000 was isolated in a pure form (Habeeb, 1978a,b) from tryptic hydrolysates of GSA and PSA. The fragment isolated from GSA inhibited the reaction of GSA-anti-GSA by 67%; that isolated from PSA inhibited the homologous PSA-anti-PSA by 79% (Table XIV). Immunoadsorbents prepared with these fragments were capable of binding antibody from ho-

Table XIV. Maximum Inhibition of the Homologous Antigen-Antibody Reaction by Serum Albumin Fragments[a]

	F2 of GSA (%)	F3 of PSA (%)	F3 of HSA (%)
Anti-HSA			
R#155 pool 1			76
R#155 pool 2			79
R#156 pool 1			91
R#156 pool 2			94
Anti-GSA			
R#157	66		
R#158	31.6		
Anti-PSA			
G#533		81	
R#215		79	
R#216		68	

[a] From Habeeb (1978a). The fragment was incubated with the homologous antiserum for 1 hr at 40°C, then for 24 hr at 4°C, after which the homologous serum albumin was added at an equivalence amount, mixed, and incubated at 40°C for 1 hr then overnight at 4°C. The amount of the immune precipitate was quantitated. The percent inhibition was calculated from the amount of decrease in immune precipitate in the presence of fragment to that in the absence of fragment. "R" refers to antisera raised in rabbits, and "G" refers to antiserum raised in a goat.

Table XV.   Adsorption of Antialbumins on a Fragment
Immunoadsorbent[a]

	Anti-GSA (%)	Anti-PSA (%)	Anti-HSA (%)
Adsorbed on Sepharose-fragment[b]	43.3	56	93.4
Second adsorption on Sepharose-fragment[c]	0	0	0
Adsorbed on Sepharose-albumin[d]	56.7	44	6.6

[a] From Habeeb (1978a).
[b] Antiserum was applied in an immunoadsorbent prepared with a fragment obtained from homologous albumin. Thus anti-GSA was applied on Sepharose-GSA fragment, anti-PSA on PSA fragment immunoadsorbent, and anti-HSA on HSA fragment immunoadsorbent. The antibody adsorbed was eluted with 5 M guanidine HCl pH 7 and then dialyzed against water followed by phosphate/saline buffer pH 7.2. The amount of total antibody was calculated from adsorbence at 280 nm using a value of 1.38 for adsorbence of 1 mg antibody/ml.
[c] Unadsorbed serum from previous step was put a second time on the same immunoadsorbent, washed with phosphate/saline buffer pH 7.2, and eluted with 5 M guanidine HCl; then the above procedure was followed.
[d] The unadsorbed serum was put on an immunoadsorbent prepared with the homologous albumin. The absorbed antibody was eluted with 5 M guanidine HCl and dialyzed, and its concentration was determined.

mologous antisera (Table XV). The GSA fragment on an immunoadsorbent bound 43.3% of anti GSA, and the PSA fragment or immunoadsorbent bound 56% of anti-PSA.

VII. Conclusion

Serum albumin, the most abundant plasma protein, has been subjected to extensive studies which resulted in a wealth of information on its chemical and physicochemical properties. Only recently has the amino acid sequence of bovine and human serum albumins become known. Prior to the availability of the amino acid sequence, immunochemical studies on BSA or HSA were hampered by the inability to assign an immunochemically reactive fragment within the sequence of the albumin molecule. With the availability of the sequence, it is becoming possible to identify immunochemically reactive fragments of known sequences. Thus fragments 11–193 and 377–571 were isolated from BSA. These fragments were shown to have rather unusual immunochemical properties. Each fragment by itself inhibited almost completely the reaction of BSA–anti-BSA, and as a result of experiments with immunoadsorbent and binding studies with fluorescein-conjugated fragments the concept that BSA has repeating identical or similar antigenic sites was advanced. This concept is new in immunochemistry, and preliminary results with HSA showed that a fragment of molecular weight 23,000 corresponding to sequence 198–389 inhibited by 91% the reaction of HSA–anti-HSA and an immunoadsorbent of this fragment bound 93% of anti-HSA. However, for localizing the amino acid residues at the antigenic reactive sites a knowledge of three-dimensional structure is mandatory.

It is hoped that the three-dimensional structure of albumin or at least of an immunochemically reactive fragment will be available for the final delineation of the antigenic sites of serum albumin.

Armed with this knowledge, controlled chemical modification at specific amino acid residues of an immunochemically reactive peptide will yield valuable information of the essentiality of a given amino acid residue at the antigenic reactive site. The final step in the localization of an antigenic reactive site is the synthesis of the site (see Chapters 3 and 4 in Volume 2 of this series). There are no shortcuts to this strategy. Scattered modification of given amino acid residues either chemically or by mutation may yield limited information about the participation of an amino acid residue at the antigenic reactive site but cannot construct an antigenic reactive site.

ACKNOWLEDGMENTS

I wish to thank Dr. M. Z. Atassi for his helpful review of the manuscript.

VIII. References

Adkins, B. J., and Foster, J. F., 1966, *Biochemistry* **5**:2579.
Andersson, L.-O., 1966, *Biochim. Biophys. Acta* **117**:115.
Andersson, L.-O., 1969, *Arch. Biochem. Biophys.* **133**:277.
Andersson, L.-O., Brandt, J., and Johansson, S., 1971, *Arch. Biochem. Biophys.* **146**:428.
Aoki, K., and Foster, J. F., 1957a, *J. Am. Chem. Soc.* **79**:3385.
Aoki, K., and Foster, J. F., 1957b, *J. Am. Chem. Soc.* **79**:3393.
Aoki, K., and Foster, J. F., 1975, *Biochemistry* **14**:3566.
Atassi, M. Z., 1969, *Immunochemistry* **6**:801.
Atassi, M. Z., 1970, *Biochim. Biophys. Acta* **221**:612.
Atassi, M. Z., 1972, *Specific Receptors of Antibodies, Antigens and Cells, 3rd International Convocation on Immunology*, pp. 118–135, Karger, Basel.

Atassi, M. Z., 1975, *Immunochemistry* **12**:735.

Atassi, M. Z., 1977a, in: *Immunochemistry of Proteins*, Vol. 1 (M.Z. Atassi, ed.), pp. 1–161, Plenum, New York.

Atassi, M. Z., 1977b, in: *Immunochemistry of Proteins*, Vol. 2 (M. Z. Atassi, ed.), pp. 77–176, Plenum, New York.

Atassi, M. Z., 1978a, in: *Immunobiology of Protein and Peptides*, Vol. 1 (M. Z. Atassi and A. B. Stavitsky, eds.), pp. 41–100, Plenum, New York.

Atassi, M. Z., 1978b, *Immunochemistry* **15**:909.

Atassi, M. Z., and Habeeb, A.F.S.A., 1969, *Biochemistry* **8**:1385.

Atassi, M. Z., and Habeeb, A.F.S.A., 1972, *Methods Enzymol.* **25b**:546.

Atassi, M. Z., and Habeeb, A.F.S.A., 1977, in: *Immunochemistry of Proteins*, Vol. 2 (M.Z. Atassi, ed.), pp. 177–264, Plenum, New York.

Atassi, M. Z., and Lee, C.-L., 1978a, *Biochem. J.* **171**:419.

Atassi, M. Z., and Lee, C.-L., 1978b, *Biochem. J.* **171**:429.

Atassi, M. Z., Habeeb, A.F.S.A., and Rydstedt, L., 1970a, *Biochim. Biophys. Acta* **200**:184.

Atassi, M. Z., Tarlowski, D. P., and Paull, J. H., 1970b, *Biochim. Biophys. Acta* **221**:623.

Atassi, M. Z., Habeeb, A.F.S.A., and Ando, K., 1973, *Biochim. Biphys. Acta* **303**:203.

Atassi, M.Z., Lee, C.-L., and Pai, R.-C., 1976a, *Biochim. Biophys. Acta* **427**:745.

Atassi, M. Z., Habeeb, A.F.S.A., and Lee, C.-L., 1976b, *Immunochemistry* **13**:547.

Behrens, P. Q., Spiekerman, A. M. and Brown, J. R., 1975, *Fed. Proc.* **34**:591 (abst.).

Bellon, F., and Lapresle, C., 1975, *Biochem. J.* **147**:585.

Bellon, F., Lapresle, C., and Escribano, M. J., 1975, *Ann. Immunol. Inst. Pasteur* **126C**:653.

Benjamin, D. C., and Weigle, W. O., 1971, *Immunochemistry* **8**:1087.

Bennhold, H., 1972, In: *Protides of the Biological Fluids*, 9th Coll. Bruges, 1961 (H. Peeters, ed.), p. 58, Elsevier, Amsterdam.

Benson, E. S., and Hallaway, B. E., 1970, *J. Biol. Chem.* **245**:4144.

Bloomfield, V., 1966, *Biochemistry* **5**:684.

Braam, W.G.M., Harmsen, B.J.M., and Van Os, G.A.J., 1971, *Biochim. Biophys. Acta* **236**:99.

Braam, W.G.M., Hilak, M.C., Harmsen, B.J.M., and Van Os, G.A.J., 1974, *Int. J Peptide Protein Res.* **6**:21.

Bro, P., Singer, S. J., and Sturtevant, J. M., 1955, *J. Am. Chem. Soc.* **77**:4924.

Brown, J. R., 1975, *Fed. Proc.* **34**:591 (abstr.).

Brown, J. R., 1976, *Fed. Proc.* **35**:2141.

Brown, J. R., Low., T., Behrens, P., Sepulveda, P., Parker, K., and Blakeney, E., 1971, *Fed. Proc. Abstr. Part II* **30**:1241.

Charlwood, P. A., and Ens, A., 1957, *Can. J. Biochem.* **35**:99.

Chen, R. F., 1967, *J. Biol. Chem.* **242**:173.

Cherry, M., 1964, Ph.D. thesis, Yale University, New Haven, Conn.

Chincarini, C. C., and Brown, J. R., 1976, *Fed. Proc.* **35**:1621 (abstr.).

Clark, P., Rachinsky, M. R., and Foster, J. F., 1962, *J. Biol. Chem.* **237**:2509.

Cohn, E. J., Strong, L. E., Hughes, W. L., Jr., Mulford, D. J., Ashworth, J. N., Melin, M., and Taylor, H. L., 1946, *J. Am. Chem. Soc.* **68**:459.

Cohn, E. J., Hughes, W. L., Jr., and Weare, J. H., 1947, *J. Am. Chem. Soc.* **69**:1753.

Colvin, J. R., Smith, D. B., and Cook, W. H., 1954, *Chem. Rev.* **54**:687.

Farr, R. S., 1958, *J. Infect. Dis.* **102–103**:239.

Feldhoff, R. C., and Peters, T., Jr., 1975, *Biochemistry* **14**:4508.

Foster, J. F., 1960, in: *The Plasma Proteins*, Vol. 1 (F. W. Putnam, ed.), p. 179, Academic Press, New York.

Foster, J. F., and Clark, P., 1962, *J. Biol. Chem.* **237**:3163.
Foster, J. F., Sogami, M., Petersen, H. A., and Leonard, W. J., Jr., 1965, *J. Biol. Chem.* **240**:2495.
Friedberg, F., 1975, *FEBS Lett.* **59**:140.
Fuller-Noel, J. K., and Hunter, M. J., 1972, *J. Biol. Chem.* **247**:7391.
Funding, L., Jacobsen, C., Steensgaard, J., Jensen, P. J., and Jelert, H., 1974, *Int. J. Peptide Protein Res.* **7**:245.
Giroux, E. L., 1975, *Biochem. Med.* **12**:258.
Goetzl, E. J., and Peters, J. H., 1972, *J. Immunol.* **108**:785.
Green, N. M., 1963, *Biochim. Biophys. Acta* **74**:542.
Griffith, O. H., and McConnell, H. M., 1966, *Proc. Natl. Acad. Sci. USA* **55**:8.
Habeeb, A.F.S.A., 1959, *Biochim. Biophys. Acta* **34**:294.
Habeeb, A.F.S.A., 1960, *Can. J. Biochem. Physiol.* **38**:493.
Habeeb, A.F.S.A., 1964, *Biochim. Biophys. Acta* **93**:533.
Habeeb, A.F.S.A., 1966*a*, *Biochim. Biophys. Acta* **115**:440.
Habeeb, A.F.S.A., 1966*b*, *Biochim. Biophys. Acta* **121**:21.
Habeeb, A.F.S.A., 1967*a*, *Arch. Biochem. Biophys.* **121**:652.
Habeeb, A.F.S.A., 1967*b*, *J. Immunol.* **99**:1264.
Habeeb, A.F.S.A. 1968*a*, *J. Immunol.* **101**:505.
Habeeb, A.F.S.A., 1968*b*, *Can. J. Biochem.* **46**:789.
Habeeb, A.F.S.A., 1969, *J. Immunol.* **102**:457.
Habeeb, A.F.S.A., 1972, *Methods Enzymol.* **25B**:558.
Habeeb, A.F.S.A., 1977*a*, *Fed. Proc.* **36**:838 (Abstr.).
Habeeb, A.F.S.A., 1977*b*, in: *Immunochemistry of Proteins*, Vol. 1 (M. Z. Atassi, ed.), pp. 163–229, Plenum, New York.
Habeeb, A.F.S.A., 1978*a*, *Adv. Exp. Med. Biol.* **98**:101.
Habeeb, A.F.S.A., 1978*b*, *Fed. Proc.* **37**:1461 (abstr.)
Habeeb, A.F.S.A., and Atassi, M.Z., 1970, *Biochemistry* **9**:4939.
Habeeb, A.F.S.A., and Atassi, M.Z., 1971, *Immunochemistry* **8**:1047.
Habeeb, A.F.S.A., and Atassi, M.Z., 1976*a*, *Fed. Proc.* **35**:753 (abstr.).
Habeeb, A.F.S.A., and Atassi, M. Z., 1976*b*, *J. Biol. Chem.* **251**:4616.
Habeeb, A.F.S.A., and Atassi, M.Z., 1977, *Immunochemistry* **14**:449.
Habeeb, A.F.S.A., and Borella, L., 1966, *J. Immunol.* **97**:951.
Habeeb, A.F.S.A, and Francis, R.D., 1976, *Vox Sang.* **31**:423.
Habeeb, A.F.S.A., and Hiramoto, R., 1968, *Arch. Biochem. Biophys.* **126**:16.
Habeeb, A.F.S.A., Cassidy, H.G., and Singer, S.J., 1958, *Biochim. Biophys. Acta* **29**:587.
Habeeb, A.F.S.A., Atassi, M.Z., and Lee, C.-L., 1974, *Biochim. Biophys. Acta* **342**:389.
Hafleigh, A.S., and Williams, C. A., Jr., 1966, *Science* **151**:1530.
Hagenmaier, R. D., and Foster, J. F., 1971, *Biochemistry* **10**:637.
Harmsen, B. J. M., De Bruin, S. H., Janssen, L. H. M., Rodriguez De Miranda, J. F., and Van Os, G. A. J., 1971, *Biochemistry* **10**:3217.
Harrington, W. F., Johnson, P., and Ottewill, R. H., 1956, *Biochem. J.* **62**:569.
Hartley, R. W., Peterson, E. A., and Sober, H. A., 1962, *Biochemistry* **1**:60.
Herskovitz, T. T., and Laskowski, M., Jr., 1960, *J. Biol. Chem.* **235**:PC 56.
Hilak, M. C., Harmsen, B. J. M., Braam, W. G. M., Joordens, J. J. M., and Van Os, G. A. J., 1974, *Int. J. Peptide Protein Res* **6**:95.
Hilak, M. C., Harmsen, B. J. M., Joordens, J. J. M., and Van Os, G. A. J., 1975, *Int. J. Peptide Protein Res.* **7**:411.
Hull, H. H., Chang, R., and Kaplan, L. J., 1975, *Biochim. Biophys. Acta* **400**:132.
Jacobsen, C., Funding, L., Moller, N. P. H., and Steensgaard, J., 1972, *Eur. J. Biochem.* **30**:392.

Janatova, J., Mikes, O., and Sponar, J., 1968a, *Collect. Czech. Chem. Commun.* **33**:788.
Janatova, J., Fuller, J. K., and Hunter, M. J., 1968b, *J. Biol. Chem.* **243**:3612.
Jirgensons, B., 1958, *Arch. Biochem. Biophys.* **78**:227.
Jonas, A., and Weber, G., 1970, *Biochemistry* **9**:5092.
Kamiyama, T., 1977a, *Immunochemistry* **14**:85.
Kamiyama, T., 1977b, *Immunochemistry* **14**:91.
Karush, F., 1950, *J. Am. Chem. Soc.* **72**:2705.
Katz, S., and Klotz, I. M., 1953, *Arch. Biochem. Biophys.* **44**:351.
Kauzman, W., Walter, J. E., and Eyring, H., 1940, *Chem. Rev.* **26**:339.
Kazim, A. L., Habeeb, A. F. S. A., and Atassi, M. Z., 1977, *Fed. Proc.* **36**:742 (abstr.).
Kazim, A. L., Habeeb, A. F. S. A., and Atassi, M. Z., 1979, *Immunochemistry* (in press).
King, T. P., 1973, *Arch. Biochem. Biophys.* **156**:509.
King, T. P., and Spencer, E. M., 1968, *Fed. Proc.* **27**:391 (abstr.).
King, T. P., and Spencer, E. M., 1970, *J. Biol. Chem.* **245**:6134.
Klotz, I. M., Burkhard, R. K., and Urquhart, J. M., 1952, *J. Am. Chem. Soc.* **74**:6178.
Kostka, V., Saber, M. A., Moravek, L. and Meloun, B., 1975, *Abstr. Commun. 10th Meet. Fed. Eur. Biochem. Soc.* No. 547.
Lapresle, C., and Doyen, N., 1975, *Biochem. J.* **151**:637.
Lapresle, C., and Goldstein, I. J., 1969, *J. Immunol.* **102**:733.
Lapresle, C., and Webb, J., 1960, *Ann. Inst. Pasteur* **99**:523.
Lapresle, C., and Webb, T., 1964, *Bull. Soc. Chim. Biol.* **46**:1701.
Lapresle, C., Webb, J., Kaminski, M., and Champagne, M., 1959, *Bull. Soc. Chim. Biol.* **41**:695.
Lee, C.-L., and Atassi, M. Z., 1976, *Biochem. J.* **159**:89.
Lee, C.-L., and Atassi, M. Z., 1977a, *Biochem. J.* **167**:571.
Lee, C.-L., and Atassi, M. Z., 1977b, *Biochim. Biophys. Acta* **495**:354.
Leonard, W. J., Jr., and Foster, J. F., 1961, *J. Biol. Chem.* **236**:2662.
Leonard, W. J., Jr., Vijai, K. K., and Foster, J. F., 1963, *J. Biol. Chem.* **238**:1984.
Luzzati, V., Witz, J., and Nicolaieff, A., 1961, *J. Mol. Biol.* **3**:379.
Maurer, P. H., Sri Ram, J., and Ehrenpreis, S., 1957, *Arch. Biochem. Biophys.* **67**:196.
Meloun, B., Moravek, L., and Kostka, V., 1975, *FEBS Lett.* **58**:134.
Moore, W. E., and Foster, J. F., 1968, *Biochemistry* **7**:3409.
Nikkel, H. J., and Foster, J. F., 1971, *Biochemistry* **10**:4479.
Oliveira, B., and Lapresle, C., 1966, *Ann Inst Pasteur* **110**:520.
Pearlman, W. H., and Fong, I. F. F., 1972, *J. Biol. Chem.* **247**:8078.
Pedersen, K. O., 1962, *Arch. Biochem. Biphys. Suppl.* **1**:157.
Pederson, D. M., and Foster, J. F., 1969, *Biochemistry* **8**:2357.
Peters, J. H., and Goetzl, E., 1969, *J. Biol. Chem.* **244**:2068.
Peters, T., Jr., and Hawn, C., 1967, *J. Biol. Chem.* **242**:1566.
Petersen, H. A., and Foster, J. F., 1965a, *J. Biol. Chem.* **240**:2503.
Petersen, H. A., and Foster, J. F., 1965b, *J. Biol. Chem.* **240**:3858.
Porter, R. R., 1957, *Biochem. J.* **66**:677.
Press, E. M.,and Porter, R. R., 1962, *Biochem. J.* **83**:172.
Putnam, F. W., 1975, in: *The Plasma Proteins* (F. W. Putnam, ed.), p. 57, Academic Press, New York.
Rangel, R., 1965, *Immunology* **8**:88.
Reed, R. G., Feldhoff, R. C., Clute, O. L., and Peters, T., Jr., 1975, *Biochemistry* **14**:4578.
Saifer, A., and Goldman, L., 1961, *J. Lipid Res.* **2**:268.
Salaman, M. R., and Williamson, A. R., 1971, *Biochem. J.* **122**:93.
Sarich, V. M., and Wilson, A., 1966, *Science* **154**:1563.

Singhal, R. P., and Atassi, M. Z., 1971, *Biochemistry* 10:1756.

Sogami, M., and Foster, J. F., 1968, *Biochemistry* 7:2172.

Sogami, M., Petersen, H. A., and Foster, J. F., 1969, *Biocehmistry* 8:49.

Spencer, E. M., and King, T. P.,1971, *J. Biol. Chem.* 246:201.

Spieker-Polet, H., and Polet, H., 1976, *J. Biol. Chem.* 251:987.

Sri Ram, J., and Maurer, P. H., 1959a, *Arch. Biochem. Biophys.* 83:223.

Sri Ram, J., and Maurer, P. H., 1959b, *Arch. Biochem. Biphys.* 85:512.

Steiner, R., and Edelhoch, J., 1961, *Nature (London)* 192:873.

Stokrova, S., and Sponar, J., 1963, *Collect. Czech, Chem. Commun.* 28:659.

Stone, T. J., Buckman, T., Nordio, P. L., and McConnell, H. M., 1965, *Proc. Natl. Acad. Sci. USA* 54:1010.

Stroupe, S. D., and Foster, J. F., 1973, *Biochemistry* 12:3824.

Tanford, C., 1950, *J. Am. Chem. Soc.* 72:441.

Tanford, C., Swanson, S. A., and Shore, W. S., 1955a, *J. Am. Chem. Soc.* 77:6414.

Tanford, C., Buzzell, J. G., Rands, D. G., and Swanson, S. A., 1955b, *J. Am. Chem. Soc.* 77:6421.

Taubman, M. T., and Atassi, M. Z., 1968, *Biochem. J.* 106:829.

Taylor, R. P., 1976, *J. Am. Chem. Soc.* 98:2684.

Taylor, R. P., and Silver, A., 1976, *J. Am. Chem. Soc.* 98:4650.

Taylor, R. P., and Vatz, J. B., 1973, *J. Am. Chem. Soc.* 95:5819.

Taylor, R. P., Berga, S., Chau, V., and Bryner, C., 1975, *J. Am. Chem. Soc.* 97:1943.

Teale, J. M., and Benjamin, D. C., 1976a, *J. Biol. Chem.* 251:4603.

Teale, J. M., and Benjamin, D. C., 1976b, *J. Biol. Chem.* 251:4609.

Timpl, R., Furthmayer, H., and Wolff, I., 1967, *Int. Arch. Allergy* 32:318.

Ui, N., 1971, *Biochim. Biophys. Acta* 229:567.

Vijai, K. K., and Foster, J. F., 1967, *Biochemistry* 6:1152.

Walker, J. E., 1976, *Eur. J. Biochem.* 69:517.

Wallevik, K., 1973, *Biochim. Biophys. Acta* 322:75.

Wallevik, K., 1976, *Biochim. Biophys. Acta* 420:42.

Webb, T., and Lapresle, C., 1964, *Biochem. J.* 91:24.

Weber, G., 1952, *Biochem. J.* 51:155.

Weber, G., and Young, L. B., 1964a, *J. Biol. Chem.* 239:1415.

Weber, G., and Young, L. B., 1964b, *J. Biol. Chem.* 239:1424.

Wilson, W. D., and Foster, J. F., 1971, *Biochemistry* 10:1772.

Wofsy, L., and Singer, S. J., 1963, *Biochemistry* 2:104.

Wong, K. -P., and Foster, J. F., 1969a, *Biochemistry* 8:4096.

Wong, K. -P., and Foster, J. F., 1969b, *Biochemistry* 8:4104.

Yang, J. T., and Foster, J. F., 1954, *J. Am. Chem. Soc.* 76:1588.

Zurawski, V. R., and Foster, J. F., 1974, *Biochemistry* 13:3465.

Zurawski, V. R., Jr., Kohr, W. J., and Foster, J. F., 1975, *Biochemistry* 14:5579.

Author Index

Subject Index